Sexuality Education

Sexuality Education
Theory and Practice

Fourth Edition

Clint E. Bruess
Birmingham-Southern College

Jerrold S. Greenberg
University of Maryland

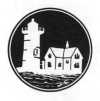

JONES AND BARTLETT PUBLISHERS
Sudbury, Massachusetts
BOSTON   TORONTO   LONDON   SINGAPORE

World Headquarters
Jones and Bartlett Publishers
40 Tall Pine Drive
Sudbury, MA 01776
978-443-5000
info@jbpub.com
www.jbpub.com

Jones and Bartlett Publishers Canada
2406 Nikanna Road
Mississauga, ON L5C 2W6
CANADA

Jones and Bartlett Publishers International
Barb House, Barb Mews
London W6 7PA
UK

Production Credits
Acquisitions Editor: Jacqueline Ann Mark
Production Editor: Julie Champagne Bolduc
Editorial Assistant: Nicole Quinn
Marketing Manager: Ed McKenna
Photo Research: Julie Bolduc and Kimberly Potvin
Composition: Interactive Composition Corporation
Cover Design: Kristin E. Ohlin
Printing and Binding: Courier Stoughton
Cover Printing: Courier Stoughton

Library of Congress Cataloging-in-Publication Data
Bruess, Clint E.
    Sexuality education : theory and practice / Clint E. Bruess, Jerrold
S. Greenberg.—4th ed.
        p. ; cm.
    Includes bibliographical references and index.
    ISBN 0-7637-4759-9 (alk. paper)
    1. Sex instruction—United States.   2. Sexual ethics—Study and
teaching—United States.   3. Hygiene, Sexual—Study and
teaching—United States.
    [DNLM: 1. Health Educators—psychology—United States.   2. Sex
Education—methods—United States.   3. Psychosexual
Development—United States.   4. Sexuality—psychology—United States.
5. Teaching—methods—United States.]   I. Greenberg, Jerrold S.
II. Title.
    HQ56.B73.B73 2004
    613.9'5—dc22
                                                        2004000682
Printed in the United States of America
08 07 06 05 04   10 9 8 7 6 5 4 3 2 1

Contents

Preface xiii
How to Use the Human Sexuality Web Site xv

Part 1
Introduction to Sexuality Education   1

1
Sexuality, You, and the Learner   3

Traditional and Contemporary Concepts
of Human Sexuality   3

The Complexity of Human Sexuality   4

Sexuality, Personal Well-Being,
and Interpersonal Relationships   6

Sexuality and the Life Cycle   7

Human Development and Issues of
Sexuality   8

Developmental Rates and Sequences   9

Masturbation   9

Homosexual Experimentation   10

Latency   11

Nocturnal Emissions and Orgasms   11

Nonmarital Versus Marital Lifestyle   11

Aging   12

Our Sexual Uniqueness   12

A Note about This Book   12

Summary   13

References   13

Suggested Readings   13

2
Foundations for Sexuality Education   15

Sexuality Education Goals and Objectives   15

A Multifaceted Definition of Sexuality
Education   18

Traditional Reasons for Sexuality Education   19

Sound Reasons for Contemporary Sexuality
Education Programs   20

Sexuality in History   22

Prehistoric Times   23

Eighth Century BCE–Fifth Century CE   23

Fifth Century–Fifteenth Century   24

Fifteenth Century–Sixteenth Century   24

Seventeenth Century–Eighteenth Century   24

Nineteenth Century   26

*Twentieth-Century–Twenty-First-Century
United States*   27

History of Sexuality Education   29

Current Trends in Sexuality Education   30

Summary   32

References   33

Suggested Readings   34

3
The Controversy   35

Background and Tactics of Movements
Against Sexuality Education   36

Background of Sexuality Education Opposition   36

Who Is the Opposition?   37

Typical Tactics of Sexuality Education Opponents   37

Characteristics and Stages of Extremist Attacks   39

Nonextremist Opponents of Sexuality Education   40

Countering Arguments Against Sexuality Education   40

Defense Against Extremist Attacks   43

Public Meetings   45

Logical Heads Prevail   45

Summary   47

References   48

Suggested Readings   48

4

Understanding Yourself   51

Sexuality Educators and Their Own Sexuality   51

Your Sexual Thoughts and Desires   51

Your Masculinity and Femininity   52

Your Body Image   52

Your Sexual Behavior   53

Your Sense of Humor   54

The Sexuality Educator's Interactions with Others   54

Interactions with Groups   54

Interactions with Individuals   54

Culture and the Sexuality Educator   55

The Sexuality Educator's Sexual Responsibility   55

Qualifications for the Sexuality Educator   56

Sexuality Education Certification   57

Everyone Is a Sexuality Educator   57

Summary   60

References   61

Suggested Readings   61

Cases for Part 1   63

Part 2

Biological, Psychological, and Sociological Aspects of Sexuality Education   67

5

A View from the Inside   69

Male and Female Reproductive Systems   69

Males   69

Females   70

Male Hormones   74

Female Hormones   75

Similarities and Differences Between Male and Female Sexual Responses   77

Similarities   77

Differences   78

Fertility Control   79

Contraception   79

Choosing a Contraceptive   88

Pregnancy, Childbirth, and Abortion   90

Pregnancy   90

Birth   91

Abortion   92

RU 486: A Method of Nonsurgical Abortion   93

Summary   94

References   94

Suggested Readings   95

6

The Cognitive and Psychological Side of Sexuality   97

Theories of Psychosexual Development   97

Freud   97

Erikson	*98*
Social Learning Theory	*98*
Self-Esteem and Sexual Maturity	99
Sexual Attitudes and Behavior	99
Sex-Role Stereotyping	100
Causes of Sex-Role Stereotyping	102
The Decision to Engage in Sexual Intercourse	102
Teenage Out-of-Wedlock Pregnancy	103
The Decision to Marry	103
The Decision to Have Children	104
Summary	*104*
References	*106*
Suggested Readings	*106*

7

Family Life and Interpersonal Relationships   107

Sexuality Education and Family-Life Education	107
Conflict Resolution	107
Communication	109
Clarify Nonverbal Communication	*109*
Plan Time to Talk	*110*
Listen	*110*
Begin with Agreement	*110*
Use "And," Not "But"	*110*
Use "I" Statements	*110*
Avoid "Why" Questions	*110*
Dating	111
Cohabitation	111
Marriage	113
The Evolving Family	113
Parenting	115
Single-Parent Families	117
Summary	*118*
References	*118*
Suggested Readings	*119*

8

The Sociological Side of Sexuality   121

People of All Ages, Types, and Conditions as Sexual Beings	122
Young People	*122*
Older People	*122*
People of Different Races	*124*
Physically Disabled People	*125*
Individuals with Cognitive Deficits	*125*
Ill People	*125*
Sexual Lifestyles	126
Marriage	*126*
Nonparenthood	*127*
Living Together	*127*
Clusters, Groups, and Communes	*128*
Contract Marriages	*128*
Sexuality and Legality	129
Legal Regulation of Sexual Behavior	*129*
Legality and Access to Treatment and Services	*130*
The Law and Sexual Discrimination	*132*
Legality, the Internet, and Information about Sexuality	*132*
Legality and Education about Sexuality and HIV/AIDS	*132*
Summary	*133*
References	*134*
Suggested Readings	*134*
Cases for Part 2	**135**

Part 3

Sexual Decision Making   137

9

Sexual Morality and Decision Making   139

Morals, Ethics, and Values	139

Value Systems and Human Potential   141

Relation of Sexual Topics to Morals, Ethics, and Values   142

Contemporary Religions and Sexuality   143

Sexual Decisions   144

Improving the Decision-Making Process   144

The Decision-Making Process and Sexuality   146

Summary   *147*

References   *147*

Suggested Readings   *147*

10

Alternative Sexual Behaviors   149

Individual Preferences and Sexual Behavior   150

Masturbation   *150*

Oral–Genital Contact   *150*

Homosexual Behavior   *150*

Heterosexual Behavior   153

Premarital Heterosexual Behavior   *153*

Are You Ready for Sex?   *153*

Marital Heterosexual Behavior   *154*

The Social Significance of Sexual Behaviors   154

Prostitution   *154*

Pornography   *155*

Other Sexual Alternatives   155

Forcible Sexual Behavior   157

The Incidence of Rape   *158*

Date Rape   *160*

Ways to Help Prevent Acquaintance Rape   *160*

Date Rape Drugs   *160*

Sexual Harassment   *161*

Summary   *162*

References   *163*

Suggested Readings   *164*

Cases for Part 3   **165**

Part 4

Conducting Sexuality Education   167

11

Education for Sexuality: Rules of Conduct   169

Ground Rules   169

Communication Skills   173

Listening Skills   *173*

Nonverbal Communication   *174*

The Sexuality Educator as a Communicator   *175*

Building Trust   *175*

Language Usage   176

Learners' Needs, Interests, and Characteristics   180

Involving Learners in the Learning Process   181

Summary   *181*

References   *182*

Suggested Readings   *182*

12

Learning Strategies for Sexuality Education   183

Learning Objectives   183

Unit Plans and Lesson Plans   185

Instructional Strategies   188

Case Studies   *188*

Critical Incidents   *188*

Brainstorming   *188*

Role-Playing   *189*

Buzz Groups   *190*

Gaming   *191*

Fishbowls   *192*

Sentence Completions   *192*

Values Clarification   *192*

Resource Speakers 193
Refusal Skills and Assertiveness Training 194
Instructional Media 195
Learner-Centered Activities 195
Summary 195
References 196
Suggested Readings 196

13

Strategies for Learning and Teaching about HIV/AIDS 197

Why a Separate Chapter on HIV/AIDS? 198
HIV/AIDS in the United States 198
HIV/AIDS and Minority Populations 200
HIV and Death 200
Prevention of HIV Infection 200
Special Considerations When Dealing with HIV/AIDS Education 202
HIV/AIDS Education 203
School HIV/AIDS Education 206
Abstinence-Only-Until-Marriage 206
Comprehensive Sexuality Education 206
Special HIV/AIDS Educational Considerations at Different Levels and Populations 207
Working with Different Levels and Populations 207
HIV/AIDS Education at Different Levels 207
Early Elementary School 207
Late Elementary School 207
Junior and Senior High School 208
HIV/AIDS Education in Different Settings 208
Religious Settings 208
Settings for Individuals with Developmental, Learning, or Mental Disabilities 211
Settings for Individuals with Sensory or Physical Disabilities 211
Teaching Suggestions 212
Program Assessment 212

HIV/AIDS Instructional Strategies 222
HIV Case Study 222
HIV Critical Incident 223
Scales and Questionnaires 223
HIV Sentence Completions 225
Role-Playing 225
Resistance Skill Training 225
Assuming Responsibility 226
Summary 226
References 226
Suggested Readings 227

14

What Should Be Taught at Different Levels and in Different Settings 229

Developmental Characteristics of Learners 229
Preschool 230
Early Elementary 230
Upper Elementary 230
Lower Secondary 230
Upper Secondary 230
Typical Questions Asked by School-Aged Learners 231
Sexuality Education for Preschool and School-Aged Learners 232
Preschool 232
Early Elementary Grades 233
Upper Elementary Grades 233
Lower Secondary Grades 234
Upper Secondary Grades 234
Sexuality Education for College-Aged and Adult Learners 235
Sexuality Education for Older Adults 237
Sexuality Education for Special Groups 238
Coronary Patients 238
Culturally Varied Groups 238
A Word of Caution 238

Summary   238
References   239
Suggested Readings   239

15

The Educator and Sexual Counseling   241

Sexuality Education and Sexual
  Counseling   241
The Domain of the Sexual Counselor   242
  Male Dysfunctions   243
  Female Dysfunctions   244
  Treatment   245
  Other Problems   245
The Sexual Educator and Quasi-Counseling   245
Referring Learners Who Need Sexual
  Counseling   247
  Summary   248
  References   249
  Suggested Readings   249

Cases for Part 4   251

Part 5

Program Implementation and Evaluation   253

16

Implementing a Sexuality Education Program   255

Achieving Support for a Sexuality Education
  Program   255
Strategies for Change   258
Group Dynamics and Sexuality Education
  Program Endeavors   260
  Group Members Play Many Roles   260

Resolving Conflict   261
Handling Concerns about Sexuality
  Education Programs   262
  Summary   266
  References   267
  Suggested Readings   267

17

Evaluation of Sexuality Education   269

Evaluation and the Continued Improvement
  of the Sexuality Education Program   269
Applying Evaluation to the Educational
  Process, the Learners, and the Sexuality
  Educator   271
  Educational Process   271
  Learners   272
  Sexuality Educator   273
The Importance of Well-Stated Objectives   273
Evaluation Can Be a Trap   274
  Cost-Benefit/Cost-Effectiveness   275
  Summary   276
  References   277
  Suggested Readings   277

18

Effectiveness of Sexuality Education and the Sexuality Educator   279

The Difficulty of Sexuality
  Education Research   279
  Learners   280
  Learning Environment   280
  Educational Strategy   280
  Sexuality Educators   280
  Content   280
  Evaluation   280
  Permission to Conduct Research   281

Encouraging Findings in Sexuality
Education Research   282

Feeling Unsure: An Encouraging Sign   286

Summary   *287*

References   *288*

Suggested Readings   *289*

Cases for Part 5   **291**

Appendix A
The National Coalition to Support Sexuality Education

293

Appendix B
State Policies in Brief

297

Appendix C
Teaching Strategies for Sexuality Education

301

Glossary   **305**

Index   **309**

Photo Credits   **317**

Preface

Many years ago the first edition of *Sexuality Education: Theory and Practice* evolved from a need for a text that approached sexuality education as the professional endeavor that it is. Since that first edition, a great deal of information about sexuality education has been published. However, it is still true that there is a lack of texts designed to help educators develop and implement comprehensive sexuality education programs.

Planners, educators, and the general public are frequently at odds concerning who should teach sexuality education and how it should be taught. At the center of this confusion are some vital questions: What is sexuality education? Why is sexuality education needed? How should a sexuality educator be prepared? How should sexuality education be implemented? This problem is compounded by *several false assumptions:*

1. The only preparation required for sexuality education is knowledge of human sexuality.

2. The function of the sexuality educator is to increase knowledge about the anatomy and physiology of the reproductive system.

3. Prospective educators today are more open and forthright and better prepared to conduct sexuality education than their older counterparts.

4. Because someone has been an effective educator in another field, he or she will be a good sexuality educator.

Certainly, potential sexuality educators need knowledge, but they need a great deal more. They also need the ability to reach learners, self-confidence in their own sexuality, skills for communicating with individuals and groups, and a feeling of comfort when dealing with the topic of human sexuality.

Many excellent separate sources of information for sexuality educators exist, but no other resource has pulled all the pieces together. The purpose of *Sexuality Education: Theory and Practice* has remained the same over the years: to provide comprehensive coverage of the many aspects of human sexuality, comprehensive coverage of information and issues related to sexuality education, and an explanation of educational skills needed to prepare sexuality educators.

Whether sexuality education is conducted in a community, school classroom, religious organization, or clinical setting, the basics are essentially the same. Therefore, the practical ideas offered in this book can be applied to almost any sexuality education program. We have selected numerous examples that emphasize this universal applicability. We have also given attention to the needs of learners of varying age groups, different races and ethnicities, different cultural and religious persuasions, and varying mental and physical capabilities.

Features of the Fourth Edition

1. **Key Concepts.** The Key Concepts at the beginning of each chapter give readers a chapter preview as well as our feelings about what is most important within the chapter. The Key Concepts can also be used as effective reminders for reviewing chapters after reading them.

2. **Insights.** The Insights prompt readers to think about issues related to the topic at hand. Each Insight has a specific purpose, contains activities to help readers learn to be sexuality educators, and helps make the learning process more interesting. Readers may be tempted to skip them, but they will miss some of the meaning and fun of this book if they do. Many of the exercises that appear in Insights can also be used later, when teaching others about human sexuality.

3. **Summaries.** The summary at the end of each chapter helps readers recall the main ideas within each chapter. When combined with the Key Concepts at the beginning, summaries give a comprehensive picture of the chapter.

4. **References and Suggested Readings.** References at the end of each chapter allow readers to easily identify the sources of information included within the text. They, along with the suggested readings, indicate where more information about topics of particular interest can be found.

5. **Cases.** Cases at the end of each section are designed to help readers think through the planning, implementation, and evaluation of sexuality education programs. All of them are based on actual occurrences that we have encountered or other sexuality educators have

related. The cases provide opportunities to integrate information from several chapters in the book into one solution.

6. **Glossary.** Understanding terminology related to sexuality is crucial for sexuality educators. Because of this, a glossary is included to help readers pinpoint meanings of words and phrases. The glossary also helps the reader focus on important points within each chapter.

7. **Web Site Access.** Access to the Web site of another of our texts, *Exploring the Dimensions of Human Sexuality, Second Edition* is provided to all users of this book. See the next section, "How to Use the Human Sexuality Web Site," for which topics we feel will be especially helpful to those preparing to be sexuality educators. Be assured that users of *Sexuality Education: Theory and Practice, Fourth Edition* have access to the entire Web site and may use as much of it as they wish.

What's New in the Fourth Edition?

Reviewers and users of the first three editions of *Sexuality Education: Theory and Practice* have been quite complimentary. Because of this, we made a conscious effort to retain those aspects of the book that readers and reviewers valued. However, a book can always be improved. In this spirit, the changes from the third edition include the following:

1. A major revision of the chapter on strategies for learning and teaching about HIV/AIDS education (Chapter 13) was done. This was obviously needed because of the many changes related to that topic in recent years. We still argue with ourselves about whether there should be such a chapter. We do this because HIV/AIDS education logically fits into an overall program of sexuality education, which should be a part of a comprehensive health education program. However, there is no other health problem related to sexual behavior choices that threatens such serious consequences. Therefore, after much deliberation, we maintained this separate chapter.

2. Although we retained the cases at the end of each section, to which readers have reacted very favorably,

we improved them. We updated, reorganized, and changed them to better reflect current sexuality education issues.

3. The organization of the book was changed. Where it seemed to make more sense, we placed chapters in different places in the book and even combined two chapters into one. This resulted in a different grouping of chapters for each section. We feel the present organization will be even more useful to users of the book.

4. Insights were also updated and changed to reflect the most current issues in sexuality education.

5. Content throughout the book was updated. Even a cursory review of dates shows that the most recent information is included.

6. Suggested readings have been updated—again to reflect the most recent information and issues in sexuality education.

7. A glossary was added to ensure sexuality educators focus on and understand important terminology.

8. As already mentioned, access to the Web site of another of our texts, *Exploring the Dimensions of Human Sexuality, Second Edition,* has been provided to the users of *Sexuality Education: Theory and Practice, Fourth Edition.*

Acknowledgments

We are proud of *Sexuality Education: Theory and Practice* and feel it will help you conduct sexuality education with confidence. We owe a great deal to Kris Ellis, editor at Jones and Bartlett Publishers, because she recognized the wisdom of revising the previous edition of the book. Her willingness to do this is much appreciated.

Finally, we acknowledge the important role that previous users of this text have played. They have helped us create a much-needed text to continue to help prepare effective sexuality educators. The need for sexuality education is as great as ever, and it must be conducted professionally and effectively. We are proud to think that this book helps to meet that need. Therefore, we dedicate it to you and all future sexuality educators who use *Sexuality Education: Theory and Practice, Fourth Edition.* Explore the book, enjoy it, and let it help you become a better sexuality educator.

How to Use the Human Sexuality Web Site

As a user of *Sexuality Education: Theory and Practice, Fourth Edition,* you have access to an excellent human sexuality Web site. This Web site is for the text titled *Exploring the Dimensions of Human Sexuality, Second Edition* that is also written by your authors. The address of this Web site is **http://sexuality.jbpub.com.**

This Web site will be very helpful when studying sexuality education. Ideally those learning about sexuality education should already have a solid foundation of human sexuality knowledge. However, this is often not the case. Using the Web site as a supplement to *Sexuality Education: Theory and Practice* can help the professor ensure that learners develop a solid background in human sexuality.

Exploring the Dimensions of Human Sexuality includes comprehensive coverage of sexuality topics as you can see from its table of contents:

Chapter 1	Introducing the Dimensions of Human Sexuality
Chapter 2	Sexuality Research
Chapter 3	Sexual Communication
Chapter 4	Female Sexual Anatomy and Physiology
Chapter 5	Male Sexual Anatomy and Physiology
Chapter 6	Gender Dimensions
Chapter 7	Sexual Response and Arousal
Chapter 8	Contraception
Chapter 9	Conception, Pregnancy, and Birth
Chapter 10	Sexual Techniques and Behaviors
Chapter 11	Sexual Orientation
Chapter 12	Sexuality in Childhood and Adolescence
Chapter 13	Sexuality in Adulthood
Chapter 14	Sexually Transmitted Diseases
Chapter 15	Sexual Disorders and Therapy
Chapter 16	Forcible Sexual Behaviors
Chapter 17	Sexual Consumerism
Chapter 18	Sexual Ethics, Morality, and the Law

The first feature of the Web site, "Want to Know More?", provides learners with a convenient way to learn more about selected topics in human sexuality. Opportunities are provided for learning additional information in every chapter.

There are Web exercises for each chapter. These are Web links with exercises for learners to complete. There are also self-assessments for each chapter. These help learners assess their viewpoints and understanding of the topics included in each chapter by participating in critical thinking activities.

The Student Study Guide includes an anatomical review and student questions. The Anatomical Review has interactive assessments of knowledge related to:

- Female External Reproductive Organs
- Organs of the Female Reproductive System
- Anterior View of the Female Reproductive Organs
- Various Positions of the Uterus
- Layers of the Uterine Wall
- The Female Breast
- Male Reproductive Organs
- Posterior View of the Male Reproductive Organs
- Testicle Cross-Section
- The Ovum from Fertilization through Implantation

Student Quizzes help learners review and evaluate personal knowledge about human sexuality by completing a practice quiz for each of the chapters. This can be a good way to determine if potential sexuality educators have the needed knowledge about human sexuality.

Finally, the Web site also includes reference links. These provide a chance for learners to explore the links included for each of the chapters to find additional information, resources, and data to complement the information within the chapters. The overall Web site for *Exploring the Dimensions of Human Sexuality* will be a great help to users of this text. We are confident that you will find that the combination of *Sexuality Education: Theory and Practice, Fourth Edition,* and the Web site will greatly contribute to the preparation of competent sexuality educators.

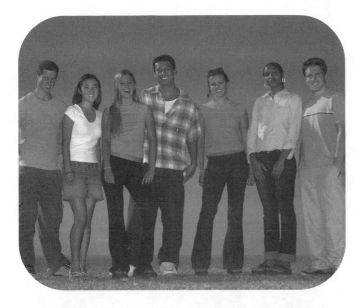
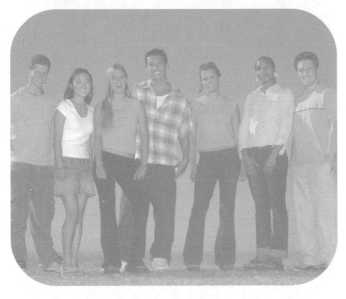
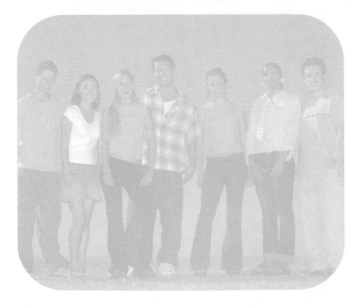
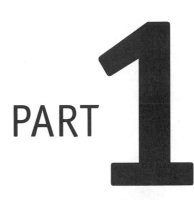

PART 1

Introduction to Sexuality Education

Chapter 1
Sexuality, You, and the Learner

Chapter 2
Foundations for Sexuality Education

Chapter 3
The Controversy

Chapter 4
Understanding Yourself

Sexuality, You, and the Learner

Key Concepts

1. There are many similarities and some differences between traditional and contemporary concepts of human sexuality.

2. Human sexuality involves a great many components and interrelationships.

3. A total view of human sexuality is basic to personal well-being as well as to interpersonal relationships.

4. People are sexual beings at all ages and stages of development.

5. As people grow and develop, they encounter a variety of topics and experiences filled with implications for total human sexuality.

6. Every individual is a unique sexual being.

Traditional and Contemporary Concepts of Human Sexuality

Sex—the word conjures up different images in each person's mind. Before you read further, reflect for a minute on Insight 1-1 on this page.

Insight 1-1

What Does "Sex" Mean?

What do *you* think of first when you hear or read the word *sex?* List the words or phrases that come to mind.

_____

_____

_____

_____

_____

The common thoughts people have when they hear or read this three-letter word usually relate to intercourse, reproduction, fun, and moral feelings. Some people associate the word with something "dirty"; some think the subject should not be discussed at all. Whatever thoughts, feelings, images, and impressions we have in regard to sexuality are the result of many different kinds of experiences we have had throughout our lives. We have learned from our parents, our relatives, our friends; from entertainment media and advertisements; from our churches and schools.

We have learned to consider sexuality in certain ways, most of them quite narrow and traditional. Think again about the list you just made. How many of the words you came up with relate mainly to a sexual act? How often do you hear people talking of "having sex" or "looking for sex"? Traditionally, human sexuality, if thought about at all, has been thought to have to do with participating in intercourse or some other sexual act, and references to sexuality have been cloaked in negative terminology. Traditional concepts imply that people participate in sexual behavior only on occasion and at other times are fundamentally asexual beings. This amounts to the view that although individuals participate in sexual acts, sexuality does not otherwise exist as part of individuals' personalities.

In the past, the word *sex* was often used interchangeably with words like *sin, dirty, unspeakable,* and *no-no.* There are some historical reasons for this negative attitude (see Chapter 2), and the influences of history and learning have affected contemporary concepts of human sexuality as well.

What do you feel people today think of when the word *sex* is mentioned? You have already identified what goes on in your own mind, but how about your friends—what do they think? And your parents? relatives? Since you are probably not about to run out and conduct a neighborhood survey at this point (although you may find it interesting to survey a few people if you get the chance), consider what you think one or two friends and one or two relatives would answer if you asked them to define the word *sex* for you. You will probably quickly realize that there are similarities between their attitudes and the narrow, negative concepts already discussed. Despite the passage of time, many people today still think about **sexuality** only in terms of sexual acts or other small pieces of the larger picture.

We found many examples of this narrowmindedness about sexuality when we started doing research for this book. It seemed appropriate to review the many books and articles on human sexuality available today to get a feeling for how they were treating the subject. It is sad to say that many contemporary books still treat the subject in a limited fashion. It is common to find books that focus on the biology of sexuality, or on the psychological aspects, or even on the decision-making components. Although some authors have written about more complete ways of viewing sexuality, it is still uncommon to find many books that deal with sexuality as something that involves the total personality and is basic to human health.

We would like to be able to tell you that contemporary concepts of human sexuality are radically different from the narrow and negative ones of the past, but unfortunately they are not. You may have already demonstrated this fact with your own list and your imagined lists for friends and relatives.

It is true that there is a trend toward a more comprehensive view of human sexuality. People today appear more willing to talk about the subject in the home as well as in educational settings. This trend toward more open interest in the subject is shown by sales of books, treatment of sexual topics in the media, and increased sexuality education programs.

While the existence of Acquired Immune Deficiency Syndrome (AIDS) has caused tremendous suffering and premature death, it has also forced a more open consideration of numerous sexual topics. Sexual practices, use of contraception, advertisement of condoms, and many moral considerations are just a few of the topics that now come up more frequently. Many people are realizing that human sexuality involves a great deal more than physical acts; however, there are still probably more similarities between traditional and contemporary concepts of human sexuality than there are differences.

The Complexity of Human Sexuality

In this book we take a broad view of human sexuality and define it as part of the total personality and thus basic to human health and well-being. This type of comprehensive view of sexuality assumes that many factors in the human makeup interact to create an individual's sexuality. The Sexuality Information and Education Council of the United

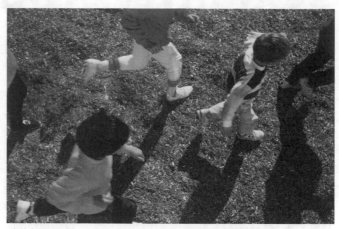

Children are not born with a concept of sexuality, rather it develops in conjunction with their experience.

States (SIECUS), whose purpose is to promote education about and for sexuality, explains human sexuality in this way:

Sexuality is more than what you do with another person sexually. That is, sexuality is not only about having sex, or taking part in sexual behaviors. Sexuality is also about the person you feel you are, your body, how you feel as a boy or girl, man or woman, the way you dress, move and speak, the way you act and feel about other people. These are all parts of who you are as a person, from your birth until you die—your whole lifetime long. . . . Our sexuality is a natural and healthy part of who we are. It's not about what you do, it's about who you are and how you live. (What is sexuality? 2000)

The Health Protection Branch of Health Canada summarizes as follows:

Sexuality is an integral part of the personality of everyone: man, woman and child. It is a basic need and aspect of being human that cannot be separated from other aspects of life. In this view, sexuality encompasses the physical, physiological, psychological, social, emotional, cultural and ethical dimensions of sex and gender. (Canadian guidelines for sexual health education, 2000)

Given the fact that many people still do have a limited view of sexuality, however, it is appropriate to take a look at what a comprehensive view of human sexuality might include. We say *might* because there is no one best or exact definition of total human sexuality. The main thing to realize is that a total view includes many components and interrelationships.

Figure 1-1 shows one view of human sexuality that attempts to encompass the main aspects that need to be considered. It is easy to see that sexuality consists of at least cultural, psychological, ethical, and biological dimensions.

---

sexuality A natural and healthy part of who we are. It is not only about taking part in sexual behaviors. It is an integral part of everyone's personality and includes cultural, psychological, ethical, and biological dimensions.

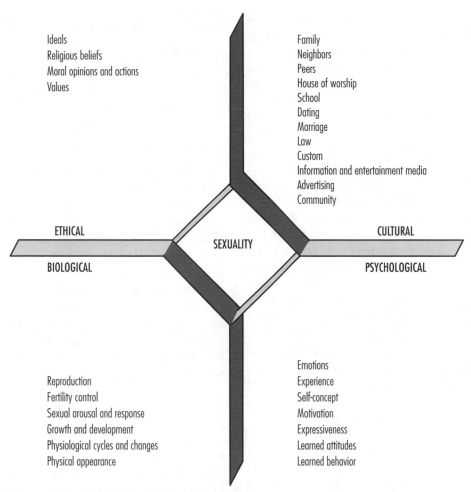

Ideals
Religious beliefs
Moral opinions and actions
Values

Family
Neighbors
Peers
House of worship
School
Dating
Marriage
Law
Custom
Information and entertainment media
Advertising
Community

ETHICAL   CULTURAL

SEXUALITY

BIOLOGICAL   PSYCHOLOGICAL

Reproduction
Fertility control
Sexual arousal and response
Growth and development
Physiological cycles and changes
Physical appearance

Emotions
Experience
Self-concept
Motivation
Expressiveness
Learned attitudes
Learned behavior

Figure 1-1 Dimensions of human sexuality.
Source: Jerrold S. Greenberg et al., *Sexuality: Insights and Issues,* 3d ed. (Dubuque, IA: Wm. C. Brown Communications, Inc., 1993).

The interrelationship of all of these dimensions results in an individual's total sexuality.

The **cultural dimension** of sexuality is the sum of the cultural influences that affect our thoughts and actions, both historical and contemporary. Historical influences become evident when one considers roles of males and females, as well as certain customs.

For example, for over 30 years (approximately 1949 to 1980) the Chinese Republic permitted virtually no information concerning sexuality to reach the Chinese people. Even since a more open attitude was adopted, Chinese women rarely inquire about sexual matters, unless they relate to pregnancy or menstruation—the only type of sexually related questions they believe are appropriate to ask (Ruan & Bullough, 1989).

Another example relates to abortion. In Greece, policies of church and state frown on most medical contraceptives, so female contraceptive methods are rejected by a great majority of Greek women. Therefore, abortion and male barrier methods are the main means of fertility control (Georges, 1996). In Ireland, however, abortion is illegal unless the mother's life is at risk. It is estimated that about 4,500 Irish women travel to other countries for abortions each year (Caron, 1998).

Among the sources of current influences are the radio, television, film, Internet and print media; social institutions, such as family, church, and school; and interpersonal relationships. Each impresses on us the culturally defined ways in which we "ought" to think as females and males and the roles our sexuality "ought" to lead us to play.

cultural dimension of sexuality Sum of the cultural influences that affect our thoughts and actions, both historical and contemporary.

The **psychological dimension** of sexuality is probably the clearest example of learned aspects of sexuality. Our attitudes and feelings toward ourselves and other people begin to develop very early in life. From the time we are born we get signals from all around us telling us how to think and act. We learn that some words are "wrong" or "dirty" and that certain parts of our body are "untouchable" and "unmentionable." We even learn to be careful about what conversational topics we enter into with certain people. If we feel one way about ourselves but think others find these feelings unacceptable, we learn to hide our true feelings and to pretend. After all, thinking or talking about sexual topics is not a good idea anyway (or so we have learned). Some of us are lucky enough to grow up with a more positive set of experiences, but regardless of whether our experiences are positive or negative, our learned responses to them become integral to our sexuality.

The **ethical dimension** might be included as part of the psychological dimension by some people, but for the sake of clarity we mention it separately here. Basically, this dimension includes questions of right-and-wrong, should-I-or-shouldn't-I, yes-or-no. Ethical aspects might be based on a particular religious philosophy, or they might have a more humanistic or pragmatic origin. Whatever the source of our ethical attitudes, each of us faces daily decisions that affect and in turn are affected by our concepts of sexuality.

The final dimension of sexuality we will mention is the one that most people usually think of first—the **biological dimension.** Just to emphasize the point that biological aspects are only one part of sexuality, we are considering them last. However, no hierarchy of sexuality dimensions can be established; it would be a mistake to assume that any one part is more important than any other.

The biological dimension of sexuality involves our physical appearance, especially the development of physical sexual characteristics; our responses to sexual stimulation; our ability to reproduce or to control fertility; and our growth and development in general. Although human reproductive functioning does not begin until puberty, human sexual-erotic functioning begins immediately after birth and lasts a lifetime. It is important to realize that biological functioning, as it relates to sexuality, is a part of the natural functioning of human beings. The biological aspects also relate to the sexuality dimensions, and the four dimensions constantly work together to produce an individual's total sexuality.

Insight 1-2

Defining Sexuality

Stop for a minute. Take a piece of scrap paper and, without looking at this book, write a two- or three-sentence definition of total human sexuality. After completing your definition, check it against Figure 1-1.

Before you read further, take a moment to complete Insight 1-2 above.

When writing your definition, you may have noticed that it is quite difficult to define the term *sexuality* in a few words. Rather than becoming frustrated over the inability to come up with a specific definition, you should realize that it is more important to get a feeling for what the concept involves. Many people find themselves using such words as *feelings, relationships,* or *decisions* to help define sexuality. We might compare the attempt to grasp a total concept of sexuality to the attempt to grasp a total concept of personality. It is extremely difficult to precisely define what personality is, but almost everyone has a pretty good idea of what it involves.

Even though it is often necessary to treat aspects of sexuality as isolated entities for purposes of clarity in discussion, it is important to remember that these aspects all combine to make up our sexuality and that our sexuality is but one part of our total personality. Our hope is that each of you will be able to consider these separate topics without losing sight of human sexuality in its totality.

Sexuality, Personal Well-Being, and Interpersonal Relationships

There has been a lot of emphasis on health education and health services by the media and by federal and state governments, but few discussions point out the importance of a total view of human sexuality to human health. Consider how much time you have spent in the past week thinking about topics related to human sexuality. How often, in the years that you were growing up, did you have questions related to human sexuality? Perhaps you have seen surveys indicating that, at any given time in a high school or college classroom, a great number of students are thinking about sexuality. This concern is natural, but if not dealt with can produce negative influences on mental health.

psychological dimension of sexuality   Learned attitudes and feelings toward ourselves and other people related to sexuality.

ethical dimension of sexuality   Includes questions of right-and-wrong, should-I-or-shouldn't-I, yes-or-no related to decisions about sexuality.

biological dimension of sexuality   Involves physical appearance, responses to sexual stimulation, reproduction, and general growth and development.

Recognizing that sexuality is a basic part of human personality and that people have numerous questions and thoughts about this topic, it makes sense to help students of all ages develop a healthy concept of human sexuality and to relieve anxieties and fears about many sexuality issues. This is an important reason for implementing sexuality education programs (see Chapter 2); health and well-being are promoted by an understanding of total human sexuality.

Of course, our personal health and our self-concept relate to our dealings with other people. Did you ever stop to think how much growing up would be facilitated if people had positive self-images and better social skills? We cannot claim that a total view of sexuality would eliminate all problems associated with interpersonal relationships, but let us consider an example or two.

As young people grow and develop, they have countless questions about their changing feelings as well as about their physical changes. A simple understanding of how these feelings and changes are common to all people, and of the biological facts, coupled with an opportunity to discuss concerns with understanding peers and adults, is definitely helpful. But how many young people do you know who experience such help?

A recognition that we are all sexual beings also contributes to positive interpersonal relationships. As we grow up, we do not realize that our parents, teachers, relatives, and everyone else around us are sexual beings. This of course does not mean they are performing sexual acts at every opportunity, but it does mean they all have sexual feelings and characteristics.

The AIDS crisis has forced increased attention on people as sexual beings. All dimensions of human sexuality come into play when dealing with the topic of AIDS. How well people can cope with the many issues and dilemmas related to AIDS can also influence their well-being.

Being comfortable with sexuality has many applications for sexuality educators. Graham and Smith (1984) developed an operational definition of sexuality comfort which includes feeling satisfaction with and pride in one's own sexuality, feeling secure about one's own sexual natures, communicating effectively about sexuality, expressing respect and tolerance for others' sexual values, encouraging others to explore sexual issues and their own sexual values, and acknowledging that sexuality is an important topic to people and therefore a legitimate topic for intellectual inquiry. They also pointed out that experiences which improve sexuality comfort include improving self-understanding, improving understanding and tolerance of divergent sexualities, improving communication skills, increasing one's knowledge base about sexuality, and being exposed to people who are comfortable with their sexuality.

Using a specific population as an example, the sexual health of adolescents can be viewed as encompassing the issues of body-image awareness, interpersonal relationships, decision making, and sexual intimacy. Specific factors related to body image might include feeling good about being male or female and feeling comfortable with bodily functions. Interpersonal relationships involve concerns such as being able to communicate feelings to others without being embarrassed and having respect for another's individuality. Decision making includes being able to decide what is right for oneself and acting in personal best interests, and having a clear sense of personal values and acting in congruence with them. Sexual intimacy might deal with such issues as understanding the difference between sexual feelings and love, and knowing that one's feelings deserve respect from others (Brick, 1989).

Removing some of the mystique that currently surrounds the topic of sexuality would certainly facilitate interpersonal communication. Cat-and-mouse games would become less prevalent, and more honesty and openness could occur. With some communication barriers lifted, the potential for more positive interpersonal relationships would be greatly enhanced.

Sexuality and the Life Cycle

Before reading further, take a minute to fill out Insight 1-3. Perhaps you already know that all people are sexual beings at all ages. In this case, you probably filled in the columns of Insight 1-3 with "birth" and "death" rather than with specific numbers. If not, why did you put down any numbers at all? Are any of the columns different from the others?

Insight 1-3 examines your feelings about sexuality as it relates to the life cycle. Actually, if you were paying attention earlier in this chapter, you realized that human sexuality is so broad that it is impossible for anyone to be an asexual being at any point unless he or she stops breathing. The idea of an absence of sexuality is similar to the idea that a person has an absence of personality. You may feel that a given person has a poor personality, but that individual still has a personality of some kind. Just as people have personalities from the time of birth, they are sexual beings at all ages and stages of development.

Dr. William Masters pointed out some facts related to sexual functioning that add an additional perspective to our picture (Masters, 1975). Dr. Masters emphasized that sexual functioning is a part of the natural functions of the body, and that it begins at birth. He told the story, for example, that as an obstetrician delivering many babies, he decided to play a little game to make things more interesting. This game consisted of seeing how often he could deliver male babies and cut and tie the cord before they had an erection. Dr. Masters reported that he won about half the time. Newborn male babies often get partial or complete erections right after birth. Dr. Masters pointed out that female babies experience vaginal lubrication early too. Obviously, penile erections and

Age and Sexuality

Consider the chart below. Note that there are six blank columns in two rows. In the top row first column, write the approximate age at which you started to be a sexual being. In the second column write the age at which you think others of your sex usually start to be sexual beings. In the third through sixth columns, do the same thing for others of the other sex, for your brothers and sisters (if you have any), for your parents, and for your grandparents.

Now, go back to the first column again (bottom row). Write the age at which you would expect to cease being a sexual being. Then do the same thing in the remaining columns for the people already considered. Before going further in this book, jot down three thoughts or feelings that came to mind while you were filling in the columns.

	You	Others (same sex)	Others (other sex)	Siblings	Parents	Grandparents
Start						
Cease						

1. _____
2. _____
3. _____

vaginal lubrication are natural functions that occur prior to any learning about sexuality.

As further support for the idea that sexual functioning is natural, Dr. Masters pointed out that all natural functions have their own rhythm. For example, most males experience an erection and females have vaginal lubrication about every 80 to 90 minutes at night while they sleep. Again, the absence of conscious control indicates that these are natural functions.

Given such information about natural functions, combined with the total sexuality concept of which it is a part, we readily see that people are sexual beings throughout life. This idea comes as a shock to some individuals, since it includes little brothers and sisters as well as older parents and grandparents, but it is simple fact that all people are sexual beings.

In spite of this fact, certain groups of people are usually seen as asexual beings: the young, the old, those individuals with disabilities, and all parents (see Chapter 8). You can readily see that this leaves us with only a select few individuals who supposedly are sexual people, expected to participate in intercourse and other physical sexual acts. In light of our total concept of human sexuality, this type of thinking simply does not make sense. Psychological, cultural, ethical, and biological forces have made their mark on all individuals. It is becoming more and more apparent that it is far healthier and more logical to consider sexuality as encompassing, not only specific acts, but attitudes, emotions, interpersonal relationships, and self-concepts as well.

Human Development and Issues of Sexuality

You may have already completed courses or parts of courses in human growth and development. In any case, you are aware of at least some of the many physical and emotional changes that take place as people grow and develop. We will cover most of these topics in greater detail later in the book, but we want to introduce their relationship to total human sexuality as part of this introductory discussion.

Looking at it a slightly different way, the National Commission on Adolescent Sexual Health asserts the following:

> *Sexual health encompasses sexual development and reproductive health as well as such characteristics as the ability to develop and maintain meaningful interpersonal relationships; appreciate one's own body; interact with both genders in respectful and appropriate ways; and express affection, love, and intimacy in ways consistent with one's own values. (Kempner, 2003)*

Many people can influence sexual health. Among them are parents, educators, religious leaders, and health care providers. All of these people can help by discussing with young people the aspects of human development that may impede optimal sexual health. For example, providing quality reproductive health care is complex and involves an open dialogue between providers and clients about issues that traditionally may not have been discussed (Smith, 2002). The same is true for parents, educators, and religious leaders in their dialogue and relationships with young people.

It is essential to realize that many aspects of development have implications for human sexuality that are usually overlooked. Let us look at some of these aspects from a more discerning point of view.

Developmental Rates and Sequences

One of the first things you learn when studying growth and development is that the sequence of development for most people is about the same. That is, we all tend to do certain things before other things—to walk before we run, for example. However, we do not all pass through this sequence at the same rate. In terms of peer acceptance and personal feelings, it might be nice if all young people grew and developed at precisely the same rate. How handy it would be not to have to explain constantly why people are different from one another.

The fact that the rates of development for different people do vary is a simple idea that leads to numerous possible problems related to sexuality. These problems can range from concerns about physical differences to difficulties understanding emotional changes and variances in oneself and in others.

Too often, educators have handled developmental topics with a degree of exactness that does not exist. Students have been told that the average girl begins menstruation at 12 years of age, that the average boy's voice changes at a certain time, and that the average young person's feelings have certain characteristics at a certain time. What many young people do not understand is that averages refer to ranges (sometimes pretty wide), not exact places on a scale. Those dealing

with young people need to emphasize the fact that while we generally all go through the same types of changes in the same order, the timing of these changes can vary widely. All we need to do is look at classrooms full of students in the upper elementary and early secondary grades to see the evidence of this variation.

It would be naive to think that an understanding of differences in rates of growth and development would solve all concerns related to human sexuality, but it would also be a mistake not to emphasize this point more than we have. Better knowledge about rate differences can only help young people to be more at ease with themselves and with their peers.

Masturbation

At this point we are not discussing **masturbation** as part of a range of sexual behavior alternatives (see Chapter 10 for this coverage), but as another area that relates to growth and development. Masturbation is a topic of concern to young people because they may have heard so much about it, they have either tried it or are interested in doing so, and they seldom have anyone to talk with who is very knowledgeable on the subject or open to talking about it.

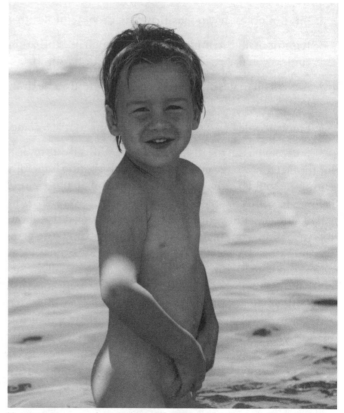

Youngsters soon learn that it feels good to touch their bodies.

---

masturbation   Self-stimulation of the genitals for the purpose of sexual pleasure.

Insight 1-4

What about Masturbation?

Stop for a minute and make a list of all of the negative things you heard about masturbation as you were growing up. Then make a list of all the positive things you heard. Compare the two lists. What do you see?

What are the facts about masturbation as it relates to growth and development? We are not making a case for or against masturbation, but we do want to put the topic into perspective within a developmental context. Here are some of the facts; perhaps you can add to the list:

1. Masturbation does not cause hair to grow on the palms of the hands.

2. Masturbation does not cause people to go insane.

3. Masturbation does not stunt a person's growth.

4. Masturbation does not cause a male's penis to fall off or a female's vagina to slam shut.

5. It is impossible to masturbate to excess.

6. It is not necessary to masturbate in order to be healthy.

7. It is impossible to injure yourself through masturbation (unless you use an instrument that can be harmful).

8. Almost all males and females masturbate at some time in their lives.

9. Some people believe it is morally wrong to masturbate.

So, what has all the fuss been about? With all due respect for the fact that some people believe masturbation is morally wrong, it would be completely honest to explain those moral feelings to young people as long as all the facts were also provided. Look back at your list of negatives and positives about masturbation from Insight 1-4 and you probably see a grim picture. Most people have been exposed to a similar view. Our point here is quite basic: Masturbation is usually a normal part of growth and development. Previously, the topic was either blown out of proportion by telling young people that nasty things would happen if they masturbated, or it was made mysterious by refusing to discuss it at all. To put young people's minds at ease, masturbation should be discussed as an aspect of growth and development. Facts can only be helpful. There is no defensible reason for scare tactics or censorship of something so important to both human sexuality and development.

Homosexual Experimentation

Anyone who reads newspapers is aware that the topic of homosexuality has received a lot of attention lately. It is not our intention to thoroughly discuss homosexuality as a sexual orientation (see Chapter 10). It is important, however, for those working with young people to realize that some **homosexual** experimentation is a perfectly natural part of growing up.

As with masturbation, many young people try different forms of sexual behavior because they are curious and because the behaviors probably feel good to them. On the other hand, it would be erroneous to give young people the impression that there is something wrong with them if they chose not to experiment.

Although some people are shocked at the idea of homosexual experimentation, a quick look at the environment of young people reveals that opportunities for such experimentation are amply provided. How would most adults react to the idea of two 11-year-old boys spending the night in a tent in the backyard or the idea of two 11-year-old girls staying over in one or the other's bedroom? How would most adults react to the idea of an 11-year-old boy and an 11-year-old girl spending the night in a tent in the backyard? Chances are, you get the point already. Socially acceptable opportunities for homosexual experimentation are all around young people, whereas similar opportunities for heterosexual experimentation are more scarce. It is realistic to accept the fact that experimentation will occur and that some of it is likely to be between members of the same sex. The fact that some people have strong moral feelings about homosexual behavior, even of an experimental nature, should be respected. We are not attempting to promote any cause except that of understanding the facts.

Speaking of facts, there are several that should be clarified about homosexual experimentation.

1. The fact that someone has experimented homosexually does not mean that person will be a homosexual for life. If it were true that one such contact makes one a homosexual, would it not follow that one drink makes an alcoholic, or one jog makes a runner? If everything we ever tried at any time in our lives is still a part of our lifestyle now, we would not have enough hours in the day to pursue all our interests.

2. Homosexual experimentation is not physically harmful. Furthermore, unless a person has been made to feel a strong sense of worry or guilt about personal behavior, homosexual experimentation is not psychologically harmful.

---

homosexual   One whose primary erotic, romantic, and affectional attraction is toward members of one's own sex.

Concerns about Sexual Orientation

Do a quick role-play with a friend. Pretend that you are a teacher and that your friend is a student who has come to you after school and told you about his or her concern about sexual orientation. What would you say to the student? What possibilities do you have? What effects might different types of responses have?

3. Some young people are not sure about their sexual orientation. This statement may seem strange, because sexual orientation is never a matter of question for most people. From the standpoint of growth and development, however, it is true that some young people are not sure whether they are heterosexual, homosexual, or a combination of the two.

In fact, a survey of 35,000 junior and senior high school students (Flax, 1992) found that 11% were unsure about their sexual orientation. The percentage of students unsure about their orientation declined with age from about 26% of the 12-year-olds to 5% of the 18-year-olds. Those working with young people should at least be aware of the possibility that adolescents' own perceptions of their sexual orientation may not conform to adult standards.

Why is the issue of sexual orientation important to the educator, nurse, counselor, or administrator? It matters because if you are a person to whom young people feel they can relate, you are likely to come in contact with a few who are concerned about the issue, and the way you react could have a significant effect on these students.

Educators need to be aware of young people's concerns about sexual orientation as they are maturing. Educators also need to be prepared to provide learners with information and responses that will be helpful, factual, and supportive rather than inaccurate or threatening.

Latency

For many years it was assumed that young people go through a period of **latency,** when sexual development and interest in sexuality are nonexistent. This period, roughly from age 5 through age 11, was supposedly a time when these "asexual" beings should be busy learning about reading, writing, and arithmetic. In fact, it was thought that teaching children

in this period about sexuality would even be harmful to them.

Recall what we have been saying about the total concept of human sexuality—that it involves feelings, self-concept, and interpersonal relationships, among other characteristics. Is it possible to conceive of children between the ages of 5 and 11 not having thoughts about their feelings, themselves, or their peers? Anyone who has worked with elementary school children knows they are filled with curiosity about these areas. It may not always show, but the interest is usually there.

Adults working with young people need to realize that the latency concept is essentially a myth—especially since this myth has often been used as the basis for establishing a case against sexuality education in schools.

Nocturnal Emissions and Orgasms

For many years there has been an emphasis on education about menstruation for females. One of the justifications for this education is the fact that all females experience a discharge from the body and that they should be prepared when it happens. This is logical enough, but what happened to the same logic when it comes to males' **nocturnal emissions**? Males experience a discharge from the body too.

Perhaps because the subject of nocturnal orgasms is closer than menstruation to the topic of human sexual response, educators have hesitated to deal with this topic. It is a fact that many young males and females experience orgasms in their sleep. They may or may not remember an orgasm the next day, but in the case of males there is evidence, in the form of semen on the bed sheets or pajamas. Young people learn directly or indirectly that, most of the time, bodily discharges are indications that something is wrong. They need to be told that menstruation and nocturnal emissions are exceptions to this rule.

Young people cannot control whether they have orgasms in their sleep. This is not a moral dilemma they can deal with consciously. Here again is a topic that involves both sexuality and growth and development and that needs to be treated naturally, for the well-being of both young males and young females.

Nonmarital Versus Marital Lifestyle

Other chapters in this book discuss nonmarital versus marital lifestyles in greater detail, but at this point we want to place this decision in perspective as a part of growth and development concerns. Everyone decides whether to get married.

latency   An alleged period of development when sexual development and interest in sexuality are supposedly nonexistent.

nocturnal emission   Emission of semen while asleep.

Perhaps the decision is made a number of times at different points in life. But whatever the decision about marriage, other decisions follow. A person choosing nonmarriage has decisions to make regarding personal sexual behavior as well as decisions regarding lifestyle in general. A person choosing marriage still has the same types of decisions to make within the context of marital responsibility and, if children are present, parental responsibility as well.

Aging

As we get older, we tend to view life differently. Sexual feelings and desires are present at all stages of life, but they may have different meanings and modes of fulfillment at each stage. We know that many forms of sexual behavior are common among people of all ages. Furthermore, concerns for self and others are constantly present, including concern about body appearance, overall health, and possible change in marital status. We all need to deal with aspects of sexuality as we age; in this way, too, sexuality is a growth and development issue.

Our Sexual Uniqueness

We will discuss sexual decision making in Chapter 9, but for now we want to point out that many personal possibilities exist when it comes to sexuality. Individual choice is important. What really matters is what *you* want to matter. Sexuality educators need to help learners arrive at a developmental level at which they can realize that it is OK to have sexual thoughts, that it might be OK to participate in sexual behavior, and that it might be just as acceptable to abstain.

Relatedly, there is a considerable time lag in the development of many children's thinking, resulting in low-level thinking and problem solving. Many children are capable of understanding quite complex sexuality concepts much earlier than most adults think. However, adults who refrain from communicating with children due to inhibitions about using correct sexual terminology and descriptions actually inhibit the children's development. Therefore, many children are well behind in their thinking and problem solving abilities compared to where they could be if adults were more at ease with sexual concepts. In other words, children can handle appropriate sexuality education—it is often the adults who cannot. There are numerous implications here for educators as well as parents.

Morals, ethics, and values influence personal decisions, as well they should; but individuals need to be comfortable with personal decisions. We cannot tell you what is right for you, and you cannot tell us what is right for us.

Some people are very interested in the topic of sexuality. Others are not terribly concerned about it. What matters is the realization that personal decisions about sexuality are both needed and welcomed. Since we are all unique sexual beings, it should not be surprising that our vast ranges of thoughts, decisions, and behaviors are also unique. And that is OK.

A Note about This Book

While we will discuss reasons for sexuality education in Chapter 2, we want to establish one important reality from the beginning. When it comes to sexuality education, the question is not whether it will occur, but rather what kind of sexuality education do we want? No sexuality education *is* sexuality education (Snegroff, 2000). We say this because adults transmit their attitudes about sexuality to young people. From the moment of birth, children observe and learn from adults' behavior in everyday life. The way adults answer questions about sexuality, the way they express affection, and the degree of comfort they demonstrate related to sexuality issues are examples of sexuality education through important informal means. The message received by young people might be positive or negative, but it is educational either way.

One of the tricky aspects of a sexuality education text is blending the content to be taught with information needed by the educator to do the teaching. Obviously, a sexuality educator must be knowledgeable about sexuality in order to be effective. However, possessing all the information in the world will not help if the educator does not know how to impart it to others. That is the secret of all types of education at all levels.

Note that in this chapter we have presented an overview of certain human developmental subject matter, offered not in isolation, but because of its relevance to accomplishing the task of sexuality education. The sexuality educator must understand latency and other aspects of growth and development in order to be an effective educator. Similarly in other chapters, we present information about selected topics because of their bearing on sexuality education. We know, and we hope you realize, that you will need more content than that detailed within this book in order to be a good sexuality educator.

Ideally, a basic course in human sexuality would be a prerequisite for a course in sexuality education. Perhaps some of you have had such a course; however, our guess is that most of you have not. That is another reason we provide as much specific sexuality content as we do. Without such background, many of you would lose sight of the educational context.

So, keep in mind that this is a sexuality *education* text and not a sexuality text. There is some sexuality content for the reasons mentioned above, but the emphasis is on planning, implementing, teaching, and evaluating sexuality education. We wish you the best as you prepare to undertake these important tasks.

Summary

In this chapter we have set the stage for many of the topics and issues to be discussed in subsequent chapters. We have seen that most people tend to think about human sexuality in very narrow terms. While traditional definitions have tended to relate only to sexual acts or to the biology of sexuality, newer approaches stress a much broader concept. Despite the development of this broader picture, the older, narrower concepts have been learned so well that they are still with us.

A comprehensive definition of sexuality could take many forms. Our definition contains cultural, psychological, ethical, and biological dimensions. Each dimension includes many aspects, but all are intertwined in a complex picture involving feelings, self-concepts, interpersonal relationships, and decision making. Although it is often necessary, for purposes of clarity, to discuss only one part of sexuality or another, it must be kept in mind that each element is part of the total picture of sexuality.

Understanding this total view of human sexuality contributes to personal well-being and enhances personal relationships. Sexuality has been an area of interest and concern for most people. Being able to place sexuality in its appropriate perspective as a part of total personality can put people's minds at ease, and it can help reduce tensions and facilitate interpersonal relationships.

People have tended to think of others and themselves as sexual beings only during certain stages of life. That is, sexual beings have been seen as those individuals between their late teens and their 30s or 40s. In fact, people are sexual beings at all ages and stages of development. Given our total concept of human sexuality, it is easy to see that people of all ages are sexual beings, just as people of all ages have personalities.

Educators, parents, counselors, and administrators need to recognize that certain topics related to both human development and human sexuality have been neglected for the most part. These topics include similarities in developmental sequences, differences in developmental rates, masturbation, homosexual experimentation, latency, nocturnal emissions and orgasms, decisions about nonmarital versus marital lifestyles, and aging related to sexuality. In each of these areas, people often have developed more anxiety than needed. If people are provided with the facts and with an opportunity to discuss and understand each of these topics as it relates to their sexuality and their growth and development, their personal well-being will be enhanced.

Many personal possibilities exist when it comes to sexuality. Each of us makes unique choices based on individual morals, ethics, and values. Sexuality educators need to help learners realize that personal decisions about sexuality are needed and welcomed. Those decisions will be facilitated by an understanding of the pervasive role sexuality plays in our lives.

References

Brick, P. Toward a positive approach to adolescent sexuality, *SIECUS Report*, 17, no. 5 (May/June 1989), 1–3.

Canadian guidelines for sexual health education. Health Canada, Health Protection Branch, Laboratory Centre for Disease Control (2000). Available: http://www.hc-sc.gc.ca/main/lcdc/web/publicat/.

Caron, S. L. *Cross-cultural perspectives on human sexuality.* Boston: Allyn and Bacon, 1998.

Flax, E. Significant number of teenagers unsure of sexual orientation, new study finds, *Education Week,* XI, no. 30 (15 April 1992), 4.

Georges, E. Abortion policy and practice in Greece, *Social Science and Medicine,* 42, no. 4 (February 1996), 509–19.

Graham, C. A. & Smith, M. M. Operationalizing the concept of sexuality comfort: Applications for sexuality educators, *Journal of School Health,* 54, no. 11 (December 1984), 439–42.

Kempner, M. E. True integration of prevention programs requires broad focus on sexual health, *SIECUS Report,* 31, no. 3 (February/March 2003), 5–7.

Masters, W. Speech presented to the American School Health Association, Denver, CO, October 11, 1975.

Ruan, F. F. & Bullough, V. L. Sex in China, *Medical Aspects of Human Sexuality,* 24, no. 7 (July 1989), 59–62.

Smith, E. J. Discussing sexuality fosters sexual health, *SIECUS Report,* 30, no. 5 (June/July 2002), 7–12.

Snegroff, S. No sexuality education *is* sexuality education, *Family Planning Perspectives,* 32, no. 5 (September/October 2000), 257–58.

What is sexuality? Sexuality Information and Education Council of the United States (2000). Available: http://www.siecus.org/.

Suggested Readings

Chilman, C. Promoting healthy adolescent sexuality, *Family Relations,* 39, no. 2 (April 1990), 123–31.

Defining sexual health. Canadian Guidelines for Sexual Health Education (2000). Available: http://www.hc-sc.gc.ca/main/lcdc/web/publicat/.

Getting it together: Integrating teen pregnancy and STD/HIV prevention efforts, Special issue, *SIECUS Report,* 31, no. 3 (February/March 2003).

Greenberg, J. S., Bruess, C. E. & Haffner, D. W. *Exploring the dimensions of human sexuality.* Boston: Jones and Bartlett Publishers, 2004.

Haffner, D. W. Toward a new paradigm on adolescent sexual health, *SIECUS Report,* 21, no. 2 (December 1992/January 1993), 26–30.

Issues and answers: Fact sheet on sexuality education, *SIECUS Report,* 29, no. 6 (August/September 2001), 30–36.

Kempner, M. A. *Toward a sexually healthy America: Abstinence-only-until-marriage programs that try to keep our youth "scared chaste."* New York: Sexuality Information and Education Council of the United States, 2001.

Mayden, B. Taking action on sexual health, *SIECUS Report,* 29, no. 6 (August/September 2001), 25–28.

Reiss, I. L. America's rendezvous with sexual reality, in *An End to Shame: Shaping our next sexual revolution,* 17–38. Buffalo, NY: Prometheus Books, 1990.

Toward a sexually healthy America: Roadblocks imposed by the federal government's abstinence-only-until-marriage education program. Advocates for Youth & Sexuality Information and Education Council of the United States (2001). Available: http://www.advocatesforyouth.org/publications/.

Foundations for Sexuality Education

CHAPTER 2

Key Concepts

1. The goals of sexuality education are comprehensive.

2. A definition of sexuality education is multifaceted.

3. Sound reasons for sexuality education programs are based on broad considerations.

4. Understanding the history of sexuality helps us understand the development of sexuality education programs.

5. The history of sexuality education programs is relatively brief and mainly involves recent decades.

6. A number of current trends and issues in sexuality education will significantly impact tomorrow's sexuality education programs.

Now that we have established a concept of total human sexuality, it is appropriate to look at **sexuality education** itself. Why should there be sexuality education programs? What are the goals of sexuality education programs? What has gone on in the past related to sexuality education? It is important to understand the answers to these questions whether a sexuality education program is being considered for a school, clinic, or other setting, regardless of the age and characteristics of the learners. Before beginning this chapter, complete Insight 2-1 to assess your thinking about reasons for sexuality education.

Insight 2-1

Justifying a Sexuality Education Program

Imagine for a moment that you have been asked to give a 15-minute presentation to the local school board on the topic "Why There Should Be a Sexuality Education Program in the Local Schools." Would you be prepared to do so at this point? Let us find out. In the spaces below, give a brief outline of the three major points you would emphasize, and a few points under each major heading that you would present.

A. _____
   1. _____
   2. _____
B. _____
   1. _____
   2. _____
C. _____
   1. _____
   2. _____

Are you satisfied with the outline for your presentation to the school board? Do you think they will be convinced that local schools should have a sexuality education program after hearing from you?

Sexuality Education Goals and Objectives

It is obvious that specific sexuality education objectives will vary from program to program. Because of this, we will present a generalized look at the types of goals and objectives likely to be included. Note that there is a mixing of statements that might be considered goals with those that might be considered objectives. At this point we are not distinguishing between goals and objectives. We just want to explore logical expectations for sexuality education programs.

---

sexuality education A lifelong process of acquiring information and forming attitudes, beliefs, and values about identity, relationships, and intimacy. It encompasses sexual development, reproductive health, interpersonal relationships, affection, intimacy, body image, and gender roles. It addresses the biological, sociological, psychological, and spiritual dimensions of sexuality.

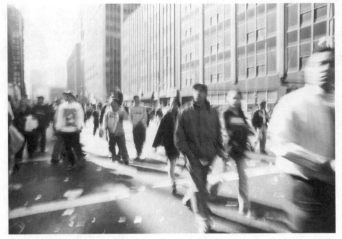

People hold many differing viewpoints about sexuality education; it is the sexuality educator's task to explore these viewpoints rationally.

Kirby, Alter, and Scales (1979, 3–4) listed the following sexuality education goals:

- To provide accurate information about sexuality

- To facilitate insights into personal sexual behavior

- To reduce fears and anxieties about personal sexual developments and feelings

- To encourage more informed, responsible, and successful decision making

- To encourage students to question, explore, and assess their sexual attitudes

- To develop more tolerant attitudes toward the sexual behavior of others

- To facilitate communication about sexuality with parents and others

- To develop skills for the management of sexual problems

- To facilitate rewarding sexual expression

- To integrate sex into a balanced and purposeful pattern of living

- To create satisfying interpersonal relationships

Tatum (1989) indicated that sexuality education is designed to help people:

1. Be prepared for life changes—puberty, adolescence, and stages of adulthood

2. Know that life changes are normal

3. Recognize their own bodies as good, beautiful, and private

4. Learn to make decisions that take into account possible consequences

5. Understand the place of sexuality in human life and loving

Some people would simply say that the objective of sexuality education should be to reduce or prevent sexual behavior. This is a variation of the "just say no" approach sometimes advocated for drug education programs. Consistent with the idea that people are sexual beings is the feeling that they also have the right to make their own sexual decisions. Haffner (1992, 1993) pointed out that we must change the dialogue around pregnancy and sexually transmitted infection (STI) prevention. She indicated that efforts would be more effective if in addition to trying to reduce the incidence of intercourse we also concentrated on reducing the incidence of *unprotected intercourse*. That means helping some people delay intercourse until they have the cognitive and emotional maturity to obtain and use contraception consistently and effectively. For others, it means helping them acknowledge that they are sexually involved, and teaching them skills to protect themselves. As you might guess, this aspect of objectives of sexuality education is controversial for many people.

The Health Protection Branch of Health Canada (Components of sexual health education, 2000) indicates that sexual health education involves a combination of educational experiences that will enable learners to do the following:

- Acquire knowledge that is pertinent to specific health issues

- Develop the motivation and personal insight that is necessary to act on this knowledge

- Acquire the skills they may need to maintain and enhance sexual health and avoid sexual problems

- Help create an environment that is conducive to sexual health

According to the Sexuality Information and Education Council of the United States (Sexuality education in the schools: Issues and answers, 2000), the primary goal of sexuality education is to promote adult sexual health. It seeks to assist people in understanding a positive view of sexuality, provide them with information and skills about taking care of their sexual health, and help them make sound decisions now and in the future. Therefore, comprehensive sexuality education programs have four main goals:

- To provide accurate information about human sexuality, including growth and development, human reproduction, anatomy, physiology, masturbation, family life, pregnancy, childbirth, parenthood, sexual response, sexual orientation, contraception, abortion, sexual abuse, HIV/AIDS, and other sexually transmitted infections.

- To provide an opportunity for learners to develop and understand their values, attitudes, and beliefs about sexuality. Opportunities should be provided for learners to question, explore, and assess their sexual attitudes in order to understand their families' values, develop their own values, increase self-esteem, develop insights concerning relationships with others, and understand their obligations and responsibilities to their families and others.

- To help learners develop relationships and interpersonal skills. Programs should help learners develop interpersonal skills, including communication, decision making, assertiveness, and peer refusal skills. Programs should also help learners develop the ability to create satisfying relationships, including caring, supportive, noncoercive, and mutually pleasurable sexual relationships.

- To help learners exercise responsibility regarding sexual relationships, including addressing abstinence, offering strategies for resisting pressures to become prematurely involved in sexual intercourse, and

encouraging the use of contraception and other sexual health measures. Sexuality education should be a central component of programs designed to reduce the prevalence of sexually related medical problems including teenage pregnancies, sexually transmitted infections, including HIV infection, and sexual abuse.

Before starting the next section, complete Insight 2-2 to summarize information about sexuality education goals and objectives. This Insight will also help determine where you stand on the goals and objectives of sexuality education.

Before leaving the topic of sexuality education goals and objectives, it is appropriate to consider that it has long been a basic right to learn about math, history, English, and other traditional subjects. Yet, the basic right to learn about the important and meaningful area of human sexuality has seldom been asserted. On the topic of individual rights and responsibilities concerning sexuality education, Haffner and de Mauro (1991) state the following:

1. All people have a right to comprehensive sexuality education.

Insight 2-2

Goals and Objectives of Sexuality Education

Now you have seen several examples of what goals and objectives of sexuality education might include. In the spaces below, list five similarities and five differences that you find among the lists as you study them again.

Similarities

1. _____
2. _____
3. _____
4. _____
5. _____

Differences

1. _____
2. _____
3. _____
4. _____
5. _____

Can you think of anything that you feel should be included in the goals and objectives of sexuality education that none of the expert sources included? Are you satisfied that you now understand the goals and objectives of sexuality education? Just to see how you are thinking at this point, list the three main goals and objectives of sexuality education from your viewpoint.

1. _____
2. _____
3. _____

2. Comprehensive sexuality education is an important part of the educational program in every grade in every school.

3. Organized religion can play a significant role in promoting an understanding of human sexuality.

4. All individuals have a right to information, education, and health care services that promote, maintain, and restore sexual health.

5. Sexual feelings, desires, and activities are present throughout the life cycle.

6. Persons with a physical and/or mental disability should receive sexuality education, sexual health care, and opportunities for socializing and sexual expression.

7. Society should give the AIDS crisis the highest priority and provide funds and strategies to combat the epidemic.

8. Sexual relationships should be consensual, with participants developmentally, physically, and emotionally capable of understanding the significance of the interaction.

9. Sexuality is a natural and healthy part of living and individuals have the right to make responsible sexual choices.

A Multifaceted Definition of Sexuality Education

If you are looking for a dictionary definition of sexuality education at this point, you are about to be disappointed. We do not know one that we like. At the same time, it is important to better understand what sexuality education is. Therefore, we offer the following understandings as characteristics of a quality sexuality education program. For example, those working in sexuality education programs need at least the following understandings:

1. Sexuality education is honestly looking at issues—not just moralizing or telling. It is often tempting to "tell" others how they ought to behave sexually. This is not what sexuality education is about today. An open and honest look at total sexuality related to groups, individuals, and decision making is appropriate and needed.

2. Sexuality education should be realistic. We need to take an honest and realistic look at what is and should be covered in contemporary sexuality education programs. Chances are, most material can be utilized with learners at an earlier age than previously thought. In addition, we need to be realistic in our recognition that all individuals are sexual beings from womb to tomb.

3. Sexuality education begins with parents. Most of the focus of this book is on planned sexuality education programs in different settings, but let us not forget that the primary sexuality educators are parents. The home is a continuous source of sexuality education. How questions are answered, how relatives act, and how total sexuality is handled are part of what sexuality education is all about.

4. Nonverbal sexuality education is at least as important as (and maybe more important than) verbal sexuality education. You can remember times when peoples' actions have spoken louder than words. This is so true in sexuality education. The person who claims to be ready to deal honestly with sexuality with young people but who squirms in his or her chair when asked about the topic of masturbation is communicating effectively nonverbally. Throughout life we see endless examples of facial expressions and other body language that serve as communication about sexuality. This is sexuality education too.

5. Sexuality education is dealing accurately with topical areas and concerns. Many studies indicate that sexual misinformation and myths are still common. Accurate information ought to help do away with many of these myths.

6. Sexuality education is not the same as sexual counseling, although the two areas may be related. We discuss sexual counseling in more detail in Chapter 15, but at this point we want you to realize that sexual counseling tends to occur in organized, one-on-one sessions between a counselor and client and is designed to lead to an adequate solution to a problem related to sexuality. Sexuality educators usually work with groups of people and do not deal directly with specific individual problems. It is sometimes tempting for educators to act as counselors, but before attempting to be a counselor, one needs to undertake appropriate additional training. This is not to imply that training is not needed to be a sexuality educator, but rather that special training is needed in both instances.

7. Sexuality education is based on the needs of the learners. Like any educational endeavor, the program goals and objectives should be derived from a needs assessment that assures the program will be relevant and appropriate to the audience. Failure to undertake this assessment often results in the inability to accomplish objectives because assumptions are made that have not been verified.

What Is Sexuality Education?

In order to consolidate the many ideas about sexuality education presented so far, complete five or six sentences beginning with: Sexuality education is . . .

1. _____
2. _____
3. _____
4. _____
5. _____

Compare the way you completed the sentences with the responses produced by one or two other people. What are the similarities and differences in your answers? Why do you feel these similarities and differences exist?

It might be helpful to consider what others have said in response to the question, "What is sexuality education?" Haffner (1990) gives this description:

Sexuality education is a lifelong process of acquiring information and forming attitudes, beliefs, and values about identity, relationships, and intimacy. It encompasses sexual development, reproductive health, interpersonal relationships, affection, intimacy, body image, and gender roles. Sexuality education addresses the biological, sociocultural, psychological, and spiritual dimensions of sexuality from 1) the cognitive domain, 2) the affective domain, 3) the behavioral domain, including the skills to communicate effectively and make responsible decisions.

According to Kirby (1997), effective sexuality education is characterized as follows:

- Uses behavioral goals, teaching methods, and materials that are appropriate to the age, sexual experience, and culture of the students

- Is based on theoretical approaches that have been demonstrated to be effective in influencing other health-related risky behaviors

- Takes places over a sufficient length of time to complete important activities adequately

- Employs a variety of teaching methods that involve the participants and allows them to personalize the information

- Provides basic, accurate information about the risks of unprotected intercourse and how to avoid unprotected intercourse

- Includes activities that address the social/peer pressures related to sexual behavior

- Provides practice of communication, negotiation, and refusal skills

- Utilizes teachers or peers who believe in the programs being implemented, and provides training for them.

Traditional Reasons for Sexuality Education

For many years the question of why there should be any sexuality education at all has been hotly debated. Unfortunately, many of those involved in sexuality education programs have immersed themselves in the program without really being able to justify why it should exist in the first place. Can you imagine the success that a sexuality education opponent would have simply by asking an unprepared educator why there should be a sexuality education program? Every person connected with sexuality education in any way ought to be comfortable responding to this often-asked question.

Although the actual statistics are pretty hard to come by, it is probably safe to say that most sexuality education programs in the country have been justified for the wrong reasons, or, at best, for some pretty shaky reasons. We still hear administrators, educators, parents, and community leaders clamoring that a sexuality education program is needed to reduce sexually transmitted infection (STI), to stop premarital pregnancy, to control promiscuity, and to eliminate all other undesirable hanky-panky. Once and for all, it would be wise to realize that it is very difficult to show that a sexuality education program is going to quickly or easily do any of these things.

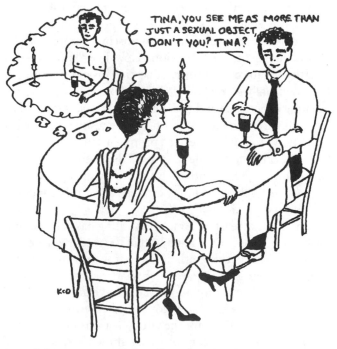

One of the purposes of sexuality education is to help people see each other as persons rather than as sexual objects.

This probably sounds like we are deserting you in the middle of the voyage, but it is true that it is almost impossible to tell whether the statistical relationships have changed as a direct result of any educational program. Let us examine briefly why this type of statistical attempt to justify a program simply does not hold up.

For example, what do STI statistics tell us? They only indicate how many people in a population are infected with certain organisms. If all students in a given classroom decided to have sexual intercourse with everyone else, assuming that no one had STI in the first place, there would still be no STI in the classroom. Even if some of them contracted STI elsewhere and did not report it, there would still be no STI according to local statistics.

It is even possible that an educational program will appear to cause a rise in STI. That is, when people understand the consequences and treatment of the disease and know about treatment facilities, they may be more likely to get treated. In this instance, the actual number of STI cases in a certain area would remain constant, but the reported cases might rise drastically. Does this mean that sexuality education caused more STI or more sexual behavior? Obviously not, but note the problem in attempting to deal with cause-and-effect relationships in a behavioral educational program.

If you are still not convinced, how about the example of promiscuity? What does the word mean? Is "responsible" sexual behavior the same as no sexual behavior? How many sexual relationships is the right number? With all these unanswered questions, it is not likely that a cause-and-effect relationship can even be considered.

If you are discouraged by this apparently dismal picture regarding the statistical success of sexuality education programs, it might make you feel a little better to realize that many of the same types of problems exist in other areas of education; they just are not as obvious. How do we know whether a math education or a history education program is successful? We usually give a knowledge and/or skills test after the learning experience and use the scores to assess success. As you will see in Chapter 18, some of the results of sexuality education programs have been promising, but it is unrealistic to expect us to be able to "prove" the results of sexuality education programs until such time as we are able to effectively demonstrate the long-term effects of other types of educational programs as well.

We hope at least one important thing has been accomplished in this section—namely, that the reader will be hesitant to use negative statistical relationships to justify a sexuality education program. Such relationships do not often hold up to a commonsense or statistical examination and can therefore backfire and jeopardize an entire program because it was justified for the wrong reasons initially.

Just because we cannot easily show these statistical relationships does not mean we should give up. Instead, let us realize that there are better reasons for sexuality education than those typically given.

Sound Reasons for Contemporary Sexuality Education Programs

Public opinion polls show that most Americans support sexuality education. While it may often be the case that people in the general public do not really understand sexuality education but support it because they think it can help decrease the negative consequences of early sexual activity, there is now more support for sexuality education than ever before. Haffner and Wagoner (1999) reported on a nationwide poll that found that more than 9 in 10 Americans (93%) support sexuality education in high school and more than 8 in 10 (84%) support it in junior high/middle school. Although the public is much more divided about sexuality education in grades 4 to 6 (48% support and 46% oppose), and largely oppose sexuality education in kindergarten through the third grade (78% oppose), those polled do support teaching early

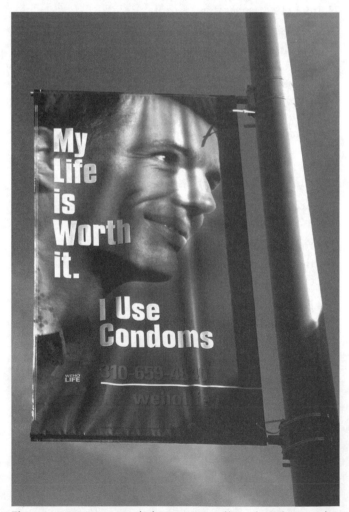

There are many ways to help meet sexuality education needs.

Insight 2-4

Major Reasons for Sexuality Education

Before reading further, list the three major reasons you would use to justify the existence of a sexuality education program.

1. _____

2. _____

3. _____

Now go back and check this list against the outline you prepared earlier (Insight 2-1) for a presentation to the local school board. What similarities and differences are there between your two lists? Has your thinking changed at all?

---

elementary students facts about sexual anatomy, reproduction, puberty, sexual abuse prevention, and sexually transmitted infections, especially HIV/AIDS.

Other studies also show strong support for sexuality education programs. For example, Lewis and others (2001) found that 91% of community members in a mid-size Midwest city favor school-based sexuality education. Additional studies have revealed that 86% of registered voters favor sexuality education for teenagers in public schools, 85% of adults agree that sexuality education should be taught in public schools, and 66% of registered voters favor increased efforts to provide sexuality education in public elementary schools (Public support for sexuality education, 2000).

By a contrast of 81% to 16%, lower income parents and guardians favor sexuality education programs that teach young people about all aspects of sexuality—including how to use birth control and how to protect against STI—over programs that focus solely on abstinence-only-until-marriage and the dangers of sexual behavior. Likewise, parents across ethnicities favor a comprehensive approach over one that only instructs about the dangers of sexual behavior and postponing sexual behavior until marriage, as shown in the following percentages: African-American (85% to 13%), White (80% to 16%), and Hispanic (80% to 18%) (National poll shows parents overwhelmingly support comprehensive sexuality education over abstinence-only-until-marriage by 5 to 1 margin, 2002).

Write your reasons for sexuality education in Insight 2-4. Now it is our turn. We would contend that there are at least three better reasons for sexuality education than those typically given. They are as follows:

1. Sexual adjustment is part of total personality adjustment. Sexuality education can *treat sexuality in its proper perspective.* Sexuality is but one part of total personality, yet it is an important part. It is necessary to understand one's sexual nature and needs as well as historically changing sex roles. Again, it is important to keep in mind our total definition of human sexuality as being part of human personality.

2. People receive a distorted view of life through the mass media—not completely false, just distorted. It is common to see sexual themes on television, in movies, and in magazines and books. Sexuality education can *place these aspects of life in their true perspective.* Promiscuity, broken marriages, illicit love affairs, and prostitution (to name a few) do happen in real life, but they are not as common in everyone's life as mass media seem to suggest. Emphasis should be on the relationship between sexuality and positive human relationships and personal feelings. Sexuality education programs can provide this perspective.

3. It has been well documented that learners receive much false information from many sources. It has generally been accepted that peers are the primary source of sexuality information; however, college students receive most sexuality information from reading. Peers are the second most common source, followed by schools and parents (Andre, Cietsch & Cheng, 1991). Sexuality education can *give factual information* that will help reduce many misconceptions. It is then possible for the learner to gain insight and understanding that will aid responsible decision making.

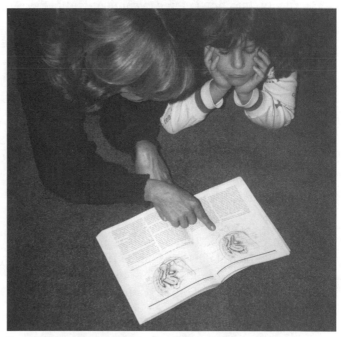

Certainly, parents ought to have a central role in the sexuality education of their children. Unfortunately, too many parents do not know how to assume this role effectively. School sexuality educators can be helpful in this regard, complementing the education received at home.

Along with these three reasons for including education about sexuality in community programs, there are a number of other reasons that might be given. Although the reasons listed below are not nearly as important as those already mentioned, they are provided in an attempt to consider all possibilities:

1. Many parents are unwilling or unable to provide the necessary education in matters of sexuality. This may be because they did not have the advantage of formal sexuality education. We are not attacking parents here; it is simply a fact that many are uncomfortable dealing with sexuality or have a difficult time relating to their own children in the area of sexuality. (And whether or not they choose to educate their children in sexuality, their attitudes and comments still serve as a foundation for more formal instruction.)

2. All children can be involved in sexuality education programs if the programs exist in schools. No other aspect of life reaches all children as the schools do.

3. Schools have the facilities and resources to provide a proper program. They are the logical place to find trained teachers, teaching aids, and a favorable environment.

4. Because of increased rates of divorce, premarital pregnancy, and STI, the community should provide education concerning sexuality. It is unrealistic to think that sexuality education is going to eliminate any of these problems. This line of reasoning is therefore weak justification for sexuality education. If we reduce misconceptions, present a total view of life, and show how sexual adjustment fits into total personality adjustment, this negative approach to sexuality education should be of secondary importance, for the reasons discussed earlier.

5. Since there seems to be more sexual freedom today, sexuality education should be taught to help people adjust to this situation. The decision-making process comes into play here, just as it does in other educational areas.

Recognizing that there are sound reasons for sexuality education programs, the Sexuality Information and Education Council of the United States (SIECUS) has called upon national organizations to join together as a national coalition to support sexuality education. To help assure that all children and youth receive comprehensive sexuality education, it (Haffner, 1990) has presented these goals:

1. Sexuality education will be viewed as a community-wide responsibility.

2. All parents will receive assistance in providing quality sexuality education for their child(ren).

3. All schools will provide sexuality education for children and youth.

4. All religious institutions serving youth will provide sexuality education.

5. All national youth serving agencies will implement sexuality education programs and policies.

6. The media will assume a more proactive role in sexuality education.

7. Federal policies and programs will support sexuality education.

8. Each state will have policies for school-based sexuality education and assure that mandates are implemented on a local level.

9. Guidelines, materials, strategies, and support for sexuality education will be available at the community level.

10. All teachers and group leaders providing sexuality education to youth will receive appropriate training.

11. New methodologies will be developed to evaluate sexuality education programs.

12. Broad support for sexuality education will be activated.

Now you should be able to justify a sexuality education program. Interestingly enough, the reasons for a program remain essentially the same regardless of the age of the learners or the setting for sexuality education.

Sexuality in History

We hope the total view of sexuality developed in Chapter 1 is still with you. You will remember that its several components are based on learning that has taken many forms. This learning is based, to a great extent, on the behavior and thinking of people who lived a long time ago. To better appreciate why many people feel as they do about human sexuality, a brief look at history is appropriate.

All of you have studied history to various degrees in school courses and on your own. Often our history books give little attention to sexual activities and thinking in previous cultures. But in more recent years, a number of sources have become available that point out countless influences on human sexuality today from past cultures. (For those historians among you, we do want to point out that whenever we generalize about people's actions and thoughts during a particular historical period, we will tend to overgeneralize; obviously, not all people at a certain time thought and did exactly the same things.)

It has only been in recent years that sexuality has been recognized as a suitable topic for open study. In fact, we are sure

Insight 2-5

Sexuality in History

If you have any history books available at home or in a nearby library, take a quick look to see if the topic of sexuality is given much attention. If references to sexuality are made, compare them to the ones you find in this chapter. Also, ask a few friends or relatives what events they can think of throughout history that are related to human sexuality. Or how about you? See how many historical events related to human sexuality you can list below.

1. _____
2. _____
3. _____
4. _____
5. _____
6. _____

you know some people today who still do think it ought not be studied. This taboo surrounding the topic is also easily seen in a historical review.

With these introductory points in mind, let us proceed with a quick look at a number of historical influences on attitudes toward sexuality in Western culture. We have broken them down by century for clarity, but we are sure you realize that they actually all ran together and that a new century did not suddenly mean everyone started thinking or acting differently.

Prehistoric Times

A look at prehistoric European cave paintings and the art of today's primitive cultures indicates that over thirty thousand years ago sexuality was already an important part of culture. Some engravings are suggestive of human intercourse, show women with exaggerated body parts, and show men with overemphasized erect penises. Prehistoric art showing human beings in physical relations with animals is thought to be evidence of bestiality.

It appears that sexual activity already had special or magical qualities in people's minds. It could have been a way to communicate with nature, participate in certain customs of a group, or relate to the supernatural. Some paintings even seem to indicate relationships between sexual activity and famine and disease.

Eighth Century *BCE–*Fifth Century *CE*

During this period, a wide variety of attitudes about human sexuality were evident. These are represented by fertility cults and the ancient cultures of the Jews, Greeks, and Romans.

1. *Fertility cults.* It has been reported that sexual behavior relating to nature and religious rites existed over six thousand years ago (Sadock, Kaplan & Freedman, 1976). For example, sexual symbolism played an important role in art. The act of intercourse was often regarded as an act of worship. Since the hymen was considered the guardian to the gateway of generation, a young woman was often ritually deflowered. There were not many restrictions on sexual behavior, except for adultery. Phallic statues played a part in religious activities.

2. *Ancient Jews.* There are many references in the Old Testament indicating that reproduction and at least a narrow form of sexuality were important to the ancient Jews. There is the covenant with God involving circumcision (Genesis 17:9–14), a declaration excluding men from the Lord's congregation if their genitals were cut off (Deuteronomy 23:1), many references to going forth and multiplying, and declarations that both menstrual blood (Leviticus 12) and semen (Leviticus 15:16) were unclean. Punishment was also specified if the male's precious seed of life was wasted.

   Significantly, there was an evident double standard for sexual behavior. That is, men and women were supposed to adhere to different standards of sexual morality. The man was the ruler of the family, and his wife was regarded as property.

   Sexual relations with a menstruating woman were taboo. A person was not supposed to expose his or her genital area to another person, even a relative. Nonreproductive sexual behavior was frowned upon, apparently a consequence of the idea that the seed was not supposed to be wasted.

3. *Ancient Greeks.* A variety of sexual behaviors were supposedly practiced by the gods worshipped by the Greeks, so they felt it appropriate to follow the example. The following Greek sexual behaviors and attitudes are illustrative of their culture (Sex in ancient Greece, 1971):

   a. The body, particularly the male body, was considered to be very beautiful. The physical was measured for its excellence, as is evident in the emphasis on athletic competition.

---

fertility cult   A group (usually in ancient times) that regards the act of sexual intercourse as an act of worship.

b. The Greeks viewed people as bisexual.

c. Worshippers of the god Dionysus tried to become possessed by his orgiastic spirit through wild dancing and sex orgies.

d. The emphasis on physical beauty led to open nudity in athletic competition and in art.

e. Women were considered to be greatly inferior to men.

f. Since the Greeks considered people to be bisexual, homosexual activity was not unusual.

g. Masturbation in the young was thought of as a useful safety valve, but it was looked down upon when practiced by adults.

4. *Ancient Romans.* In the early years of Rome, women bore the burden of sexual morality. Chastity before and fidelity after marriage was the rule, and it was better to die than to be dishonored. (Do you see any resemblance between this philosophy and current thinking?) Again, there was a double standard, since men were allowed to enjoy prostitutes. Because homosexual behavior was a Greek practice, the Romans considered it an insult. There was no divorce; in fact, there was no legal process by which to obtain one.

Later in Roman history, many sexual restrictions were abandoned, and divorce became a fact of life. Orgies were common, and the penis became a religious object. A certain crudeness and directness marked this period. Lust was a major satisfaction. Abortion was common, but as the birth rate fell there were attempts to stop the practice (Sex in ancient Rome, 1971).

Fifth Century–Fifteenth Century

During these centuries, the main influence on sexuality was early Christian morality, which in turn led to the growth of belief in witchcraft.

1. *Early Christians.* For many early Christians, the highest form of moral achievement was a complete rejection of the body except for the minimum satisfaction of needs required for maintaining life. Since sexual behavior was viewed as primarily physical, it was considered sinful and inferior to all things of the spirit. Even within the sanction of marriage, sexual intercourse was a shameful thing. The glory of everlasting virginity was the highest state for women.

There was not supposed to be any pleasure associated with sexual activity. In fact, the only official reason for intercourse was reproduction.

It appears that Jesus advocated a single standard against adultery, rather than the earlier double standard. Paul urged people to remain celibate, but it must be remembered that he felt the end of the world was near. In this regard, faithful people should have been concerned with preparing themselves for the end rather than with such earthly matters as sexual needs.

2. *Witchcraft.* Since people had learned to disguise sexual feelings, the fact that some sexual feelings still existed caused interesting reactions. For example, some individuals punished themselves physically by sleeping on hard wooden beds or by purposely wearing extremely uncomfortable clothes. Others never completely satisfied such physical desires as hunger and thirst since they felt it was better to deny physical pleasures.

Anything that could not be explained was attributed to the supernatural. Strong emotional feelings, especially lust and passion, supposedly came from evil spirits. Since women inspired lust, they were sometimes seen as agents of the devil. Such women were tortured to drive out the devil in them. Bewitchment was said to account for the mysterious and overwhelming emotional effect that women have on men, sometimes driving them to commit irrational acts (Sadock, Kaplan & Freedman, 1976).

Fifteenth Century–Sixteenth Century

In the early fifteenth century, life seemed to take on a new meaning. In Renaissance Europe the individual was seen as important, and the existence of desires and impulses was recognized. There was greater recognition of emotional relationships between people. Of course, the fact that emotional relationships could exist led to a gradual uplifting in the status of women; they could be valued, and they were acknowledged to have feelings too.

As part of the movement away from some of the constraints of the past, more attention was given to human sexuality in literature, art, and daily living. Once again it began to be acceptable to enjoy sexual behavior.

Modesty in dress declined. Women dressed in such a way as to make their breasts more visible, and men wore a codpiece that covered an opening in the front of their breeches. Some men even padded the codpiece to add more emphasis to their genital area.

As New World explorations became relatively common, the incidence of syphilis soared. This led to attempts to decrease the incidence of prostitution, as it was believed that prostitutes were a major source of the disease.

Seventeenth Century–Eighteenth Century

Many scientific discoveries occurred in the seventeenth century that influenced thinking about sexuality. Throughout previous years, religious scriptures had been the main source of information for answering questions. Because scientific discoveries provided explanations for things not previously

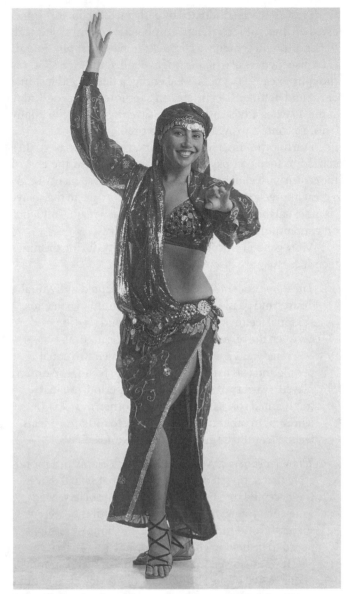

Sexuality and culture is a topic that sexuality educators should explore.

understood, intellectuals turned away from reliance on scriptures. In fact,

> *faith in reason, belief in absolute truth, and the concept of natural laws marked all aspects of later 17th and 18th century life. With the mystery of sex diminished and the fear of supernatural retribution for sexual transgressions all but eliminated, the Age of Reason became, as well, the age of license. Laissez-faire, laissez-passer, live and let pass, an attitude toward economic matters, became applicable to sexual behavior and mores. (Sadock, Kaplan & Freedman, 1976, 42)*

1. *Seventeenth-century England.* This time period marked the transition from Puritan thinking to relatively unrestrained thinking about sexuality. Queen Elizabeth I

wanted to be known as a lifelong virgin. Shakespeare's plays, however, had countless references to direct sexual behavior; of course, the Puritans spoke against the immorality of the theater and immoral conduct in general.

The Puritan influence was responsible for legislation designed to prevent amusements such as dancing, singing, and the theater. Women were treated like prostitutes if they wore long hair or makeup. On Sundays, any activities not related to worship were banned.

The austere Puritan period did not last long in England, and during the Restoration many people participated in sexual acts of many kinds to a degree probably not seen before in history. The king (Charles II) set the tone by participating in sexual activities with a number of mistresses himself. The theater again used sexual themes successfully and quite openly. And homosexual behavior was not censured.

Rational sexuality, defined as reason used in physical and emotional relations between the sexes, was a concept that came about as a result of the new emphasis on reason and science. Daily activities were supposed to be controlled by the mind and the will. For some people, proper sexual behavior was to be learned almost in an educational situation, and refined manners were to be used while passion was suppressed. Passion was then viewed as an opposite force to logic.

2. *Puritan New England.* As it became difficult for some of the English Puritans to practice their beliefs, many fled to American shores for freedom. The culture of Puritan New England contributed greatly to the shaping of sexual thinking in the early days of the new United States. Puritans believed in the supreme sovereignty of God and the totally sinful nature of man. The patriarchal family structure was the rule, and the father made all important decisions, even those related to future mates of children.

Premarital chastity was the rule for both males and females, but church records indicate that premarital intercourse was the most popular sin in Puritan New England. There were strong restrictions against sexual pleasure, and, even within marriage, intercourse was allowable only as a means designated by God for reproduction of the species.

3. *Eighteenth-century England.* This century again marked rapid changes in sexual thinking. Certain standards for behavior developed by the end of the century that had not existed at all at the beginning. Sexual behavior became more subdued, and spontaneous behavior gave way to inhibitions. Open sexual affairs became a thing of the past as people started to conduct their lives more privately.

Negative attitudes toward homosexuality developed, and there are numerous reports of putting homosexuals to death during this period. People asking for leniency for those convicted of sodomy were thought to have a personal interest in the behavior themselves.

It is interesting to note that by the end of the eighteenth century, many sexual restrictions were similar to those desired earlier by the Puritans. Perhaps this is evidence that social changes can evolve naturally but cannot be forced.

4. *American southern colonists.* We would miss an important influence on American sexual attitudes if we did not note the sexual attitudes and behavior of the southern colonists. These colonists still believed in a patriarchal family structure, and the male was considered superior to the female. The status of the female was relatively high for the times, though, since she had some property rights, and sometimes her sentiments would be considered in mate selection.

Perhaps the most significant social characteristic with regard to sexuality was the double standard for sexual behavior. This philosophy influenced American sexual thinking for many years. In its simplest sense, the double standard meant that males had sexual freedom not shared by females. Promiscuity by husbands was condoned, whereas the purity of upper-class white females was closely guarded. The women were warned to accept the double standard and to avoid showing jealousy. In fact, they were to conceal knowledge of their husbands' infidelity.

Of course, wherever there is a double standard, the question must be posed: Who are the males going to participate with if females are not supposed to participate? In this case, the males had sexual access to lower-class white women and to black female slaves. Some historians feel that this situation is responsible for the beginning of problems related to sexuality and racism. Since white males had sexual access to black female slaves but white females were not supposed to have contact with other males, a social system arose to justify this situation. In effect, there were two double standards at the same time—one between the sexes and the other between the races. To support the racist structure, myths related to racial differences in genital size, sexual abilities, and sexual desires were created. Some of these myths still exist today and have continued to be a source of personal, social, and legal conflict.

Nineteenth Century

While research into the area of sexuality was for centuries not acceptable to many people, during the eighteenth century some research was conducted by early medical doctors interested in the subject. Their emphasis was physiological. Expenditure of semen was thought to have vast physiological consequences. Particularly if expended to "excess," it was thought to cause dryness, weakening, a decay of the spinal cord, and aching. It is interesting to note that even today some coaches advise athletes to "save themselves" sexually before a contest to avoid being too tired.

During the nineteenth century, research on sexuality started to focus on psychological areas. Toward the end of the century, psychoanalytic interpretations of sexuality made a great impression on society. A clinical approach to the analysis of sexual thoughts and behavior still has a major influence on contemporary thinking about sexuality.

More general attitudes toward sexuality during the nineteenth century are discussed below.

1. *The Romantic era.* The Romantics accepted individual desires and passions as important to human behavior. Personal feelings were emphasized, and relations between the sexes were supposed to be natural. Marriage was viewed as a union between two equal people and was to be based on mutual feelings. Women played a variety of roles during this period, not just a fragmented role as either a wife, mother, mistress, or whore, as in other times. According to romantic ideals, feelings should be guides to choices and behavior.

2. *The Victorian era.* Around 1840, Victorianism, a moral ethic that supported the suppression of sexual drives, was accepted by a large part of English society. Men were encouraged to delay marriage until they were successful and financially stable. Passions were supposed to be held in check before and after marriage.

It was believed that men had natural and spontaneous sexual desires but that women's drives were not spontaneous and were dormant unless subjected to undue excitation. Children were thought to have no sexual feelings.

Many efforts were made to protect people from being placed in danger of sexual excitation. Sexual references in literature and surroundings in general were suppressed. Masturbation was viewed as a negative behavior and was called "the secret sin," "self-pollution," and "the solitary vice." Devices were even developed to place around the male's penis at night to prevent "spermatorrhea," or wet dreams.

3. *The United States in the nineteenth century.* In its usual way, the United States served as a sort of melting pot, representing a variety of activities and thoughts originating in other, much older countries. The family was still strongly patriarchal, and the double standard for sexual behavior was quite common. In fact, it was often believed that a man could not be expected to restrict

his sexual needs to marriage. For many women, even within marriage, sexual relations were an unspeakable and unpleasant duty necessary for reproduction and for satisfying their husbands' "animal" needs.

Women were not supposed to experience sexual pleasure; if they did, it led to suspicion from husbands and guilt on the part of wives. To help meet the male need, prostitution emerged as an important social institution. Then the male could turn to the prostitute to satisfy his strong drives and also protect the "good" women from his uncontrollable desires.

Many social changes were occurring in the United States that contributed to rather rapid changes near the end of the nineteenth century and particularly in the early twentieth century. Examples of these changes are the Industrial Revolution, the westward expansion, and a great deal of immigration. These factors influenced thinking about male-female roles, family styles, and sexual behavior in general. It is also significant to note that in 1848 the first organized meeting took place to formulate a statement on the rights of women. As sexuality started to be a legitimate area of study, researchers collected evidence that indicated varieties of sexual behavior were much more common than had been thought. This led to the questioning of traditional moral viewpoints.

Thanks to the activities of Anthony Comstock, birth control became a public issue. Comstock, an official of the New York Society for the Suppression of Vice, was able to persuade the U.S. Congress in 1873 to pass a law prohibiting the mailing across state lines of obscene material. Birth control information and devices were specifically defined as obscene.

Before leaving the nineteenth century, we should pause to consider the thinking of two men, Havelock Ellis and Sigmund Freud. Their ideas have had a significant impact on the thinking of many others about human sexuality.

Ellis (1859–1939), who decided to become a physician and study human sexuality, grew up in fear of what might happen to him because of what he had been told about the danger of nocturnal emissions. He was also concerned about his general ignorance of human sexuality. Between 1896 and 1910 Ellis published a six-volume series, entitled *Studies in the Physiology of Sex,* that contained the following beliefs:

1. Masturbation is common for both sexes.

2. Orgasm in males and females is very much the same.

3. Homosexuality and heterosexuality are a matter of degree.

4. Women do have sexual desire, contrary to Victorian thought.

5. There is no one norm for human sexuality. Thoughts and acts vary between individuals and among cultures.

6. There should be sexual education for both sexes starting at early ages (note how radical this one was).

7. There should not be laws against contraception or private sexual behavior.

It is clear that Ellis's ideas were very controversial and way ahead of their time. In fact, some people today would still have difficulty accepting them. His work was influential on the later pursuits of many sexuality researchers and writers.

Freud (1856–1939), a psychological researcher, developed theories about human development, personality, and psychopathology that have influenced later thinking. In order to develop into a well-adjusted person, according to Freud, one has to progress successfully through a number of psychosexual stages.

Freud viewed sexuality and sexual pleasure as a central part of human life and felt that people naturally sought to have as much pleasure and as little pain as possible. He indicated that sexual activity was natural, that procreation was secondary to pleasure, and cautioned against too severe restriction on sexual instincts. People, he maintained, could become neurotic if they were denied natural expression.

One of Freud's important contributions was his suggestion that children are sexual beings and that early childhood experiences have strong consequences for adult functioning. Largely owing to Freud's work, sexual thoughts and behaviors are still considered to be major influences on contemporary life in general.

Twentieth-Century–Twenty-First-Century United States

As traditional moral viewpoints were questioned, people began to wonder whether any one standard of morality could apply universally. Social scientists talked about people being definers of their own morality, while religious leaders saw morality as being determined by a higher order than mere humans.

1. *1900–1945.* As traditional religious morality began to slip, there were secular attempts to legislate morality. Censorship, prohibition, and the revival of old statutes against certain sexual behaviors were the next step. The role of the female underwent significant change. Women had more social freedom, as shown by less parental control in choosing a mate, and they had more bodily freedom, as shown by changes in styles of dress.

   World War I had a social impact too. It forced large numbers of people to come into contact with other societies, which led to a further questioning of traditional sexual mores. Family roles were questioned and altered as well.

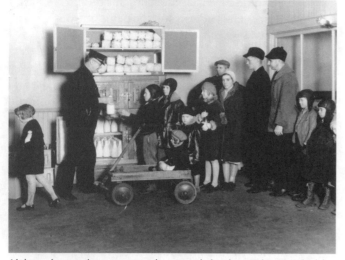

Although people are apt to be nostalgic about the good old days, a closer look reveals that they were not always so good. Students should be encouraged to make decisions in the here and now.

Many social forces resulted in new patterns of thinking about sexual behavior. There was a decrease in the "sinful" view of sexual behavior, and there were arguments for sexual expression as being natural and meaningful. The increased knowledge and reliability of contraceptives led to the view that there must be a reason for intercourse other than reproduction. This meant that people were admitting that they were participating in sexual behavior for enjoyment and as part of a relationship.

In the 1920s and 1930s Margaret Sanger's work gave a push to the development of the birth control movement. She wrote about the need to give women more control over their own bodies and emphasized the fact that happiness in marriage was related to the ability to control births. In addition, she opened clinics designed to make birth control information and services more readily and widely available.

The family structure started to shift from a patriarchal style to a companionship style, involving more democracy and recognition of the rights and feelings of all members. The sexual rights of women were held to be important, and it was even believed that female sexual drives existed and needed to be satisfied.

The spontaneous invention of dating influenced mate selection and provided countless opportunities for people to better know themselves as well as others. Romantic stories became a part of the mass media as improved technology facilitated the establishment of the media as a significant social force. The early movies and soap operas presented a variety of stories of love and romantic experiences.

The nineteenth amendment to the Constitution gave women the right to vote. The presence of the automobile gave people a bedroom on wheels and great mobility. Toward the end of this period, World War II again caused a social upheaval that tested and changed thinking about lifestyles and sexuality.

2. *1945 to the present.* During this time it has become accepted that early childhood experiences are important in relation to the development of a child's future sexuality. (Note that this probably came about because of Freud's work, which was already mentioned.) This idea is in direct contrast to earlier thinking that children should be treated as asexual beings, and it has ramifications for sexuality education of children of all ages.

Theoretically, in the United States there is a separation of church and state, but legal debates about such subjects as abortion, access to sexual services, homosexuality, and other sexual behaviors have prompted some people to wonder about the separation. The formal restrictions on sexual behavior are much the same as they have been for a long time, but the behavior of many people indicates that the formal restrictions are no longer effective—if they ever were.

Kinsey's research on human sexual behavior in males and females provided a look at proportions of people engaging in many different sexual behaviors. The existence of such research findings had social influences that are still being felt.

Sexual themes in the mass media have become prominent. Almost any type of product can apparently make one more attractive, make one smell better, have psychological benefits, or in some other way influence one's sexuality. Magazines, TV, and radio all use sexual themes to sell products. In addition, a variety of magazines of the *Playboy* type have published written and visual images about sexuality quite openly.

More reliable contraceptives, especially birth control pills, have been developed and accepted by large numbers of people. Today there are so many reliable and relatively safe contraceptive means that planning for conception or contraception has become a simple matter for motivated people.

The work of Masters and Johnson on human sexual response greatly contributed to knowledge about how we work sexually and what might go wrong. In addition to providing needed basic information about human functioning, their research has become the foundation for sexual counseling and methods for dealing with human sexual inadequacy.

Various experiments in living have been common, including communes, swinging, extended families,

A Historical Comparison

You have been exposed rather quickly to different descriptions of how sexuality has been regarded in Western history. If you were able to live in a different time period than today, which of the previously described historical eras would you choose? List three advantages and three disadvantages of your choice as it relates to your sexuality.

Period: _____

Advantages

1. _____

2. _____

3. _____

Disadvantages

1. _____

2. _____

3. _____

contract marriages, and trial marriages. Depending upon one's viewpoint, these experiments may be signs of decaying family relationships or signs of the search for more positive, more vital human relationships. Numerous researchers contributed to our knowledge of human sexual behavior.

You probably noticed that there was little if any mention of sexuality education in our historical overview. This is because throughout most of history there was little provision for sexuality education of people at any age. The history of sexuality education is comparatively brief; while we are still in a historical mood, let us take a look at it.

History of Sexuality Education

As we have seen in our brief trip through history, sexuality has been intermingled with other social factors for centuries. Although it could be interpreted that sexuality education in an extremely broad sense was present at various times, as an educational concern it can be traced back about a century. Carrera (1971) pointed out that as early as the 1880s, groups such as the American Purity Alliance, the YMCA, the YWCA, and the Child Study Association sponsored lectures and panels on sex-related topics. He also indicated that the National Education Association and the National Congress of Parents and Teachers discussed sexuality education in the schools in the early 1890s.

It was not until the early twentieth century, however, that sexuality education started to appear somewhat regularly

as a topic in educational literature. Most of the early references to sexuality education involved school settings, but they contained implications for other settings as well.

A number of writings and events relevant to the early development of sexuality education were outlined by Means (1962). These included references as early as 1900 to the importance of instruction in sexual hygiene as well as preparation for marriage and parenthood. Provision for sexuality instruction in the schools was stimulated by the 1919 White House Conference on Child Welfare, at which it was stated that "the problem of [sex] instruction becomes more properly a task of the school" (Means, 1962, 134). Also in 1919, the U.S. Government Printing Office issued two publications relevant to sexuality education. One, with an obvious physiological emphasis, was titled *A High School Course in Physiology in Which the Facts of Sex Are Taught;* a second, titled *The Problem of Sex Education in Schools,* was more broadly based.

Means also pointed out two interesting surveys conducted in the early 1920s. In one, which represented 224 of the largest school systems in the United States, it was found that less than 26% made provision for social hygiene and sexuality instruction. In the other, a survey of courses of study in the 48 states, only three stated curricular outlines stipulated suggestions for teaching "sex hygiene."

There are periodic references to sexuality education in a few sources throughout the late 1920s and 1930s. In most instances, they consist of simple statements indicating that it would be a good idea to provide some instruction related to sexuality. For example, as a result of the 1930 White House Conference on Child Welfare, a statement was made that the school should provide instruction in "social hygiene, including sex; and in the preparation for potential parenthood" (Means, 1962, 260). Leibee (1937) stated: "We in America are just beginning to realize that if our aim for education is to develop the whole child, then we must not and cannot neglect the education of his sex life." He further indicated that sex education does not mean merely instruction concerning sex organs. The fact that it has been thought of only in such a narrow light has been the greatest barrier to its development. In 1940, the U.S. Public Health Service produced a pamphlet entitled *High Schools and Sex Education,* which broadly covered methods, materials, planning, organization, and integration of sexuality education in many fields. It also contained a suggested outline of a course for teachers on sexuality education in secondary schools.

The American Social Health Association (ASHA) deserves mention as an important group in the history of sexuality education. It was founded in 1910 as the American Federation for Sex Education and eventually evolved to its present name. In the process, other organizations joined with it to attempt to improve community conditions, point out the need for sexuality education, help reduce venereal diseases, and repress commercialized prostitution. As a result, in 1953

ASHA launched a nationwide program for family-life education (Means, 1962).

In 1950, delegates to the Mid-Century White House Conference on Children and Youth also emphasized the importance of family-life education. They indicated that well-prepared teachers should avoid emphasis on sex facts and give proper attention to the total topic. They felt that sexuality education should be psychologically and humanistically oriented.

In 1955, the Joint Committee on Health Problems in Education of the National Education Association and the American Medical Association published five pamphlets that were referred to as the sex education series. These included *Parents' Privilege* and *A Story About You* for upper-elementary grades, *Finding Yourself* for junior-high grades, *Learning About Love* for later teenagers, and *Facts Aren't Enough* to assist adults in understanding sexuality education.

Manley (1964) reminded educators that the home should be the source of children's first sex education, and that children should receive as much approval on their discovery of their genitals as of their toes. She further indicated that the schools were lagging because of fears on the part of administrators. She also gave an example, however, dating from as early as 1930, when a teacher recognized the need for a sexuality education unit and added the material to the curriculum without excitement or commotion. (Perhaps there is a lesson here for us today.)

As individuals and groups became more interested in sexuality education programs in the 1960s, groups opposed to sexuality education came into being. Also in the 1960s, two important groups in support of sexuality education were created. The first was the Sexuality Information and Education Council of the United States, and the second was the American Association of Sex Educators, Counselors, and Therapists. Both of these groups remain strong in their contributions to sexuality education literature and programs.

A few more recent events related to sexuality education have been outlined by Schiller (1973). In the early 1960s it was apparently the policy of the U.S. Office of Education to encourage and support family-life and sex education programs at all levels, as well as teacher-training programs. These programs were to focus on psychological, sociological, economic, and social factors that affect personality and individual adjustment and were to be included in school programs in a variety of ways. This policy did not immediately change teacher-preparation programs, as shown by the fact that a 1967 survey of teacher-preparation institutions determined that only 21% of the 250 responding institutions offered a specific course or courses designed to prepare teachers to teach sexuality education.

Initially, the sexuality education and family-planning movements developed separately. In fact in many sexuality education programs, the subject of contraception was often avoided. In the early 1970s, however, it was realized that sexuality education and family planning are interdependent for reasons related to personality, education, and behavior.

In more recent years a wealth of information has been learned about sexuality education programs. Probably because of greater visibility and controversy, most of this information has been related to the school setting. For example, Kirby, Alter, and Scales (1979) reported extensively on sexuality programs around the United States as well as their effects. The Alan Guttmacher Institute (1983) developed a statement on school sexuality education in policy and practice. A number of researchers have provided us with reliable information about the effects of sexuality education programs (Kirby, 1985, 1997).

As of 2000, 19 states and the District of Columbia required schools to provide sexuality education (Sexuality education in the schools: Issues and answers, 2000). In some of the remaining 31 states, there are still content requirements for schools where sexuality education is taught. In addition, 34 states and the District of Columbia require STI or HIV/AIDS education. There have always been people opposed to sexuality education programs. Yet, because of the existence of many strong sexuality education programs, we can now justify them and describe their probable effects (assuming that the programs are well planned and implemented) with a great deal of confidence.

Current Trends in Sexuality Education

It is obvious that the early history of sexuality education was very fragmented, inconsistent, and limited in its focus. Today there is a trend toward a more total approach to sexuality education. This has brought about a broadening of program objectives and an obvious emphasis on such things as the total person and decision making as opposed to earlier educational efforts aimed mainly at the acquisition of knowledge.

Many different types of organizations now play an important role in sexuality education. The schools have remained a basic potential source of sexuality education programs, but churches, voluntary agencies, health departments, professional schools, and even clubs now contribute to overall sexuality education efforts.

While certainly not true everywhere, a more open atmosphere in which to handle sexuality education has developed. In many places the subject of sexuality can usually now be handled much like other subjects. It is not always considered a sacred subject that requires many different guidelines and approaches.

Approaches to sexuality education have been expanded. In the past, sexuality education programs often consisted of a lecture or two on physiology or body care by a doctor or a nurse. A variety of teaching methodologies are used today: entire courses are sometimes required of students, elective programs are available, and sexuality education may be found as a part of many different programs and subjects.

Planned courses of study have become common. They exist for parents, administrators, counselors, physicians, nurses, and other professionals as well as for elementary- and secondary-school students.

Better literature and audiovisual materials have become available. Not too many years ago it was difficult to find good books, pamphlets, and audiovisuals to use in a sexuality education program. This is no longer the case; in fact, today, the problem is often in wading through the many resources to evaluate them and decide which are most useful.

There is a trend away from the use of euphemisms in sexuality education. Terminology tends to be more accurate and direct, and there is less need to skirt so-called sensitive issues.

Sexuality education is provided for children at earlier ages today. In many school districts, programs exist for students from kindergarten through the twelfth grade, and are available in some form even in nursery school. The need for establishing a strong educational foundation has been recognized.

Training of sexuality educators has improved greatly. Colleges and universities offer single courses, combinations of courses, and even entire degree programs designed to prepare people to be sexuality educators. Some voluntary agencies and professional training programs also contribute to the training of sexuality educators.

The gender of the students and the educators is usually no longer much of an issue in sexuality education. It used to seem important to separate males and females for sexuality education, but such segregation is less common today. In

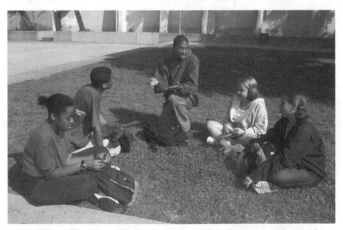

Sexuality education does not end at the classroom door. The trend now is for groups to respond to the sexual education needs of people long after formal sexuality education has ceased.

---

addition, it used to be felt that only males should teach other males and females should teach other females, but this is now seen as less important than the ability of the educator to relate to the learners.

There is a trend away from treating sexuality education solely as something necessary for marriage or childbearing. It is more widely recognized that people of all ages living any lifestyle are sexual beings in a total sense. They have important choices to make related to human sexuality. In this context, marriage and childbearing are important issues, but they are not by any means the only ones.

In some places, we have seen school-based clinics (or a clinic based elsewhere in the community) used in conjunction with a sexuality education program. Nurses, physicians, counselors, and others in the clinic are available to help people learn more about sexuality and perhaps receive sexuality-related services, such as contraceptive information, counseling, and even the actual contraceptives.

Diverse titles are still given to sexuality education programs—family-life education, sex education, human growth and development, family life and human development, etc. The old term "sex education" is problematic because it gives the image of a class focused on sexual behavior or perhaps the "plumbing" related to reproduction. "Sexuality education" is preferable because it conveys a broader meaning—education about the human condition, being male or female, feelings, roles, communication, as well as sexual functioning. The title "family-life education" is often chosen in schools because it sounds less controversial since it implies the importance of family life and family relationships.

Despite all of the improvements and potential for quality sexuality education, many obstacles remain that inhibit the realization of successful programs. In many communities, certain (and sometimes all) sexuality content is banned;

poorly prepared teachers often have responsibility for the program; book companies are reluctant to include sexuality as a chapter (it is often relegated to a supplement); and educators often fail to plan a comprehensive approach to teaching about sexuality.

In addition, controversies about sexuality education are all around us (Kempner, 1999). They include the following:

- Controversies stemming from complaints that curricula, presentations, and materials expose young people to inappropriate information. Debates include arguments over books, videos, speakers, and information about, or availability of, condoms and contraception.

- Educators coming under attack, not only for what they said and did in classes, but also for reasons related to their own sexuality (though unrelated to their teaching).

- Issues revolving around abstinence-only-until-marriage education. This includes many examples of people feeling that programs should only emphasize the importance of refraining from sexual activity until marriage.

The trend toward abstinence-only sexuality education is controversial. Public school sexuality education teachers report that the focus on abstinence-only instruction increased markedly during the 1990s. In 1999, 23% of teachers taught abstinence as the only way of preventing pregnancy and sexually transmitted infections (STI), compared to only 2% in 1988. Many topics are still taught less often and in later grades than many teachers think they should be. For example, instruction in all grades is less likely to cover birth control, abortion, how to obtain contraceptive and STI services, and sexual orientation than it was in the late 1980s (Trend toward abstinence-only sex ed means many U.S. teenagers are not getting vital messages about contraception, 2000).

Most research studies indicate that abstinence-only sexuality is not effective (see Chapter 18 for more about this). In some cases, however, even though teachers, parents, and students want young people to receive far more comprehensive information, politicians still want to fund and promote abstinence-only education (All but politicians seem to agree that teens need more than abstinence-only education, 2002). Abstinence-only-until-marriage programs enjoy substantial economic and political support, but evidence of the effectiveness of this approach is scarce (Goodson, et al., 2003).

Today's sexuality education trends will greatly affect future programs. Many issues related to these trends will be discussed in more detail in other chapters of this book.

Summary

In this chapter we have discussed the foundations for sexuality education. The goals and objectives of sexuality education vary depending upon the desires of the community and those handling the program. Similarities and differences exist among approaches, but generally the need for learners to have adequate knowledge, understanding, and decision-making abilities is the basis for any program. In addition, it is important to recognize the basic right of people to learn about human sexuality.

It is sometimes difficult to define sexuality education in precise terms. An explanation of sexuality education should include such terms as honesty, realism, and accuracy, and should emphasize the parental role, nonverbal sexuality education, and differences between sexuality education and sexual counseling.

Traditionally, the justification of sexuality education programs has been based on inappropriate interpretations of statistical relationships. To expect that these relationships will be altered quickly or dramatically as a result of sexuality education programs is unrealistic. It cannot be assumed that a direct cause-and-effect relationship exists when so many variables are involved.

More positive reasons should be used for the justification of sexuality education programs. These reasons should emphasize the need for factual information and a broad perspective on sexual behavior, and an attempt to treat human sexuality as one important part of total personality.

Some understanding of the historical development of attitudes toward human sexuality and sexuality education is important. We have given many examples of past thinking about sexuality not usually found in history books.

Cave paintings reveal the magical qualities associated with sexual activity during prehistoric times. From the eighth century BCE until the fifth century CE, a wide variety of views of human sexuality were evident. Fertility cults and phallic statues were common over six thousand years ago; the ancient Jews followed many stringent laws related to sexuality in the Bible; the ancient Greeks much more freely practiced many sexual behaviors and celebrated physical beauty; and the ancient Romans shifted from a very conservative to an indulgent attitude toward sexual behavior.

From the fifth century to the fifteenth century, the early Christians rejected physical pleasure and believed the reason for sexual intercourse was reproduction only. People learned to disguise sexual feelings, and witchcraft was blamed for inflaming sexual appetites.

With the fifteenth and sixteenth centuries came a greater recognition of emotional relationships between people. More attention was given to human sexuality in literature, art, and daily living.

The many scientific discoveries of the seventeenth century led to questioning of traditional beliefs. Intellectuals turned away from the scriptures as their source of knowledge; the Puritan influence became rather strong as a countermeasure. Since many Puritans did not feel free in England, they imported their beliefs to America. In their view, intercourse was solely for reproduction, and there was to be no pleasure in sexuality.

The American southern colonists contributed an obvious double standard to our thinking about sexual activity. In addition, the foundation for later problems related to sexuality and racism developed within the southern colonies.

Eighteenth-century medicine brought an emphasis on the physiological aspects of sexuality and warned about sexual excesses, while nineteenth-century research focused more on psychological aspects of sexuality. The nineteenth century saw wide swings in sexual attitudes, from the Romantics, who regarded passion as important in human behavior, to the Victorians, who wanted to suppress sexual drives.

The twentieth century has seen the development of many social forces that have influenced thinking about human sexuality, including two world wars, the beginning of sex research, changes in family living and lifestyles, and the expanding influence of the mass media. A significant change was the recognition of the importance of early childhood experiences in the development of sexuality.

The history of sexuality education itself relates to our overall historical picture but in its truest sense does not begin until the early twentieth century. Many references to the importance of sexuality education are found throughout the twentieth century, but it has only been in the past 20 years or so that programs have become common.

Contemporary trends in sexuality education include a total approach to sexuality education, a more open learning atmosphere, more planned courses of study, expanded approaches to sexuality education, better literature and audiovisual materials, and improved training of sexuality educators. It can easily be seen that many changes have occurred in thinking about human sexuality and in sexuality education programs throughout the years.

References

The Alan Guttmacher Institute: school sexuality education in policy and practice. *Public Policy Issues in Brief,* 1983, 1–6.

All but politicians seem to agree that teens need more than abstinence-only education. The Alan Guttmacher Institute News Release (2001). Available: http://www.agi-usa.org.

Andre, T., Cietsch, C. & Cheng, Y. Sources of sex education as a function of sex, coital activity, and type of information, *Contemporary Educational Psychology,* 16 (1991), 215–40.

Carrera, M. A. Preparation of a sex educator: A historical overview, *The Family Coordinator* (April 1971), 99–108.

Components of sexual health education. Health Protection Branch, Health Canada (2000). Available: http://www.hc-sc.gc.ca/main/lcdc/web/publicat/.

Goodson, P., Suther, S., Pruitt, B. E. & Wilson, K. Defining abstinence: views of directors, instructors, and participants in abstinence-only-until-marriage programs in Texas. *Journal of School Health,* 73, no. 3 (March 2003), 91–96.

Haffner, D. W. *Sex education 2000. A call to action.* New York: Sex Information and Education Council of the United States, March 1990.

———. From where I sit, *Family Life Educator,* 11, no. 2 (Winter 1992/1993), 14–15.

——— & de Mauro, D. *Winning the battle: Developing support for sexuality and HIV/AIDS education.* New York: Sex Information and Education Council of the United States, March 1991.

——— & Wagoner, J. Vast majority of Americans support sexuality education, *SIECUS Report,* 27, no. 6 (August/September 1999), 22–23.

Kempner, M. E. 1998–99 sexuality education controversies in the United States, *SIECUS Report,* 27, no. 6 (August/September 1999), 4–14.

Kirby, D. Sexuality education: A more realistic view of its effects, *Journal of School Health* (December 1985), 421–24.

———. School-based programs to reduce sexual risk-taking behaviors: A review of effectiveness, *Public Health Reports,* 190 (1997), 339–60.

———, Alter, J. & Scales, P. Executive summary, in *An analysis of U.S. sex education programs and evaluation methods.* Atlanta: U.S. Department of Health, Education, and Welfare, 1979.

———. *An analysis of U.S. sex education programs and evaluation methods,* Rep. CDC-2021-79-DK-FR. Washington, DC: U.S. Department of Health, Education, and Welfare, 1979.

Leibee, H. A sex education program, *Journal of Health and Physical Education* (November 1937); reprinted in *Health Education* (April/May 1985), 18–19.

Lewis, R. K., Paine-Andrews, A., Custard, C., Stauffer, M., Harris, K. & Fisher, J. Are parents in favor or against school-based sexuality education? A report from the Midwest, *Health Promotion Practice,* 2, no. 2 (April 2001), 155–61.

Manley, H. Sex education: Where, when, and how should it be taught? *Journal of Health, Physical Education, and Recreation* (March 1964); reprinted in *Health Education* (April/May 1985), 24–27.

Means, R. K. *A history of health education in the United States.* Philadelphia: Lea & Febiger, 1962. Data used with permission of Lea & Febiger.

National poll shows parents overwhelmingly support comprehensive sexuality education over abstinence-only-until-marriage by 5 to 1 margin. *SIECUS Press Release,* October 1, 2002. Available: http://www.SIECUS.org/media/press.

Public support for sexuality education, *SIECUS Report,* 28, no. 5 (June/July 2000), 29–32.

Sadock, B. J., Kaplan, H. I. & Freedman, A. M. *The sexual experience.* Baltimore: Williams & Wilkins, 1976. Excerpts used by permission.

Schiller, P. *Creative approach to sex education and counseling.* New York: Association Press, 1973. Data used by permission of Follett Publishing Co., a division of Follett Corporation.

Sex in ancient Greece, *Sexual Behavior* (June 1971), 61–67.

Sex in ancient Rome, *Sexual Behavior* (July 1971), 82–87.

Sexuality education in the schools: Issues and answers. Sexuality Information and Education Council of the United States (2000). Available: http://www.siecus.org/pubs/.

Tatum, M. L. Overview: A perspective on school programs, in *Sexuality education: A resource book,* Cassell C. & Wilson P. M., eds. New York: Garland Publishing, Inc., 1989.

Trend towards abstinence-only sex ed means many U.S. teenagers are not getting vital messages about contraception. The Alan Guttmacher Institute News Release (2000). Available: http://www.agi-usa.org.

Suggested Readings

Bullough, V. L. History and the understanding of human sexuality, *Annual Review of Sex Research,* Society for the Scientific Study of Sexuality, 1 (1990), 75–92.

Common questions about sexual health education. Sex Information and Education Council of Canada (2000). Available: http://www.sieccan.org/.

Darroch, J. E., Landry, D. J. & Singh, S. Changing emphases in sexuality education in U.S. public secondary schools, 1988–1999, *Family Planning Perspectives,* 32, no. 5 (September/October 2000), 204–11 & 265.

Donovan, P. School-based sexuality education: The issues and challenges, *Family Planning Perspectives,* 30, no. 4 (July/August 1998), 188–93.

Murray, B. Debates over sex education may put teen health at risk. American Psychological Association (2000). Available: http://www.apa.org/monitor.

Positive sexual health promotion through comprehensive sexuality education. Minnesota Organization on Adolescent Pregnancy, Prevention, and Parenting (2000). Available: http://www.cyfc.umn.edu/moappp/comprehe.htm.

Teens weary of mixed messages about sex, want accurate info, *Intelihealth Health News* (May 25, 2001). Available: http://www.intelihealth.com/.

The Controversy

Key Concepts

1. The tactics involved in movements against sexuality education need to be understood.

2. Not all individuals or groups opposed to sexuality education can be classified in the same fashion.

3. Attacks from extremist groups have identifiable characteristics and stages.

4. People are opposed to sexuality education for a variety of reasons, but there are many factual ways of dealing with these objections.

5. Sound suggestions for defense against extremist attacks do exist.

6. Cool and logical heads usually prevail in the sexuality education controversy.

SEX EDUCATION

Parents no longer have to worry about instructing their children in sex education. Big Brother knows the correct way to raise your family and he is going to take care of that for you.

Find out how he's going to do it! Come to the meeting of the Statesville School Board when the committee of 18 makes its report on Sept. 15, 8:00 P.M., Jackson High School.

Come out and meet the new members of your household.

TAXPAYERS FOR DECENCY

SEX EDUCATION
FAMILY LIVING
HUMAN GROWTH AND DEVELOPMENT

Don't be misled by a title; they all mean the same thing.

The whole concept of public or group education in sex knowledge and practices is a bestial and degrading monstrosity.

Come to Jackson High, Sept. 1, 8:00 P.M. and let the School Board know that you intend to retain your God-given right to raise your children in the manner you see fit.

TAXPAYERS FOR DECENCY

These two newspaper advertisements appeared at the time when one community was considering introducing a local school sexuality education program. They are not atypical of statements you are likely to hear regarding sexuality education. Do they represent an accurate picture? Are they based on fact? Do they appeal to logic or to emotions? The sexuality education controversy has been around for a number of years. Strangely enough, the facts and feelings related to it have not changed a great deal during the past 25 to 30 years.

In fact in the early 1990s, in Clayton County, Georgia, local members of the Christian Coalition challenged the film *Am I Normal,* used in grades 9 to 12, for its discussion of sexual development, masturbation, and homosexuality. The objectors also questioned the entire sexuality education program for not promoting abstinence. In Kern County, California, a group of parents at a school board meeting objected to a seventh grade sexuality education class for allegedly promoting promiscuity, discussing anatomy, teaching abstinence as a choice instead of a goal, and being coeducational. Some parents urged adoption of the abstinence-only curriculum *Sex Respect* in its place (Sedway, 1992).

It is also significant to note that in recent years the sexuality education controversy has centered more on the *content* and *methodology* of programs, rather than whether there should be a program. For example, some groups say they have nothing against sexuality education; however, they will only support abstinence education that makes no mention of contraception or responsible sexual behavior. Still others might not want abortion or homosexuality discussed unless the topics are presented in a manner that discourages them. Even though the push is not necessarily to do away with sexuality education—but instead to mold it to the liking of the very active and verbal minority, the basics for understanding and dealing with the controversy remain similar.

Trevor (2002) reported that recently there have been fewer controversies relating to sexuality education than in previous years. She pointed out, however, that this does not indicate a widespread acceptance of comprehensive sexuality education, but rather a tendency of school personnel to adopt conservative policies to avoid controversy. Many debates were based on efforts to restrict the scope and content of sexuality programs. Attempts to institute strict abstinence-only-until-marriage programs remained one of the most popular ways to do this. Opponents also worked to limit topics, exclude materials, and prevent discussions. Other attempts to restrict sexuality education involved mandating specifically what words to use when talking about sexuality.

Background and Tactics of Movements Against Sexuality Education

Background of Sexuality Education Opposition

In the late 1960s, the Sexuality Information and Education Council of the United States summarized the history of the campaign against sexuality education (*A brief history of the current campaign against sex education,* n.d.). A few highlights from this summary are relevant to an understanding of the sexuality education controversy.

In 1968, the Christian Crusade, led by the Reverend Billy James Hargis, launched a direct-mail promotion campaign to raise money through the distribution of a 40-page booklet entitled *Is the School House the Proper Place to Teach Raw Sex?* by Dr. Gordon V. Drake, Educational Director of the Christian Crusade. The promotion letter indicates that the overall scheme of sexuality education programs is to demoralize youth and repudiate Christian morality, and that it is part of a giant Communist conspiracy. The letter asserts that those responsible for sexuality education programs are all part of the "rotten liberal establishment." The letter appeals for funds to run the Christian Crusade so that the "vicious sex in schools campaign" can be stopped.

This campaign had an influence on citizens in many states. Local committees opposed to sexuality education formed quickly, and groups already in existence became more vocal. Other groups joined in the theme. The John Birch Society *Bulletin* attacked sexuality education as a "filthy Communist plot." The society also formed its own organization to help fight sexuality education: the Movement to Restore Decency (MOTOREDE). A system of recorded telephone messages called "Let Freedom Ring" supported the campaign in many cities.

A number of citizens' groups appeared on the scene during what could be termed an "alphabet soup" time. They had such names as MOMS (Mothers Organized for Moral Stability), POSSE (Parents Opposed to Sex and Sensitivity Education), PAUSE (Parents Against Unconstitutional Sex Education), ACRE (Associated Citizens for Responsible Education), POPE (Parents for Orthodoxy in Parochial Education), and CHIDE (Committee to Halt Indoctrination and Demoralization in Education). Interestingly enough, a group of students also got together and formed a group called SPAAM (Students for the Prevention of Asinine Adult Movements), conceived to counteract the formation of adult organizations that were contrary to the idea of educational freedom.

Even though there was a local flavor to the campaigns against sexuality education, there were generally three main objectives that appeared in the nationwide pattern (*Brief history,* n.d., 3):

1. By attacking the Sex Information and Education Council, the Education Association and other groups, and by attempting to link officials of these organizations in a sinister and vaguely defined "conspiracy," the campaign seeks to discredit the concept of family life and sex education.

2. In this way, without ever really examining the merits and flaws of an existing local program, the campaign aims to eliminate family life and sex education from the schools.

3. As a long-range goal, at least in some areas, the forces behind the campaign appear to be seeking control over parent-teacher associations and school boards. For this purpose, family-life education serves merely as a useful interim target. By launching attacks on officials who support the program, these forces try to undermine their position and drive them from office.

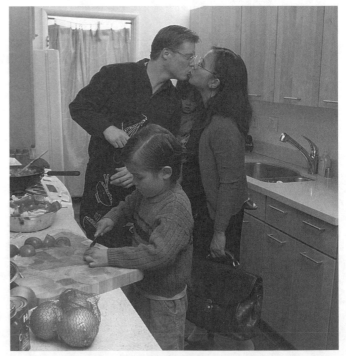

Sexuality education occurs informally in many ways. Even observing adults being affectionate is a form of sexuality education.

Following the flare-up of attacks on sexuality education in the late 1960s, movements sprang up in some states in the early 1970s to inhibit and even legislate against sexuality education programs. There were examples of reduced as well as greatly expanded programs all during the 1970s. In general, it can be said that there are now many more quality sexuality education programs existing in schools, churches, and other institutions than ever before, but a great deal remains to be done.

Because the late 1970s were a relatively quiet time on the sexuality education controversy scene, it would have been easy to become too complacent and feel that the controversy was over. However, as was seen in New Jersey in the early 1980s, those who opposed the family-life education mandate were vocal and well financed (Knowlton, 1986).

In the 1990s, there was a growing wave of censorship ravaging sexuality education in communities and states around the nation. In an ever-expanding campaign, grassroots groups backed by national far-right organizations waged a war on textbooks and programs (Sedway, 1992).

More recently, the Christian Right has dominated the public conversation about sexuality education (Talk about sex: The battle over sex education, 2002). Although people often assume that bitter debates about sexuality education are spontaneous uprisings of outraged citizens, they are usually not. They are public arguments that are provoked by conservative national advocacy organizations that are actively committed to shaping sexual values and influencing education policies in communities throughout the United States. National Christian Right groups succeed on the local level mainly through arguments resulting in gridlock and intimidation. They have paralyzed many community debates and constrained programs by depicting sexuality education as being transgressive and immoral.

Complacency could lead to an inability to deal with strong opposition when it does arise—and it often does. It is essential to be aware of extremist groups and tactics commonly used when attacking sexuality education programs.

Who Is the Opposition?

Parents, administrators, and teachers are usually not the ones opposed to sexuality and HIV/AIDS education. Instead, citizen's groups, which typically have not been involved in education decision making, are the most likely opponents. They range from local conservative groups to national organizations with formal platforms of opposition. Their goal is often to curtail freedom of expression and academic freedom as well as the right to one's privacy, the right to sexual information, and the right to a healthy sexual life (Haffner & de Mauro, 1991).

It is wise to find out whether those opposing a program are operating individually or as representatives of a larger, organized group. If a group is involved, it should be publicly known. It can be helpful to find out about the organization, what it stands for, and how it works and then publicize the information. Common national organizations in the 1990s that were opposed to sexuality and HIV/AIDS education were the American Family Association, the American Life League, Concerned Women for America, Eagle Forum, Focus on the Family, and the National Association for Abstinence Education (Haffner & de Mauro, 1991).

Opponents of sexuality education take many forms, from large, nonprofit organizations with the broad mission of promoting conservative values, to small for-profit distributors of abstinence-only-until-marriage curricula and materials. In recent years the abstinence-only-until-marriage message and its supporters have received media attention and have developed a presence on the Internet. Existing organizations have become more visible, and new organizations have formed (Opponents of comprehensive sexuality education, 2003). A list of these organizations can be found at http://www.siecus.org/pubs/fact/fact0016.html.

The Christian Right opponents have some powerful advantages. Their infrastructure is large, rich, and very well organized. Christian Right national organizations have served as strong allies to residents in communities across the United States who oppose comprehensive sexuality education programs (Talk about sex: The battles over sex education, 2002).

A good example of groups opposed to comprehensive sexuality education is the Coalition for Adolescent Sexual Health. Its members include the Christian Coalition of America, Concerned Women for America, Eagle Forum, the Family Research Council, Focus on the Family, the National Abstinence Clearinghouse, and the Traditional Values Coalition. In 2003, a major effort of the coalition was to claim that proponents of comprehensive sexuality education have been evasive and deceptive (*Deception uncovered: An analysis*, 2003).

Typical Tactics of Sexuality Education Opponents

In most instances, extremist groups are not interested in objectively evaluating a sexuality education program but instead want to wipe it out and prevent an objective evaluation. In fact, sexuality educator Sol Gordon said that "virtually all opposition to sex education is based on the assumption that knowledge is harmful" (Should sexologists lobby for sex ed in school, 1986). A number of tactics have been used in attacks on sexuality education plans and programs. The following list, although not exhaustive, gives an indication of possibilities (*Brief history*, n.d.; *Extremist groups*, n.d.):

1. *Blacklisting and labeling.* The backgrounds of those connected with the program are studied, and labels such as "un-American" and "radical" are applied to anyone whose beliefs are different from those of the extremist group.

2. *Church support.* The local group opposed to sexuality education may be based on the thinking of a fundamentalist religious denomination. Those disagreeing with their views may be labeled as "antireligious" or "anti-God."

3. *Coercion, intimidation, and suspicion of teachers.* Opponents try to drive a wedge between parents and school officials by declaring that educators cannot be trusted. In addition, investigations of school officials and others supporting the program are threatened.

4. *Disruption of meetings.* Extremists appear to be more interested in disrupting meetings than participating in them. Ignoring the rules of order, shouting down other speakers, and asking "loaded" questions are common.

5. *Distribution of publications.* Pamphlets and fliers are distributed, the contents of which are based upon other tactics listed here.

6. *Divide and conquer.* Irrelevant discussions of broad issues and programs are encouraged in an attempt to discredit state and national organizations. Then it is easier to isolate local groups and control them.

7. *Formation of a committee.* Not all committees are extremist groups, but it is crucial to look at the objectives of a committee and its employment of other tactics.

8. *Free speakers or outside speakers.* The services of local or national speakers may be offered in order to showcase "authorities" who will help discredit the program.

9. *Front groups.* Extremist groups sometimes set up front organizations with patriotic-sounding names to promote their anti-sexuality-education views.

10. *Half-truths and dubious documentation.* Arguments based on rumor, out-of-context quotations, and incidents in "other schools" that no one has the chance to check are common. These help plant suspicion in people's minds.

11. *Hysteria and fear.* Highly emotional charges can create fear and insecurity that contribute to doubts about the program.

Insight 3-1

Opponents of sexuality education will sometimes resort to bizarre means to thwart a program. Who knows what caption these opponents would write for this simple picture of a box of disposable diapers in the trash. List possible captions that an opponent of sexuality education might write for this photo.

1. _____

_____

2. _____

_____

3. _____

_____

4. _____

_____

5. _____

_____

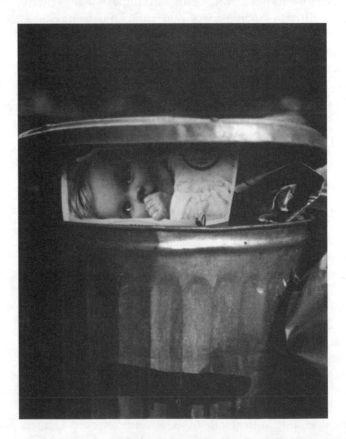

12. *Infiltration.* Respectable and accepted organizations, such as the PTA, are targets for infiltration, which allows opportunities to capture key positions, prolong meetings, and send "prepared" representatives to meetings.

13. *Letter writing.* Common themes and charges run through letters-to-the-editor and other materials. These charges are directed at individuals connected with the program.

14. *Pressure on public officials.* By means of letters, visits, and other pressure tactics, opponents try to pressure public officials to introduce legislation against sexuality education or to restrict programs.

15. *Radio and TV.* Just like newspaper campaigns and letter writing, talk shows and panel discussions provide opportunities for extremist views to be presented in a dominant way.

16. *The "foot in the door" argument.* If programs are nonexistent or planned, extremists claim that educators are attempting to start a program and "get a foot in the door" with pilot programs.

In the 1990s, challengers used tactics such as flooding school board meetings, threatening and sometimes pursuing costly litigation against schools, and pressuring teachers and administrators. The fear of attacks, disruption, controversy, and costly lawsuits led more and more teachers, administrators, and school boards to yield to the demands of censors (Sedway, 1992).

There are still clear patterns in the strategies of sexuality education opponents. One common tactic is the use of provocative language in community debates. This might include calling a curriculum a "sodomy" curriculum or "pornographic." They also use provocative language to stigmatize sexuality educators themselves. For example, sexuality educators have been called perverts or pedophiles. Opponents distort and misrepresent comprehensive programs, saying that learning about birth control will encourage students to participate in sexual activity. Studies indicate otherwise, but that does not stop them from making the claim. Opponents also tell scary stories, which could be called "depravity narratives." One such story indicated that a teacher took off her clothes to teach her students about anatomy. Another tale alleged that a teacher had sexual intercourse in front of her class. Neither of these incidents ever happened, but some people still believe they did. These strategies are incredibly effective, because they are difficult to refute and cast suspicion upon comprehensive sexuality education (Talk about sex: The battle over sex education, 2002).

At this point you may be getting a little tired of all of this negative talk. You might even be thinking that it would not be possible for these kinds of things to happen. If you know someone who has worked in sexuality education programs for 5 to 10 years, ask them if they have ever seen any occurrences such as those described above in movements against sexuality education. We strongly suspect that most of those involved will be able to relate a number of "horror" stories for you. It is precisely for this reason that this background information is pertinent today.

Characteristics and Stages of Extremist Attacks

The characteristics of extremist attacks on sexuality education have been explained in the PTA pamphlet, *Extremist Groups* (n.d.). It should be noted that most of the characteristics are contrary to basic democratic principles.

Extremist groups try to stifle free consideration of views that differ from their own, try to have publications that they do not like removed from local libraries, and put pressure on schools to utilize courses and textbooks that reflect their views. They may espouse democratic principles while at the same time ignoring the rights of others to express different views, suppressing free access to information, and proposing the indoctrination of students to their own views.

Extremist groups use coercion and even violence to force change, believe there are simple and fast solutions to complex problems, and believe in rule by their own minority. By contrast, those supportive of a democracy believe that social change is best brought about by democratic procedures, that patience and cooperative effort are needed to deal with complex problems, and that the majority should rule with consideration for minority opinion.

Typically, an extremist attack against sexuality education occurs in four stages (*Suggestions for defense against extremist attack: Sex education in the public schools,* n.d., 8–9):

- *Stage 1: Sowing the seeds of doubt.* The intent is to arouse the public by informing them of the supposed dangers inherent in sexuality education. This stage might involve meetings, demonstrations, and rallies held at the local and state level.

- *Stage 2: Internal incubation.* Front groups are likely to be used to identify opponents of sexuality education within the community. The group sponsors speakers, sends letters to the editor, makes telephone calls to talk programs, advertises in periodicals, circulates petitions, and performs other activities designed to build momentum against sexuality education.

- *Stage 3: Outbreak.* Front-group programs are well under way. Local meetings are disrupted and materials opposing sexuality education are distributed. The public is also primed for any upcoming elections.

- *Stage 4: Shift to real goals: the power grab.* The public is led to believe that the answer to the "problem" is to elect a new slate of school board members or other elected officials. At this point the energies of the attackers become focused on taking over control instead of the actual sexuality education issue.

It should be remembered that most of the foregoing activities are legitimate in a democratic society. This is why they might be successful for sexuality education opponents. It is only when the activities involve questionable tactics that parents, educators, and administrators need to mobilize their own forces against an obvious extremist attack. Failure to recognize these tactics, characteristics, and stages could result in the elimination of one or more sound educational programs.

Nonextremist Opponents of Sexuality Education

It would be a serious mistake to think that anyone opposed to sexuality education must be in an extremist group. Some people have legitimate concerns about sexuality education programs unrelated to extremist views. For example, there are those who feel that sexuality education is a basically sound idea, but not before a certain age, or only in certain circumstances, or only if teachers have a certain type of preparation, or only if moral issues are handled in a certain way, or only if certain topics are covered and other topics are not. In most instances these people will listen to reason and are able to objectively consider many sides to a question.

In New Jersey (Knowlton, 1986), it was found that those who opposed family-life education generally fell into three categories. The first group (about 5% of the population of New Jersey) believed that sexual matters should not be mentioned or discussed in public, because it is immoral to do so. These people generated the bulk of meetings, letters, and political or legal opposition to the family-life education requirement. The second group (also estimated at 5%) were convinced that young people who were informed about sexuality will promiscuously indulge in premarital sexual intercourse and become pregnant. The third group did not trust schools to do a good job of sexuality education and thought that if schools did it, then parents, churches, and other socially responsible persons would not.

Informed educators may be able to help many kinds of sexuality education opponents understand that people of all ages have needs related to sexuality education, that sexuality education occurs constantly whether we want it to or not, and that it is not educationally sound to censor certain topics. Certainly, it is appropriate to deal with topics differently with various age groups, but taboo topics have an unrealistic aura around them that inhibits rather than promotes learning.

Insight 3-2

Dealing with Opposing Viewpoints

As you read this section, do the following things: (1) Cover up the suggested response to the typical item of opposition, (2) read the typical item of opposition, (3) decide how you would answer the opposition item, and (4) compare your answer to our suggested response. Remember, no peeking at our suggestions until you have thought about your own!

Before assuming that someone opposed to a sexuality education program is automatically an extremist, it would be wise to assess the person's reasons for opposition. In many cases it may be possible to turn these types of opponents into some of your most avid supporters after they better understand the total program.

Countering Arguments Against Sexuality Education

Are you now ready to deal with viewpoints that are opposed to all or part of sexuality education activities? Let us find out.

1. *Opposition argument.* Sexuality education will cause sexual experimentation.

   Suggested response. It seems that some sexual experimentation is natural. No amount of education is likely to affect it one way or the other. However, in many cases it seems that those who are the *least* informed about sexuality are the most likely to experiment. In addition, if sexual experimentation does occur, sexuality education experiences may result in a healthier experimentation. For example, people may be more considerate and take fewer risks. Through proper sexuality education programs, people can learn wholesome attitudes and correct information about sexuality that will help them attain a healthy approach to human sexuality.

2. *Opposition argument.* Sexuality educators are not trained to handle sexuality education.

   Suggested response. This is probably the most logical complaint against sexuality education, but it is one that is easily overcome. There should be more concern shown for the qualifications of the sexuality educator (see Chapter 4) than there has been. A sexuality educator who is not prepared to handle the topic of sexuality is likely to do more harm than good. The same can be said for group leaders for individuals of all ages. Today, however, there are many excellent opportunities for in-service programs for sexuality educators and leaders as well as undergraduate and graduate courses concerned with sexuality. Therefore, there is no longer any valid reason why sexuality educators should not be prepared.

3. *Opposition argument.* Some sexuality education programs are started too quickly.

    Suggested response. This complaint is probably also justified in some cases, but again it is one that is easily remedied. Any new or existing program in the community should be carefully planned, well taught, and constantly evaluated. If these steps are followed and if the community is informed about progress, this criticism will have no foundation.

4. *Opposition argument.* Parents should handle sexuality education for their children.

    Suggested response. The fact that parents play a major role in the sexuality education of their children is not denied. Churches also contribute to education about sexuality. No organizations should attempt to replace parents in educational pursuits. They simply assist parents. We do not expect parents to be able to teach their children math, English, history, or science. It makes no more sense to expect them to teach sexuality education. Parents cannot be expected to know current research, to have a wide variety of resources, or even to be able to handle the topic objectively with their own children.

5. *Opposition argument.* Sexuality education is too controversial for schools and other institutions.

    Suggested response. If sexuality education is properly planned and the community is well informed, it is no more controversial than history or social studies. The controversy seems to arise concerning moral values. It is not the job or the right of the school or other community organizations to make value judgments concerning sexuality. This is the job of the home, the church, and the individual.

6. *Opposition argument.* A moral attitude toward sexuality is not developed in sexuality education programs.

    Suggested response. See response for number 5.

7. *Opposition argument.* It is improper to teach young children all the details of sexual intercourse.

    Suggested response. This is a legitimate argument, but anyone using this or similar arguments does not understand sexuality education. Sexuality education programs do not teach sexual techniques in schools or other institutions at either the elementary or secondary level. It might be appropriate to teach this subject to older individuals in nonschool settings, but claims such as this can readily be handled by properly informing citizens about the program.

8. *Opposition argument.* Sexuality education will undermine a person's moral and patriotic concepts.

    Suggested response. As stated earlier, sexuality education should not greatly concern itself with moral judgments. This is the job of the home and the church. Again, a proper public-relations program will help alleviate this fear. If the community understands the program, they will know that morals and patriotic concepts will not be undermined.

9. *Opposition argument.* Sexuality education is needed only in culturally deprived areas, since that is where sexual problems exist.

    Suggested response. This is, again, a very narrow view of sexuality education (the promiscuity, STI, and premarital-pregnancy approach). Problems relating to sexuality can occur in any cultural group.

10. *Opposition argument.* The school curriculum is overcrowded.

    Suggested response. In most situations, a separate sexuality education course should not be the means for basic handling of the topic. Sexuality education should be included as a part of a health education or similar course that already exists in most schools and that is already geared toward total personality development. This demands some additional training for teachers, but it requires no more time from the crowded curriculum. If a separate course can be fit into the curriculum in addition to this basic coverage, great; but that will not be the case in most schools.

11. *Opposition argument.* Sexuality education is simply a plot to make money.

    Suggested response. It is naive to say that there is no money involved in sexuality education. There are financial gains to be found in all educational areas. It is, however, interesting to note that the strongest supporters of sexuality education are educators, physicians, and counselors who are primarily interested in human well-being and who reap no monetary gain from sexuality education programs.

12. *Opposition argument.* All material published by the Sexuality Information and Education Council of the United States (SIECUS) is evil and should be banned along with sexuality education itself.

    Suggested response. Remember that one common tactic of extremist groups is to condemn an organization and by so doing drag down a cause too. SIECUS was established in New York in the early 1960s to act as a clearinghouse for sexuality education materials. Since its origination, SIECUS has been an excellent source of information, but the organization has never advocated particular curricular materials or specific types of sexuality education. If some material associated with SIECUS is objectionable in a given situation, then it should not be used. Any other objectionable material should likewise be discarded. Each book, film, or picture should be evaluated on its own merit and not condemned because it is associated with a certain organization. To use the terms "SIECUS" and "sexuality education" synonymously is also an error. There are many other organizations interested in sexuality education as well as other fine resources.

SIECUS believes that all people should receive comprehensive sexuality and HIV/AIDS education. SIECUS endorses comprehensive sexuality education as an important part of the educational program in every school. SIECUS believes that classes conducted by specially trained educators complement the sexuality education given by families and religious and community groups (Haffner & de Mauro, 1991).

13. *Opposition argument.* The SIECUS curriculum in sexuality education is undesirable.

    Suggested response. Related to response for number 12, there is no "SIECUS curriculum" in sexuality education. SIECUS consultants themselves emphasize the importance of individualized approaches to sexuality education as well as community involvement in curriculum planning to meet the needs of a given community.

14. *Opposition argument.* Sexuality education is not needed for older or married people.

    Suggested response. The need for sexuality education is not decreased simply because one has lived longer. People of all ages need sexuality education even though their needs may be different. It is a fallacy to think that just because one has made it "this far" one does not need sexuality education (or other forms of education too, for that matter).

15. *Opposition argument.* Sexuality education is not needed for those with different sexual preferences.

    Suggested response. Regardless of sexual preference, the basic reasons for sexuality education remain. In fact, a recognition that one is a little "different" from the apparent majority might even increase the need for information and understanding.

16. *Opposition argument.* Sexuality education is simply a plot to promote homosexuality and other sick behaviors.

    Suggested response. It is a basic tenet of education that it is helpful to learn about differences. It is not the intent to push people toward experimentation, but to help them better understand themselves and others. To avoid discussions about a variety of sexual behaviors would be like avoiding studying other cultures in a geography class. It is frequently (if not always) the case that a lack of knowledge is far more dangerous than being educated.

17. *Opposition argument.* Sexuality educators are in favor of promoting sexual behavior. They do not preach enough about abstinence.

    Suggested response. It is logical for sexuality educators to stress abstinence from sexual activity for young people—especially with the serious AIDS threat. However, it must be borne in mind that most young people who eventually have sexual intercourse have already been strongly encouraged, by their parents and their schools, to believe in abstinence and avoid sexual intercourse. The fatal error is that we ignore the fact that vows of abstinence break far more easily than do condoms (Reiss, 1991).

    We know that many young people are already sexually active, and others will decide to become sexually active—no matter what we say. Therefore, educating about responsible sexual behavior is not only necessary, it may save lives. Teaching people to "just say no" is not the only answer in drug education, and it is not in sexuality education either. Also, we must remember that there is a great difference between promoting sexual behavior (which good sexuality educators do not do) and educating about responsible decision making.

18. *Opposition argument.* There is too much emphasis on sexual pluralism (often either undefined by opponents or defined as something very evil).

    Suggested response. The heart of pluralism is to tolerate a broad range of choices by others and try not to impose one's personal choices on other people. Pluralism is the way Americans view religion and politics, marriage partners, and occupational and educational choices. However, many still believe that in sexual matters there is but one moral path.

    Sexual pluralism does not indicate that all forms of sexual behavior are legitimate. Nor does it mean that if it feels good, you should do it. It totally rejects the use of force or manipulation and encourages concern for self and others. Sexual pluralism indicates that honesty, equality, and responsibility are essential ingredients in any sexual relationship (Reiss, 1991).

    While there is some overlap with the list of arguments already presented, here is a list of some relatively recent examples of arguments, along with suggested responses (Responding to arguments against comprehensive sexuality education, 2000):

- *Comprehensive sexuality education has not worked.* Comprehensive sexuality education has not been tried. For example, only 5% of typical students receive comprehensive sexuality education during every year of school.

- *Teaching children about sexuality before the age of 12 interferes with the latency period and disturbs children's natural modesty.* Modern experts agree that humans are sexual beings from birth until death and that no latency period exists. People of all ages are curious about issues related to sexuality and need accurate, age-appropriate information.

- *Schools are spending so much time teaching about health that kids don't even know how to read and write.* It is important to teach people basic skills. However, they also need information about health and relationships.

- *People who want sexuality education are saying, in effect, that young people are going to have sexual intercourse anyway, so we might as well tell them how to make it a little safer.* Good sexuality education programs give people skills to make responsible decisions. Researchers have found that these programs help young people delay having sexual intercourse and to use contraception effectively if they do.

- *Teaching young people that they can have sexual intercourse encourages promiscuity.* This is not true. Programs that teach about both abstinence and safer sexual activity can help young people to postpone having intercourse.

- *Teaching that abstinence is the expected standard and leaving out any mention of contraception will set a strong ethical guideline for young people.* Programs most effective in helping young people to abstain discuss both abstinence and contraception. This is why providing comprehensive sexuality education is so important.

- *Courses in sexuality education teach young people how to "do it."* Comprehensive sexuality education gives information about a broad variety of topics and teaches young people the skills they need to make responsible decisions. Classes do not include teaching about sexual techniques.

- *If fear convinces young people that sexual intercourse is not a good idea, then I'm all for it.* Fear-based health education has never worked. Early smoking campaigns emphasizing that cigarettes can kill did not work. Effective education is based on presenting accurate information and helping people learn strategies for changing their behavior.*

Once the reasons typically given for and against education about sexuality have been compared and explained, it is hoped that common sense and reason will prevail. It must be remembered, however, that rationality and objectivity often go out the window when it comes to human sexuality. Program planners must sometimes deal rationally with people who are subjective and emotionally overstimulated. It has been said that as a person's emotional level rises, the functional-intelligence level drops. Our desire might be to handle emotionalism with more of the same, but our best ammunition is still the objective facts supportive of sexuality education.

Defense Against Extremist Attacks

Now that you understand the viewpoints of those opposed to sexuality education, you can see why some severe confrontations can occur. Recognizing the types of individuals opposed to sexuality education, the characteristics and stages of extremist attacks, and the many possible reasons some people might be opposed to sexuality education will help during a confrontation; but a defense against extremist attack needs to be planned too. What should you do when you hear an argument like the following (Woodworth, n.d., 3)?

> *A modern drive for all-out, tell-all sex instruction from kindergarten through high school is now on! It is a carefully designed program of sex without morality to guide children from infancy to adultery. Christians need to know just exactly the* intents *and* contents *of this new mania for school children.*

There are a number of things that can be done to defend against an extremist attack. It is important to keep in mind that the vast majority of citizens are concerned, perhaps misinformed, and will respond to reasoning and common sense.

In a Michigan handbook for establishing sexuality education programs (Bensley, 1986), several suggestions for confronting anti-sexuality education groups are given. The first is to state your position in an understandable way and to avoid arguments with the opposition. There is no way of winning an argument in a public meeting with a person opposed to sexuality education. The second is to try to agree with something an opponent is saying that you can support. If you can agree with part of what is being said, the opponent is more likely to feel you are not totally against him or her and that individual rights are being respected. The third (in school situations where this is the policy) is to explain that parents have the right to withdraw their children from sexuality education classes. The law provides for this opportunity just as it provides the opportunity for school districts to develop sexuality education programs for the vast majority of children whose parents are supportive.

---

* Reprinted with permission of the Sexuality Information and Education Council of the United States. 130 West 42nd Street, Suite 350. New York, NY 10036.

For reasoning citizens, the most effective way to counter the opposition is to do a good job in sexuality education. Programs should be properly planned and implemented. Showing that sound planning and educational procedures are being followed can be a good defense in itself.

It can be helpful to remind people that, as already indicated, a number of national and local polls show a great degree of parental and general citizen support for sexuality education programs. Different polls have shown that from 70% to 90% are supportive.

It might be helpful to remind people that a large number of national groups have gone on record as supporting sexuality education. As of 2002, there were 135 groups in the National Coalition to Support Sexuality Education (see Appendix A for a list of the members). These organizations represent a broad range of child development specialists, educators, health care professionals, parents, physicians, religious leaders, and social workers whose combined work reaches more than 30 million young people. The mission of the coalition is to assure that comprehensive sexuality education is provided for all children and youth in the United States. The coalition's goals include advocating sexuality education at the national and state levels, developing strategies for facilitating national and local implementation of sexuality education initiatives and efforts, and providing proactive strategies to address the activities of those who oppose comprehensive sexuality education (The National Coalition to Support Sexuality Education, 2002).

Any given group might be criticized by someone who dislikes particular people or causes, but such an impressive list of groups supportive of sexuality education is often convincing to people who are willing to be rational. In any local community, it ought to be easy to add appropriate groups or to make up a more relevant list for local use.

Putnam (n.d.) gives suggestions for what those outside the school system can do to support activities of administrators and educators against an attack. He points out that the first thing needed is to get someone to coordinate the program against the attack. He suggests that this might be done by inviting prominent community leaders and civic groups known to support the schools to a meeting. This meeting can be used to alert the audience to the apparent dangers and to seek their assistance. A brief program describing opposition points and tactics would be informative.

The representatives should be invited to a second meeting after they have had a little time to discuss the problem with their respective groups. At the second meeting, they should be able to indicate backing from their groups for a coordinated movement against the opposition. It must be emphasized that absence from the second meeting, when more specific assignments will be given, will be interpreted as a lack of support and an inability to be counted upon. Obviously, there should not be a great deal of time between the first and second meetings.

During the second meeting, specific assignments can be given out, which might include (1) preparation of materials to be used in the community, (2) mass mailing of appropriate materials, (3) establishment of a telephone tree so people can be alerted to what is taking place, and (4) securing speaking opportunities for speakers knowledgeable about sexuality education programs. It does not take many people to carry out this type of community-support program. Particularly if the problem is dealt with in the early stages, the task is to throw the spotlight on accurate information and truth.

The National Education Association (NEA) describes a variety of strategies for defense and suggestions for what a local group can do (*Suggestions for Defense*, n.d.). The importance of establishing a broad base of community support for sexuality education programs is emphasized. Committee responsibilities would include legislative action, press relations, a speakers' bureau, a direct-mail campaign, materials development and distribution, and such other activities as telephone calls to talk shows in support of sexuality education, letters to the editor, and informal neighborhood meetings.

In addition, the NEA has given suggestions for what a school system can do. They suggest that since the best defense is a good offense, the most effective strategy is preventing attacks or thwarting them before they achieve much momentum. Preventing an attack or rendering it harmless depends on an active public relations department and an immediate response to the first unjust attack on the curriculum. Public relations activities cannot be emphasized too heavily; too often, people (especially influential people) are not properly informed about a program. Negative statements sound much better if you do not know about the positive.

Extremist groups, employing the tactics discussed earlier in this chapter, have been successful when there has been no community- or school-organized opposition to their activities and when school systems have not had or followed sound procedures for planning and implementing

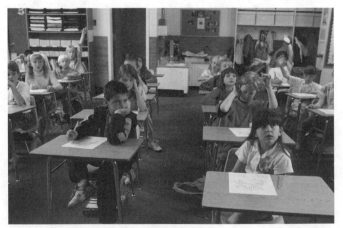

The innocence of youth should not be synonymous with the ignorance of youth. Sexuality is a topic that individuals of all ages profit from studying.

Insight 3-3

Conducting a Public Meeting

Since sexuality education is controversial, it is common to have a public meeting to discuss it. If you were in charge of conducting such a meeting, how would you plan the meeting? What would you do before and during the meeting? Make a list of these items. After you have made your list, compare it with the suggestions given in this chapter.

---

educational programs, selecting teaching materials, and selecting teachers. A great deal of progress has been made along these lines in recent years, with the emphasis on accountability and the movement toward spelling out everything more clearly. Nonetheless, the basic suggestions for dealing with opponents of sexuality education remain essentially the same. We cannot afford to become too complacent just because vocal sexuality education opposition has not appeared in our locality. Preventing problems is always better than dealing with them after they develop.

In summary, Sowers and Associates have provided tips for dealing with negative resistance (*Tips for dealing with negative resistance,* 1992). In order to help prevent resistance it is important to (1) do your homework, (2) assure broad-based planning at the local level, (3) state goals clearly, (4) seek support, (5) select articulate spokespersons, (6) make the community aware of the need, and (7) be positive. In spite of all of your efforts, if opposition surfaces it is important to (1) know your goals and be able to communicate them positively and effectively, (2) listen and find common ground, (3) do not get defensive, (4) keep supporters informed and involved, (5) step up your information campaign, (6) be honest and aboveboard, (7) respect differences, and (8) remain positive.

Public Meetings

Greater success is likely when public meetings are focused on a comprehensive health education program of which sexuality education should be a part. In this way, individuals can see how sexuality education fits into the broad range of health decision making.

Whether the meeting focuses on the entire health education program, or just on a sexuality education program, a public meeting can bring out individuals with many varied opinions. Since the topic is potentially explosive, and in order to guarantee success of the public meeting, consideration of the following ideas is highly recommended (adapted from Bensley, 1986).

1. Prepare a meeting agenda with clearly defined purposes. This should be a written statement, so that everyone can be reminded of the purpose if necessary.

2. Clearly define sexuality education. All program planners should agree with this definition and constantly refer to its meaning when communicating to others.

3. Have one person chair the meeting. A person who has respect and skill in conducting a public meeting should do this.

4. Allow all people to speak on the issue, but rules should be established that are understood by the attendees. For example, there might be a time limit, one person might be allowed to speak only once until everyone has had a chance, and people might clearly state their name and address before speaking.

5. Introduce those associated with the program, such as advisory board members, administrators, or educators.

6. Make sure that those attending the meeting realize that their input is needed and appreciated.

7. Have a recorder present so that comments can be recorded for future use. If a tape recorder is used, or if someone is taking minutes, everyone present should be told about this.

8. Try to avoid long statements and answers to the attendees' questions. There should be an opportunity to express opinions without excessive time being used in answering questions.

9. Inform the attendees as to what will happen with the information that has been expressed at the meeting.

10. Always maintain a positive atmosphere during the meeting.

11. Start on time and end on time.

12. At the end of the meeting, the chairperson or recorder should summarize what has been said.

13. Be sure that people leave the meeting feeling that it has been worth their time.

A public meeting can be a great help to program planners and can give the public confidence that the program is sound. If not run properly, however, the meeting could become a disaster and the program could be destroyed.

Logical Heads Prevail

Remember that as the emotional level goes up, the level of functioning intelligence tends to go down. This bit of information can come in handy when one is confronted with arguments about sexuality education. Of course, it is not always easy to be cool and logical, since the topic of sexuality often stirs up people's emotions, but cool and logical heads usually do prevail.

Let us look at an example from a classic court case in the state of Kansas (Gendel, 1970). A group of people attempted to stop a local program of sexuality education with legal action based on arguments that (1) the program violated the personal liberty of a parent to determine the subjects taught to children, (2) the schools had not been empowered to carry out such a program, (3) the use of tax money to conduct the program without authority was an unlawful diversion of such money, and (4) the program resulted in the violation of constitutional rights. It is an understatement to say that these claims could easily be the foundation for some rather emotional arguments. In addition, they came about after several months of controversy in a local community.

The judge in the case set some ground rules. He indicated that the focus would be on broad legal issues and that no hearsay (undocumented evidence) or evidence not examined in pretrial hearings could be introduced. This, in effect, eliminated the name calling and insinuations so common in a sexuality education controversy.

An objective examination of the sexuality education program was made, and the above-mentioned legal arguments were considered. As a result, the judge ruled that the "defendant is authorized by constitutional and statutory authority to conduct programs of education in the promotion of the public health, welfare, and morals"; that "the program of sex education being conducted by the defendant is a reasonable exercise of its constitutional and statutory authority"; that the "defendant's program of sex education does not unreasonably restrict the liberty of the plaintiff"; and that the "defendant's program of sex education is not conducted in violation of the [United States or Kansas constitutions]."

In short, the sexuality education program continued just as it had, because things were in order. An objective examination showed that the program was based on sound educational principles and that it was properly planned and conducted. Clearly, these last facts are crucial too, but the important point from the Kansas example is that cool heads did prevail.

Fortunately, logical heads have prevailed in most court cases related to sexuality education. In fact, the courts have generally continued to support state and local school authorities in cases dealing with sexuality education programs (Whitson, 1992).

Now let us take a look at an example of logical versus illogical thinking when dealing with criticism of sexuality education programs. One comparison often made in the sexuality education controversy is between the United States and other countries—particularly Sweden since sexuality education has been required there since 1956. Sexuality education critics often like to point to statistics from other countries to support their claim that many evils will result from the program.

While the example is now over 30 years old, it is related in a classic fashion that still deserves attention today. As a supposed result of the Swedish sexuality education program, Fulton (1972, 127) pointed out the following:

We are informed that thirty-five percent of all Swedish brides are pregnant on their wedding day, venereal disease has increased catastrophically and is now more widespread than in any other country in the civilized world, twenty percent of those reaching adulthood never marry (for whatever implications it might have), reported rapes have risen fifty-five percent in a two-year period, "hard core" pornography is flourishing, the Swedish divorce rate is one of the highest in the world, the suicide rate is the highest in the world, and promiscuity is the social norm.

First of all, the old saying that "you can't compare apples and oranges" is appropriate to remember here. Anyone who has looked at different cultures knows that it is usually impossible to make accurate cross-cultural statistical comparisons because of given cultural variances. To attempt to use these statistics to establish a cause-and-effect relationship is even more ludicrous. Since our present emphasis is on logical thinking, however, let us look at the claims.

Fulton pointed out a logical response to each claim regarding the Swedish statistics:

1. At first glance, the figure of a 35% pregnancy rate for brides seems to be awfully high, but U.S. statistics do show numbers in the same general range. If we wanted to be smug about it, we could claim that we should be proud that the United States has reached this situation without the "benefit" of sexuality education, but that would be missing the real point.

2. High STI rates are a public health concern in every major country today. To say that in Sweden this is a result of sexuality education is illogical. In addition, it should be remembered that rates of infection reflect behavior other than promiscuity—mainly sexual contact with infected persons (not with those not infected) and to some extent reflect educational efforts, since those who are educated are more likely to seek treatment. Therefore, higher rates may be a healthy sign that people are dealing with the problem.

3. In the case of rape statistics, a logical examination of Swedish statistics shows that the claims are false. While rape is never a positive event and should not be condoned, the Swedish rape rate is one of the lowest in the world.

4. Regarding pornography, it has been said that pornography, like beauty, is in the eye of the beholder. This complicates the issue, because it is difficult for people to agree on what is pornographic and what is not. Again, the cross-cultural comparison leaves us with situations that cannot accurately be compared.

5. Divorces are of concern to all societies. Lest we think that Swedish sexuality education has been the reason for divorces, however, we must consider that the U.S. divorce rate is much higher than the Swedish rate. Again, we have achieved this distinction without the "benefits" of sexuality education.

6. That Sweden has the highest suicide rate in the world is false information. There are about eight other countries that have higher rates.

7. Comparing rates of promiscuity or premarital sexual activity is a perfect example of difficulties when trying to utilize cross-cultural data. It has been known for a long time that in the Scandinavian countries premarital sexual activity tends to be socially accepted (and even expected). Given this norm, how is it possible to compare rates with a country such as the United States that has traditionally not held this belief?

We hope that this example of statistical comparisons will show you why logical thinking can prevail. Each of the claims made about the effects of sexuality education in Sweden has emotional implications and the potential for real problems, but a logical look at the facts and relationships can provide effective answers.

As further support of the fact that logical heads can prevail, it is wise to remember that an overwhelming majority of people do support sexuality education. Occasionally, there is a chance to show this support. In Wisconsin, opponents of sexuality education attempted to bar sexuality educator Sol Gordon from speaking at a local high school on "How can you tell if you're really in love?" A group called Citizens Concerned for Our Youth held a series of public meetings, blitzed the media, and appeared to have circumstances in their favor. A wise school principal, however, ascertained that there was sufficient community support to allow the program to continue. When Gordon finally did speak, out of the town's 18,000 people, about 2,500 were in the high school fieldhouse waiting to hear him—1,800 students and hundreds of adults along with reporters and TV cameras. Outside stood the opposition: some 10 or 15 lonely pickets (Gilgun & Newman, 1982).

It might also help to point out that a free exchange of ideas in the classroom and the complete and accurate presentation of issues ensure that educators do not impose one particular viewpoint on learners, thereby preserving the rights of parents to transmit their own values to their children. This approach reflects the interest of *all* people rather than denying the interests of *many* people by sanctioning only one view (Sedway, 1992). Cool and logical heads can and must prevail to appropriately evaluate each sexuality education program on its individual merits.

In spite of controversy, there are reasons for optimism. It may be easy to think that sexuality education opponents have succeeded, but this is not true. For example, sexuality education advocates have (1) introduced new legislation in the United States Congress that supports such education, (2) defeated attempts to increase federal funding for abstinence-only-until-marriage programs, (3) sparked debates about the federal government's abstinence-only-until-marriage programs that were not thought possible previously, and (4) advanced comprehensive sexuality education in many states (Smith, 2002).

Summary

In this chapter we have explored claims and facts surrounding the sexuality education controversy. Since school systems have been the usual object of criticism, many of the points within the chapter relate to schools; however, the same ideas have been applied to sexuality education programs in other settings.

Many of the facts and feelings related to the sexuality education controversy have not changed much during the past 25 to 30 years. Statements still need to be evaluated from the standpoint of whether they are accurate, are based on facts, appeal only to emotions, or appeal to logic.

A look at the history of campaigns against sexuality education shows that many of them were based on claims related to supposed negative moral and patriotic effects. In some communities, organized groups formed to prevent or combat sexuality education. As a result, many communities hesitated even to consider a sexuality education program. In some states, there were also attempts to legislate against sexuality education programs. In spite of this opposition, today there are many excellent sexuality education programs throughout the United States.

Tactics utilized by extremist groups opposed to sexuality education have not usually been based upon objective evaluation of programs but instead have been geared to prevent such an evaluation. These tactics have included blacklisting, coercion, disruption of meetings, distribution of publications, use of front groups, assertion of half-truths, infiltration, and the use of hysteria and fear.

There are identifiable characteristics of attacks from extremist groups. These include attempts to stifle free consideration of all views, to have certain publications removed from local libraries, and to utilize courses and textbooks that reflect extremist views. Most of these characteristics are directly contrary to the characteristics of a democratic society.

Attacks on sexuality education typically occur in four stages: sowing the seeds of doubt, internal incubation, outbreak, and shift to real goals—the power grab. Although these are perfectly legal activities in a democracy, if they involve questionable tactics, then educators, parents, and community leaders need to mobilize their own forces.

It would be erroneous to think that all people opposed to sexuality education, or with hesitations about it, use the same tactics as the extremists. In many instances concerned parents and members of the community simply need to be adequately informed about the program to understand it and become supporters. Before assuming that someone with questions about a program is an extremist, it is wise to assess his or her reasons for opposition.

There are many reasons commonly given for opposition to sexuality education. In every instance, however, there are many factual refutations of arguments against sexuality education.

Sound suggestions for defense against extremist attacks do exist. We need to remember that a large majority of parents, professional and lay organizations, and community leaders are in favor of good sexuality education programs. Organized community efforts in support of sexuality education that focus on facts related to program planning, implementation, and content can go a long way in eliminating many negative claims. Public meetings about sexuality education can bring out individuals with many varied opinions. If run properly, such meetings can give the public confidence that the program is sound.

In the final analysis, cool and logical heads usually prevail in the sexuality education controversy. As long as we remember that there are emotional issues involved, that the resistance of some people is based on years of negative learning about human sexuality, and that functioning intelligence goes down as the emotional level goes up, the final result of a controversy will usually be a better program. An objective examination is good for any planned or implemented program and should only make it stronger.

References

Bensley, L. B. *A handbook for establishing sex education programs in Michigan schools.* Mt. Pleasant, MI: Michigan School Health Association, 1986.

A brief history of the current campaign against sex education. New York: Sexuality Information and Education Council of the United States, no date.

Deception uncovered: An analysis. New York: Coalition for Adolescent Sexual Health, February 13, 2003.

Extremist groups. Chicago: National Congress of Parents and Teachers, no date.

Fulton, G. B. Sex education: Some issues and answers, in *Readings in marriage, sex education, and human sexuality,* Conley, J. A. & Huffman, W. J., eds. Champaign, IL: Stipes Publishing, 1972.

Gendel, E. S. Sex education lawsuit in Kansas—impressions and implications, *SIECUS Newsletter* (October 1970), 1–4.

Gilgun, J. & Newman, L. Democracy triumphs in Wisconsin Rapids, *Impact,* no. 4 (1982), 6–7, 10.

Haffner, D. W. & de Mauro, D. *Winning the battle: Developing support for sexuality and HIV/AIDS education.* New York: Sexuality Information and Education Council of the United States, March 1991.

Knowlton, R. Co-opting the opposition, *Family Life Educator* (Spring 1986), 14.

The National Coalition to Support Sexuality Education. Sexuality Information and Education Council of the United States (2002). Available: http://www.siecus.org/pubs/fact/fact0005.html.

Opponents of comprehensive sexuality education. Sexuality Information and Education Council of the United States (2003). Available: http://www.siecus.org/pubs/fact/fact0016.html.

Putnam, P. *The involvement of the schools.* Washington, DC: National Education Association, no date.

Reiss, I. Sexual pluralism, *SIECUS Report,* 19, no. 3 (February/March 1991), 5–9.

Responding to arguments against comprehensive sexuality education. Sexuality Information and Education Council of the United States (2000). Available: http://www.siecus.org/advocacy/kits0005.html.

Sedway, M. Far right takes aim at sexuality education, *SIECUS Report,* 20, no. 3 (February/March 1992), 13–19.

Should sexologists lobby for sex ed in schools? *Sexuality Today* (April 28, 1986), 1.

Smith, W. Reason for optimism about comprehensive sexuality education, *SIECUS Report,* 30, no. 6 (August/September 2002), 35–36.

Suggestions for defense against extremist attack: Sex education in the public schools. Washington, DC: National Education Association, no date.

Talk about sex: The battles over sex education, *SIECUS Report,* 30, no. 6 (August/September 2002), 20–21.

Tips for dealing with negative resistance. Hampton, NH: Sowers and Associates, 1992.

Trevor, C. Number of controversies decline as schools adopt conservative policies, *SIECUS Report,* 30, no. 6 (August/September 2002), 4–17.

Whitson, J. A. Sexuality and censorship in the curriculum, in *Sexuality and the curriculum,* Sears, J. T., ed., 59–77. New York: Teachers College, Columbia University, 1992.

Woodworth, R. T. *From infancy to adultery.* Baltimore: Open Bible Broadcasts, no date.

Suggested Readings

The controversy report. Sexuality Information and Education Council of the United States (2004). Available: http://www.siecus.org/controversy.

Gordon, S. Values-based sexuality education: Confronting extremists to get the message across, *SIECUS Report,* 20, no. 6 (August/September 1992), 1–4.

Greenberg, J. S. Opposition to sexuality education, in *Sexuality education within comprehensive school health education,* 33–40. Kent, OH: American School Health Association, 1991.

Haffner, D. W. & de Mauro, D. Responding to the opposition, in *Winning the battle: Developing support for sexuality and HIV/AIDS education,* 17–29. New York: Sexuality Information and Education Council of the United States, March 1991.

Irvine, J. *Talk about sex: The battle over sex education in the United States.* Berkeley, CA: University of California Press, 2002.

Kaiser Family Foundation national survey of public secondary school principals: The politics of sex education. Menlo Park, CA: The Henry J. Kaiser Family Foundation, December, 1999.

Peter D. Hart Research Associates, Inc. *Teaching sex education in public elementary schools.* Washington, DC: Children's Research and Education Institute, 1999.

Stayton, W. R. A theology of sexual pleasure, *SIECUS Report,* 20, no. 4 (April/May 1992), 9–15.

Understanding Yourself

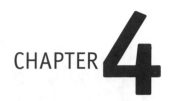

CHAPTER 4

Key Concepts

1. A sexuality educator should accept himself or herself as a sexual being.

2. A sexuality educator should be comfortable interacting with others about sexuality.

3. A sexuality educator should be committed to sexual responsibility.

4. A sexuality educator should have certain qualifications to be effective.

5. In certain respects, everyone is a sexuality educator.

Kevin was a second-year teacher of a class of mainstreamed junior high school students who was expected to teach a sexuality unit. Wanting to be responsive to students' needs, Kevin had a policy of allowing students to ask whatever questions they wanted, and Barry took him up on that offer one day. While discussing contraception, Barry raised his hand and asked, "A friend of my older sister got pregnant even though she took the Pill, but she was able to get an abortion. Why do I need to worry about contraception if abortions are available? I just want to focus on having fun." Kevin believed strongly that abortion was taking a life and was, therefore, immoral. How was he to respond? He wanted to be nonjudgmental, but that would be opposed to his view of morality.

In this chapter we discuss in more detail the concept that all of us are sexual beings and that our sexuality is rooted in who and what we are rather than in what we do. You will have an opportunity to consider how qualified you are to be a sexuality educator, for not everyone can effectively teach sexuality education. As we discuss the qualifications that are needed and the importance of these qualifications, you will have an opportunity to consider your feelings about your own sexuality and how they are related to your role in educating others.

Sexuality Educators and Their Own Sexuality

An important consideration regarding your qualifications to be a sexuality educator is your degree of comfort with your own sexuality. It is necessary for you to accept your own sexuality before helping others accept theirs. Let us explore this concern by considering such topics as your sexual thoughts and desires, your masculinity and femininity, your body image, your sexual behavior, and your sense of humor.

Your Sexual Thoughts and Desires

A nationally renowned sexuality educator was heard to say that every time he saw an attractive woman walking down the street, he had intercourse with her right then and there! She did not know it and continued on her way without so much as a glance. He, on the other hand, broke out in a grin and was a little happier than prior to the "experience." The point of relating this story is to emphasize that sexual thoughts and desires in themselves are not wrong. They are natural (though some may be unusual), and one should not feel guilty about having them. It is the translation of thoughts and desires into behaviors that can cause problems. If the sexuality educator had actually harassed, attacked, or in some other way infringed on the rights of the women to whom he was attracted, his behavior would have been unacceptable. In such an instance, the appropriate societal institutions would have come into play. He might have been arrested by the police, or referred to a mental health counseling program. Notice that we do not have a "thought-preventing" societal institution that punishes people for sexual desires. Even if we could, in some way, determine what people were thinking, it is doubtful that we would be willing to punish people for thoughts alone. And yet people often *are* punished for their thoughts and desires, not by a societal institution, but rather

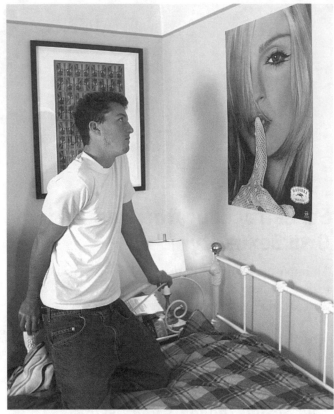

Guilt about sexual thoughts can be devastating to one's self-esteem and ability to function. Accepting that sexual thoughts do not equal action is important to leading a fulfilling life.

by those who should know better—themselves. It is not the thoughts that are the problem, it is the guilt people allow themselves to feel because of those thoughts. Guilt is so devastating that it undermines people's self-esteem and their ability to function.

It is interesting to notice the reaction of the American people and press to Jimmy Carter's admission in 1976 to having "lusted" for women other than his wife. The public hue and cry about his admission of sexual desires was enough to cause concern that he might lose the presidential election. This reaction evidences the guilt some people are willing to ascribe to sexual thoughts. This kind of guilt or punishment is absurd. We do not have control of many of our thoughts. They erupt. They are there. To punish ourselves for them, when they have not been acted out, is to be less than accepting of who and what we are. If we allow ourselves to feel guilty about our sexual thoughts and desires, we have not accepted our own sexuality. If this is the case with you, you are advised to work this out prior to attempting to participate in the sexuality education of others.

Your Masculinity and Femininity

Certainly, an important aspect of understanding ourselves is being in touch with our masculinity and femininity. Notice that the phrase is "masculinity *and* femininity," rather than

"masculinity *or* femininity." Each of us has both feminine and masculine qualities. Although this topic is discussed in more detail later in this book, mention needs to be made of it here. Too many people have limiting and stereotypical views of what is masculine and what is feminine, even in the face of tremendous changes in these attitudes over recent years. We have learned that women can perform any job men can. We have also learned that men can perform jobs that have traditionally been held by women. The notion that men are not to cry during times of great sorrow, great joy, or whenever feeling touched or tender, does a disservice to men. In fact, it is downright unhealthy to suppress these emotions. Likewise, perpetuating an environment where women are not to take charge of situations without being perceived as a "bitch," or are not to win when bowling or playing golf with dates in whom they are interested, or are not to show their competence in other situations without believing the other person will be offended and made to feel inferior is unconscionable. Sexuality educators need to be aware of these perceptions that may be ingrained in their psyches, because they can interfere with the effectiveness of the sexuality education they conduct. Our students and we ourselves have the right to actualize who we are, not what we are presumed to be by stereotypical thinking associated with our gender.

The point of this description is that we are often shackled by others' conceptions of who and what we should be sexually, rather than allowed to evolve into who we are *naturally*. The root of the word naturally—nature—is important here. If we do not develop into who we naturally are, we become unnatural.

Your Body Image

Understanding and accepting one's sexual thoughts and masculinity and femininity are important for a sexuality

Insight 4-2

Evaluating Your Body Image

In the blanks below, place the number that best represents your thoughts and feelings about each body part.

1 = very satisfied

2 = OK

3 = not very satisfied

4 = very dissatisfied

——— *hair*	——— *nose*	——— *mouth*
——— *face*	——— *ears*	——— *chin*
——— *neck*	——— *buttocks*	——— *thighs*
——— *shoulders*	——— *hands*	——— *arms*
——— *hips*	——— *chest*	——— *knees*
——— *legs*	——— *eyes*	——— *genitals*
——— *fingers*	——— *toes*	——— *elbows*
——— *abdomen*	——— *back*	——— *calves*
——— *ankles*		

Now sum up the numbers in the blanks. The greater your score, the more dissatisfied you are with your body; conversely, the lower your score, the more satisfied you are with your body. Since we know that satisfaction with one's body is related to one's general self-esteem, a sexuality educator with a negative self-image may not be as confident, relaxed, non-threatened, or effective as one with a positive self-image, *all other things being equal.*

---

educator to be effective. Having a positive **body image** (accepting one's body with its attractiveness and uniqueness) is another characteristic desirable in a sexuality educator. If you are self-conscious about the shape of your body, you will not be able to discuss body development adequately. Your discomfort will be conveyed either verbally or nonverbally. You may rush through the topic, may be unable to objectively answer questions, and so forth. Our point here is that you should accept your body for what and how it is, not that you should like all parts of it, nor that you must think it is sexually attractive. To determine your body image, complete the exercise in Insight 4-2.

If your score on Insight 4-2 indicates to you that you are generally dissatisfied with your body and you desire to be a sexuality educator, there are two things you can do:

1. You can work to change those parts of your body with which you are dissatisfied. You could exercise, go on a diet to lose or gain weight, and so forth.

2. You can work on becoming more accepting of those parts of your body with which you are dissatisfied. You could stress their uniqueness or dress to maximize other attributes.

Probably a combination of both of these is best. That is, identify those body parts that can be changed for the better and go about changing them; at the same time, work on being more accepting of those parts that cannot be changed. Remember, though, we are speaking of your being more *satisfied* with your body, not of making it more attractive per se. There are many attractive people who have poor body images, as well as many unattractive people who have positive ones. The main point is that sexuality educators should be satisfied with their bodies so that negative thoughts and feelings regarding their body parts do not interfere with the task at hand—educating others about sexuality.

Your Sexual Behavior

There is a story told of a mother who entered her son's room only to find him masturbating. Not knowing what to do, but disapproving of her son's behavior, she said with a sense of exasperation, "What are you doing? Stop that immediately! Don't you know that could make you blind!" The son looked up sheepishly, contemplated for a moment on the predicament in which he found himself, and with all the courage he could muster asked, "But it feels so good. Couldn't I do it just 'til I need glasses?"

This story serves well to illustrate the misinformation surrounding sexual behavior. We investigate this matter in some detail elsewhere in this text. For our purposes here, however, let us consider the effect of one's sexual behavior, and thoughts regarding this behavior, on one's effectiveness as a sexuality educator.

The first point worth making is that we are human, and as such are fallible. The sexuality educator who is burdened by guilt feelings surrounding his or her sexual behavior is one who might inappropriately moralize in the instructional setting, who might not be objective in approaching the subject, or who might eliminate instructional content or material that resurrects these guilt feelings. Consequently, if you want to be a sexuality educator and yet are burdened with guilt feelings surrounding your sexual behavior, you should seek some means of working out these feelings. Perhaps a counseling center could help. Maybe some introspection and realistic thinking are all that is needed. How about talking with a close friend or a member of the clergy?

The second point is that sexual inexperience is no reason to shy away from preparation to be a sexuality educator.

---

body image   One's view of one's body; may be positive or negative.

One need not have committed suicide in order to instruct others about that topic. Some excellent sexuality education programs are conducted by priests and nuns, ministers, and rabbis for instance.

Although it seems absurd that a sexuality educator would be hired *because of* sexual experience, although illegal in most states, marital experience has been a hiring consideration on the part of some organizations in both school and community settings. Some employers argue that a married person is more mature, more experienced (there is that word again), and more familiar with marriage and family. To generalize from one situation to all marriages and families is ridiculous. What is needed in a sexuality educator is a person who is willing to learn about marriages and families and gay and lesbian relationships by immersing himself or herself in the literature and research on these topics. Marital status is an irrelevant consideration in the effectiveness of a sexuality educator.

Similarly, age is an irrelevant consideration in the effectiveness of a sexuality educator. We all know some young people who interact well with others and some older ones who do not. Conversely, we also know of some older people who interact well with others and some younger ones who do not. The important factor here is not age but the ability to interact well with others. Regardless of the age of the learner, the sexuality educator of any age can be effective. The popular stereotype is that a younger sexuality educator is sexually active and more "with it," whereas the older sexuality educator is more sensible and stable. As is the case with most sterotypes, this one does not make any sense. Being "with it," sensible, and stable is not a function of age.

Your Sense of Humor

As can be other enjoyable parts of life, sexuality can sometimes be funny. A sense of humor will help the sexuality educator to demythologize sexuality and place it into a meaningful context in relation to the whole of life. Sexuality should be no more serious a matter, nor any less, than any other aspect of living. A sexuality educator who cannot be comfortable with humor about sexuality or who cannot find humor in funny questions or situations that may arise in the instructional setting will probably not be able to relate well to his or her students.

The Sexuality Educator's Interactions with Others

A young boy asked his older brother where babies come from. The older brother told him that babies come from the stork. Seeking verification for this shocking revelation, the boy asked his father where babies come from. His father said that babies come from the stork. Not wanting to be impolite but not completely satisfied, the young boy approached the sage of the family, his grandfather, and asked him where babies come from. The grandfather, following the party line, told him that babies come from the stork. In school the next day, the young boy related his conversations with his brother, father, and grandfather to the teacher and his classmates and concluded that there had not been normal sexual relations in his family for three generations.

Obviously, the brother, father, and grandfather had more information about the origin of babies than they were revealing (or at least we assume they did). The reason they did not tell the boy where babies come from was that they did not know how to conduct such a conversation, how much or how little to reveal, or whether a frank answer would provoke a "Well, how did the sperm get in the mother?" type of question. In other words, they felt uncomfortable as well as unprepared for this teaching opportunity.

Interactions with Groups

The sexuality educator should feel comfortable talking to groups of people about sexuality. Questions emanating from a group should not embarrass you as a sexuality educator, regardless of the topic or the language used. Some learners will attempt to embarrass you and will learn much from your reaction.

Other learners may seem to be attempting to embarrass you but are actually expressing themselves in the only way in which they know how. They may not know the proper name of a body part and so call it by its slang name, for example. Your responsibility in such instances is to identify the correct terminology, without embarrassing the person asking the question, and then answer the question. The important thing to remember is that you want to educate those with whom you are working. To inhibit their questions by requiring certain language or by identifying some topics as off-limits is to limit the amount of learning that can occur. If you remain focused on open and clear communication and are careful to avoid reinforcement of a student's inappropriate behavior, then the stage will be set for learning. Certainly, there may be limits placed on you by others who administer your institution, school, or organization, and you will have to function within these limits. However, you should not create further unreasonable limits because you are uncomfortable discussing sexuality in group settings.

Interactions with Individuals

Embarrassment and discomfort are of concern not only in group settings but in one-on-one settings as well. Because of the nature of the subject matter, an effective sexuality educator is likely to be approached by individual students who have questions or requests for help. When it is realized that people do not usually discuss sexual matters with others in any serious manner (and that includes their physicians), it is understandable that such an opportunity would provoke a desire for discussing previously undisclosed problems. When such a discussion is inappropriate in a group setting, the learner might approach the sexuality educator individually to seek help or answers to questions left unanswered. The sexuality educator should be comfortable discussing such sexual concerns with students on an individual basis.

Culture and the Sexuality Educator

There are many influences on the development of sexual attitudes, values, and behaviors—not the least of which is the culture in which people grow up and reside. Several obvious examples illustrative of the influence of culture come to mind. In some Latin American countries, males are accepted as being dominant. That is where the term "macho" (for machismo) derives. In other cultures, it is the female that assumes a dominant role. For example, approximately two-thirds of African-American families with children in the United States are headed by a single-parent female. In that setting, women assume a role relationship, develop values and attitudes, and adopt behaviors quite different from the women in Latin American cultures.

In some other cultures, homosexuality is a socially accepted identity. In fact, in the large area in the Pacific between Sumatra through Papua New Guinea and Melanesia, homosexuality is actually institutionalized (Greenberg, Bruess & Mullen, 1993). Males between the ages of nine and nineteen move out of their families' homes into the long houses in the center of the village. There, they engage in homosexual activity until they are ready for marriage (at about age nineteen). After marriage, homosexuality activity ceases or is kept to a minimum.

Recognizing the influence of culture (here we include such factors as **gender, ethnicity, race,** religion, and **societal mores**) on sexual attitudes and values, the sexuality educator needs to introspectively identify these influences on his or her own sexual development. Once that is done, the same should be attempted for the people participating in sexuality programs conducted by this sexuality educator. In this way, a greater understanding, appreciation, and

In some cultures, women are expected to cover their bodies from head to toe. Willing compliance with such restrictions can be difficult for Western cultures to understand.

acceptance of different points of view will more easily be achieved, and the education offered will be more effective and meaningful.

The Sexuality Educator's Sexual Responsibility

The place of **morality** in sexuality education is difficult to determine. Whose morality is to be taught? There are certain aspects of morality, though, upon which everyone can agree. One point of agreement is that people should demonstrate responsibility in their sexual behavior. This moral conclusion holds several implications for the sexuality educator.

---

gender   Traits associated with acting, behaving, and feeling like a female or a male.

ethnicity   Designation of a subgroup of people having a common cultural heritage consisting of customs, characteristics, language, or common history.

race   Designation of a subgroup of people distinguished by physical traits (such as hair, eyes, skin, color), blood types, genetic

code pattern, and unique inherited traits. Primary divisions are Caucasoid, Negroid, and Mongoloid.

societal mores   A set of practices deemed to be acceptable and others deemed to be unacceptable by a large group of people or a society.

morality   A designation of what is right or good (moral) or what is wrong or bad (immoral).

First, one of the criteria for making a decision about sexual behavior must be its effect on other people. To behave in a manner that infringes on the rights of others, or is in some manner detrimental to others, is to behave irresponsibly. The sexuality educator, while affording learners their own choices regarding how they will behave sexually, must therefore insist upon a consideration of the effect of the chosen behavior on other people. That is, any decisions made by students in sexuality education should be viewed in terms of their effects on parents, lovers, friends, and so forth. For example, someone with a sexually transmitted infection should be responsible enough to refrain from sexual intercourse until it is treated and to inform any past sexual partners that they too might be infected. As you can see, being sexually responsible is not always easy.

Second, sexual responsibility must include a consideration of effects of decisions on society in general. A sexually active teenager who does not use some method of contraception, for example, might be considered socially irresponsible by some. A resulting pregnancy might entail the need for medical services at public expense (for abortion, prenatal care, obstetrical services, postnatal care) or public support for the child through social services or welfare agencies. In addition, children born to teenage mothers stand a greater chance than average of having a birth defect, perhaps requiring medical care that might otherwise have been available to someone else. You can see that this irresponsible sexual behavior has far-reaching societal implications.

Sexual behavior that is detrimental to the self can also be classified as irresponsible. How could this possibly occur? Consider the teenager who is pressured by peers to be sexually active but who is morally and religiously opposed to sexual activity before marriage. If such a person succumbs to peer pressure, his or her needs and best interests would not be served. In such a case the behavior could be labeled sexually irresponsible.

To summarize, we would argue that sexual responsibility entails consideration of the effects of sexual choices upon oneself, one's immediate family and friends (including one's sexual partner), a potential child, and the society in which the sexual choice occurs. Further, the sexuality educator should be committed to sexual responsibility and should include it as an integral component of any sexuality education program.

Others have added to the definition of sexual responsibility by including the need for relationships. They argue that sexual relationships, to be responsible, must include caring and consideration by the partners. Others maintain that marriage is needed for sexual behavior—in particular coitus—to be responsible.

The purpose of this section is not to argue for any moral view of sexual behavior but rather to advocate the inclusion of the teaching of sexual responsibility in sexuality education programs. To assure this inclusion, the sexuality educator should be committed to sexual responsibility and should understand its implications.

Qualifications for the Sexuality Educator

Although many people attempt to teach education for sexuality, not all are qualified. In fact, this is probably the most valid criticism made by opponents of sexuality education. Not many years ago, it was impolite to discuss sexuality other than to recall a bawdy incident or to tell an off-color joke. Consequently, professional preparation programs for sexuality educators were nonexistent. With increasing recognition of the need for sexuality education and the subsequent implementation of such programs, there developed a need for educators with necessary competencies. Responding to this need, colleges and universities began courses to train the sexuality educator, private and public organizations developed workshops on human sexuality and sexuality education, and sexuality books started rolling off the presses. Usually, professional preparation programs in sexuality education train health educators, home economists, counselors, nurses, or physicians to teach some sexuality education. The rationale for preparing such other professionals to teach sexuality education will soon become clear.

Now look back at the three criteria for a sexuality educator that you listed in Insight 4-3. Compare your recommendations with those obtained from high school health and sexuality teachers, when they were asked what they needed to be competent in the area of human sexuality (Munson, 1976, 31). Although this study was conducted some time ago, the findings appear relevant for today's sexuality teachers.

All the teachers surveyed felt that it was not essential for the sexuality educator to be married or to have been married, nor to be a parent, nor to have any particular church affiliation to be effective.

Insight 4-3

Qualifications to Teach Sexuality Education

Consider for a moment the qualifications you think are important. List at least three of these.

1. _____

2. _____

3. _____

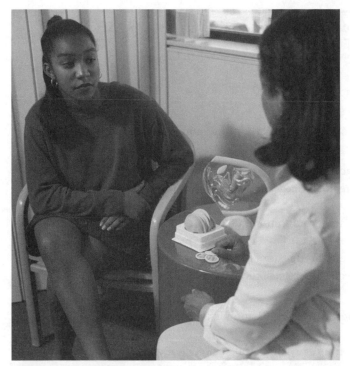

Nurses and physicians are usually trained to educate patients about sexuality. How can you be sure you are trained to be a competent sexuality educator?

In what academic and subject matter areas did teachers feel sexuality educators should be well-versed? Over 90% of the teachers felt that knowledge of reproduction and human anatomy, venereal disease (sic—sexually transmitted infections), and contraception was essential. Masturbation, abortion, and the role of marriage in family life was rated by 89% as essential. More than 85% of the teachers felt that knowledge of the psychology of adolescence, menstruation, pregnancy and childbirth, guilt and conflict over sexual behavior, sex differences and roles, and homosexuality should be regarded as essential. And over 80% of the teachers felt that knowledge of premarital coitus, nocturnal emissions, dating, courting and marriage was essential background for effective sexuality teaching.

Of the teachers surveyed 80% felt that sensitivity work was essential to their preparation. This fact may be interpreted as a call from such teachers to help them feel right about themselves and their sexuality feelings (sexuality concept) before entering the classroom to teach in what may be regarded by many teachers as an emotionally charged area.

About half of the teachers (56%) felt that knowledge of aging and sexual response, along with trends and issues

in human sexuality, was to be regarded as essential in sexuality education preparation for teachers.

Less than half of the teachers surveyed felt that knowledge of multiple births, sexual aberrations, biological anomalies, heredity and sex determination, and cultural differences was essential to human sexuality teaching. . . . Close agreement existed between teachers and experts as to essentiality of a wide background of communication, evaluation techniques, research techniques, group dynamics, curriculum aids and development, dealing with the community and parents, and individual counseling skills.

Sexuality Education Certification

The American Association of Sex Educators, Counselors, and Therapists (AASECT) has set forth requirements in order for them to certify a person as a sexuality educator. These requirements are shown in Table 4-1.

It is important to differentiate between **certification** and *qualification*. Although a state or national agency may certify someone as a sexuality educator, that does not ensure that the person is qualified to teach sexuality education. Conversely, the fact that someone does not possess a particular requirement to be awarded certification (for example, a bachelor's degree) does not mean that the person is not qualified to be a sexuality educator. Of course, we hope that in most cases certification does attest to qualification. Without certification, anyone could claim to be a sexuality educator. At least certification evidences that some responsible agency has reviewed the sexuality educator's credentials and has found them adequate.

Everyone Is a Sexuality Educator

If you are a parent, you are certainly already a sexuality educator. While learners are young and impressionable, they spend most of their time with their parents. Consequently, parents are a very important component of any learner's sexuality education. For example, parents who demonstrate affection for each other and their children teach that it is OK to express one's love for another (be it sexual or otherwise). Furthermore, parents often are the first to have to answer questions about sexuality asked by their children: What is growing in Mommy? How are babies made? Where did I come from? Not only are the answers to these questions important, but *how* they are answered is also significant. Does the parent hesitate, stammer, and otherwise demonstrate discomfort in discussing sexual topics? Or does the parent react the same way to these questions as to any others? The child

certification   Designation by some overseeing group of an applicant's having met the minimum requirements to perform a job.

Table 4-1 The American Association of Sex Educators, Counselors and Therapists (AASECT) Requirements for Certification as a Sex Educator

I. Membership in AASECT:

The applicant may hold Full, Institutional, Retired, or Life Membership in AASECT.

II. AASECT Code of Ethics:

The applicant will have read the AASECT Code of Ethics. By signing the certification application form, the applicant agrees to be bound by the AASECT Code of Ethics.

III. Academic and Professional Experience as a Sexuality Educator:

The applicant will have earned an academic degree from an accredited college or university and acquired professional experience as follows:

A. A Bachelor's degree plus four years of professional experience as an educator (1,000 hours per year), or;

B. A Master's degree plus three years of professional experience as an educator (1,000 hours per year), or;

C. A Doctorate degree plus two years of professional experience as an educator (1,000 hours per year).

D. Applicants from outside the United States must document equivalent academic and professional experience.

IV. Human Sexuality Education:

The applicant will have completed a minimum of ninety (90) clock hours of education in the following core areas:

A. Sexual and reproductive anatomy/physiology.

B. Developmental sexuality (from conception through old age) from a psychological, sociological, and biological perspective.

C. Dynamics of interpersonal relationships.

D. Gender-related issues.

E. Sexual orientations and gender identities.

F. Sociocultural factors (ethnicity, culture, religiosity, socioeconomic status) in sexual values and behavior.

G. Relationship and family dynamics.

H. Health factors that may influence sexuality including illness, disability, drugs, abortion, pregnancy, contraception, fertility, HIV/AIDS, sexually transmissible infections, and safer sex practices.

I. Sexuality research principles.

J. Sexual exploitation, including sexual abuse, sexual harassment, and sexual assault.

K. Learning theory and application.

L. Presentation skills.

M. Diversity in sexual expression.

It is expected that the applicant document at least three clock hours for each content area listed above (A–M) with the additional hours to be spread as desired with a maximum of twenty hours in any one area. Please refer to Section VIII of this document for examples of acceptable documentation sources.

V. Attitudes and Values Training Experience:

A. The applicant will have participated in a minimum of twelve (12) clock hours of structured group experience in which the major focus is on a process-oriented exploration of the applicant's own feelings, attitudes, values, and beliefs regarding human sexuality and sexual behavior (e.g., a SAR). Such training may not be personal psychotherapy nor an academic experience in which the primary emphasis is on cognitive information. It is strongly recommended that this experience occur early in the applicant's training to be most beneficial.

B. The applicant will submit a one-page comprehensive statement of his or her professional philosophy and goals of sex education, including how the SAR affected that philosophy.

VI. Professional Experience Specific to Sexuality Education:

A minimum of two (2) years of work experience involving sexuality education (minimum 100 student-teacher contact hours), which must be documented. Such education may be conducted in various settings such as public or private clinics, classrooms, social service agencies, colleges or universities, religious institutions, and/or family planning centers.

The experience may include participating in professional development seminars, training, conferences, and courses: designing and conducting workshops, courses, and seminars; contributing to the sexuality education literature, developing curriculum; planning and administering programs; delivering lectures and/or providing one-on-one client education sessions. This paid or volunteer experience may have been obtained prior to or following the receipt of the highest degree earned.

Table 4-1 (*Continued*)

VII. Consultation:

The applicant will have completed a consultation of at least 25 hours with an AASECT Certified Sex Educator, or be able to document competence as a sexuality educator. The minimum duration of the consultation will have been at least three months (one semester).

The twenty-five (25) hours of consultation required for those seeking Certification as a Sex Educator must be provided by a consultant with a minimum of three (3) years as an AASECT Certified Sex Educator. Some experience in the consultation role is recommended, but not required.

Consultation should occur with some regularity once initiated (once a week or twice a month for a minimum of one hour per consultation session), should take place over a minimum of six (6) months, and would include but not be limited to:

1. Development of an educational/learning philosophy;
2. Curriculum and syllabus development;
3. Direct observation of teaching/training activities;
4. Discussion and development of pedagogic styles and strategies.

In the event there is no AASECT Certified Sex Educator within a reasonable geographic location, an alternative method of consultation may be proposed to the AASECT Sex Educator Certification Committee.

The consultant will review and evaluate the applicant's academic preparation, professional experience, and educational/facilitation skills. Through the provision of a sexuality education program developed and implemented by the applicant, the consultant will seek to determine the applicant's ability to:

A. Assess educational needs;
B. Define goals and objective;
C. Match teaching strategies with proposed outcomes;
D. Design and effectively use instruments which assess the performance (knowledge, behavior, attitude changes) of program participants and program effectiveness;
E. Utilize evaluation feedback;
F. Apply educational research findings;
G. Access and use other human and material resources;
H. Implement and effectively utilize educational methodologies which address the cognitive and affective dimensions of sexuality.

The following do not meet the consultation requirements:

A. Consultation with a family member or a significant other;
B. Consultation with a colleague with whom one is involved in a professional partnership;
C. Management or administrative meetings with an organizational director or executive.

VIII. Documentation:

The following documentation must be submitted in four (4) sets, for review by the Sex Educator Certification Committee. The material will become the property of AASECT. Each document should be clearly marked so as to identify the requirements to which it applies.

A. Completed formal application for AASECT Certified Sex Educator that is signed and dated.
B. Official transcripts of programs(s) in which degree(s) was earned (Item II).
C. Official documentation of ninety (90) hours of education in the designated core areas of human sexuality. Documentation must include the dates, sponsors, faculty, and content of the educational experience, transcripts of course work, certificates of attendance, continuing education (CEU) certificates, or other credible evidence (Item III). Dates of attendance, official sponsor, and faculty must be included on all non-academic materials.
D. Official documentation of participation in a structured group experience focused on personal attitudes, beliefs, and values (e.g., SAR) (Item IV-A).
E. Statement of philosophy of sex education (Item IV-B).
F. Letter(s) from employer(s) and/or supervisor(s) documenting a minimum of two (2) years experience in providing comprehensive sex education (Item V).

(*Continued*)

Table 4-1 *(Continued)*

G. Signed Certificate of Endorsement from consultant attesting to the applicant's having received twenty-five (25) hours of supervised consultation (Item VI) (Use AASECT provided form).

H. Signed Certificate of Endorsement from a professional colleague (Use AASECT provided form).

I. The appropriate certification fee.

IX. Miscellaneous:

A. Upon the approval of the Sex Education Certification Committee, the successful applicant will receive a certificate in recognition of having met the AASECT requirements for certification in the area of sexuality education. This certificate will be subject to renewal after three (3) years, and subsequent renewals every five (5) years.

B. Membership in AASECT must be maintained on an annual basis to retain the AASECT certification status. If membership in AASECT lapses, certification will also lapse.

X. Implementation of New Certification Requirements:

Individuals currently involved in the process of becoming certified by AASECT are subject to the requirements outlined in the document.

Reprinted with permission from the American Association of Sex Educators, Counselors, and Therapists.

may learn that it is OK to be concerned with and openly discuss sexuality, or the child may learn that sexuality is a topic to be suppressed and only discussed in locker rooms and behind closed doors. Parents who establish good rapport with their children provide an environment conducive to their children's willingness to seek their advice and guidance in sexual matters throughout their lives. What better sexuality education role could anyone hope to fulfill?

Even if you are not a parent, however, you are already a sexuality educator to the people around you. As a matter of fact, everyone is! When your masculinity and femininity are appropriately expressed, others about you learn something regarding masculinity and femininity. When you express your behavior with some degree of acceptance and responsibility, others learn from that. When you are caring and loving in relation to other people, still other learning occurs. When you demonstrate to others that you are accepting of your sexuality, that you believe sexuality is all right to discuss, that you believe information about sexuality is not harmful, and that you are able to allow others their sexual ethics, you are conveying much to those about you.

The converse of these behaviors and attitudes will also result in learning, but this learning will have negative consequences for the learner. The result may be a person who is incapable of accepting his or her sexuality, misinformed and uncomfortable with the topic, or intolerant of sexual expressions other than those that he or she adopts.

We all learn from each other, and since our sexuality is such an integral part of ourselves, our sexuality is always evident. We are all models of sexuality from whom others learn. However, though we are all sexuality educators, clearly we are not all good sexuality educators!

Qualified sexuality educators are professionally prepared for that role. They are knowledgeable regarding human sexuality and competent in the educational process. They are comfortable with the topic and can discuss sex and sexuality with individuals and small and large groups. They care about those whom they are educating, they believe in sexual responsibility, and they are unwilling to attempt the inculcation of their personal morals into their students' lives. They often are certified health professionals with experience as students in formalized sexuality instructional courses, workshops, or programs. They are continually updating their sexual knowledge and their educational process skills.

Now is the time for you to consider whether you are committed to making the personal changes and educational efforts necessary to become a qualified sexuality educator.

Summary

This chapter was designed to point out that although all of us, to some degree, are sexuality educators, there are certain unique characteristics of truly qualified ones. Sexuality educators need to accept themselves as sexual beings. They need to recognize and accept their sexual thoughts and desires. They need to recognize aspects of themselves traditionally categorized as feminine and masculine, and they need to realize that each of us has both of these traits. Furthermore, sexuality educators need to accept their bodies, whatever their physical assets and liabilities; they need to evidence a lack of guilt associated with their own sexual behavior; and they need to demonstrate a sense of humor regarding sexuality.

Sexuality educators should be comfortable interacting with both individuals and groups of people about sexuality. This becomes important if the sexuality educator expects to be effective when instructing in group settings as well as when responding to the concerns of inquisitive or motivated individuals after group instruction.

Sexuality educators also need a sense of sexual responsibility. Although the teaching of one set of values or morals relative to sexual behavior is inappropriate for sexuality education, there are some common elements of morality on which consensus can be reached. One of these common elements is that sexual behavior should be responsible—that irresponsible sexual behavior is undesirable. The sexuality educator's role is to include a consideration of sexual responsibility in sexuality education programs.

Among sexuality education authorities and professional organizations there is both agreement and disagreement regarding necessary qualifications for sexuality educators. No definitive studies are available to recommend one particular set of qualifications. Some argue for a knowledge base, others stress comfort with one's own sexuality and the topic, and still others emphasize a genuine concern for the welfare of those being educated. We suggest that all of these characteristics are necessary for a qualified sexuality educator.

If you recognize some deficiencies in your own readiness to be a sexuality educator, do not be alarmed. This book is devoted to aiding you in your preparation. A recognition of your shortcomings is a vital first step in this preparation. Remember, though, a commitment to becoming an effective sexuality educator begins with a commitment to self-understanding.

References

Greenberg, J. S., Bruess, C. E. & Mullen, K. *Sexuality: Insights and issues.* 3rd ed. Dubuque, IA: William C. Brown Communications, 1993.

Munson, H. E. What teachers think they need to be sexuality educators, *Health Education,* 7 (March/April 1976), 31.

Suggested Readings

Cornog, M. & Perper, T. *For sex education, see librarian: A guide to issues and resources.* Westport, CT: Greenwood Publishing Group, 1996.

Drole, J. C. & Clark, K., eds. *The sexuality challenge: promoting healthy sexuality in young people.* Santa Cruz, CA: ETR Associates, 1994.

Greenberg, J. S., Bruess, C. E. & Haffner, D. W. Body image, in *Exploring the dimensions of human sexuality.* 2nd ed. 172–95. Boston: Jones and Bartlett, 2004.

Kirby, D. *Emerging answers: Research findings on programs to reduce teen pregnancy.* Washington, DC: National Campaign to Prevent Teen Pregnancy, 2001.

Koch, P. B. & Weiss, D. L., eds. *Sexuality in America: Understanding our sexual values and behavior.* New York: Continuum, 1999.

Maddock, J. W., ed. *Sexuality education in postsecondary and professional training settings.* Binghamton, NY: Haworth Press, 1997.

Cases for Part 1

The cases in this section are designed to utilize the information included in Chapters 1, 2, 3, and 4. Case 1 is concerned with justifying a school sexuality education program. Although this case focuses on a school setting, there are similarities to other potential settings for sexuality education. Chapter 2 contains specific information that is helpful in preparing a justification, but Chapters 1 and 4 also contain useful background information.

Case 2 relates to a common problem—who should handle the sexuality education program? Chapter 4 provides some possible answers to this dilemma, but again the other chapters in Part I provide additional background information that should aid in the decision.

Case 3 forces us to consider the common problem of helping others realize what total sexuality is all about, as well as the role of sexuality education in different settings. In this case we are considering a situation in a medical school, but it could just as well be an elementary school, a rap session, or a conversation with friends. Chapter 1 provides the ammunition to deal with the problem specifically, but Chapters 2, 3, and 4 should also be useful.

Case 4 helps us get close to common feelings of uncertainty about being comfortable with our own sexuality. Chapters 1 and 4 provide most of the information needed to deal with this case; however, some of the facts in Chapter 2 may help as well.

Case 5 gives you a chance to use some of the historical information in Chapter 2. It demonstrates how a basic understanding of historical information can be helpful when working with sexuality education programs.

Case 6 gives you a chance to figure out how to make plans for dealing with groups opposed to sexuality education. Chapter 3 provides an understanding of some of those opposed to sexuality education, as well as suggestions on how to deal with them. In addition, Chapter 16 contains information related to obtaining support and bringing about change.

Case 1

Undecided Unified School District: Justifying a School Sex Education Program

Dr. I. M. Sure, the curriculum coordinator for the Undecided Unified School District, has been attempting to start a sexuality education program in the district for a number of years. Despite her efforts, the program is essentially nonexistent. She is still convinced that there should be a program, but her ideas seem to fall on deaf ears.

During the past school year, several things happened that stirred up concerns on the part of parents and other school administrators. Twelve girls—eight senior-high students and four junior-high students—dropped out of school because they were pregnant. Representatives from the local health department approached Dr. Sure about wanting to come into the schools to tell students about sexually transmitted infection. In addition, a group of 50 students wrote letters to the superintendent of schools about the local need for birth control information as well as services.

One day the superintendent called Dr. Sure into his office. He indicated that he was aware of her long-time interest in sexuality education. He was still undecided about whether to institute a program in the district, but he asked Dr. Sure to prepare a presentation for the board meeting to be held the following month. He wanted the presentation to be no longer than 20 minutes; it must provide the board with a justification for a district sexuality education program, along with an overview of what should be in the program.

Dr. Sure left the superintendent's office pleased that the opportunity to justify a program had finally come. As she started to think about it, however, she realized that the future of a sexuality education program in the Undecided Unified School District rested solely on what she could present in a 20-minute period.

1. What should Dr. Sure say about the need for a district sexuality education program?

2. What do you think the board and the school administrators want to hear?

3. What should Dr. Sure say about course content emphasis in a sexuality education program?

Case 2

Will the Real Sexuality Educator Please Stand Up? Deciding Who Should Teach a Sexuality Education Program

After lengthy deliberations, the Planit Well Unified School District has finally approved a sexuality education curriculum for its elementary and secondary schools. The planning and writing process covered a 3-year period, during which school administrators were oriented about the new curriculum.

Mrs. Lotta Gutz is the principal of one of the junior high schools in the district. Since the program will begin next fall, she must decide which teachers will handle sexuality education. The curriculum is designed to relate to the total school curriculum, but the principal has the option of choosing which teachers will be used and what subject-matter areas will be implemented.

1. How should Mrs. Gutz decide which three teachers will handle the sexuality education program?

2. After her decision is made, what should she tell the teachers, the rest of the faculty, and district supervisors about why she decided the way she did?

Case 3

The Narrow-Thinking Board: Overcoming Traditional Thinking about Sexuality

The local medical school board recently discussed the need for a sexuality education program as part of the training of doctors. The board decided that sexuality education training is not needed, because doctors already know a great deal about reproductive physiology. In addition, the board felt that the public should learn about sexuality only from their families and that additional sources of information about sexuality would only confuse the issue.

Dr. Neva Givup wants to make one more attempt at convincing the board that their decision is not in the best interest of either medical education or society. She has decided that the major issues are based on three questions:

1. What is a total concept of human sexuality, and how does it relate to the training of medical personnel?

2. Where does sexuality education currently occur in society?

3. What role can institutions such as medical schools play in sexuality education in society?

Answer these questions for Dr. Givup so that she can present the best case to the board.

Case 4

Being Concerned about Handling Sexuality Education: Understanding One's Own Sexuality

A friend of yours, U. N. Certain, has been asked to provide sexuality education services as part of his job at the county health department. He knows that sexuality education is needed, but is concerned about how he feels about some sexuality topics as well as how comfortable he will be dealing with the subject.

1. What can he do to better understand his own sexuality?

2. What hints will you give him to help him feel more at ease?

3. How will he know when he is ready to handle sexuality education at the health department?

Case 5

Consolidated Counselors Convention: Looking at Sexuality in History

Dr. I. Will Helpu, the program planner for the Consolidated Counselors Convention, has received several requests for convention programs related to the topic of human sexuality. He is in the process of putting together the overall plan for the forthcoming annual convention and calls you in for a discussion.

Dr. Helpu indicates that he is getting fed up with the talk about sexuality today. He says he is tired of seeing references to sexuality in advertising, on TV shows, and in the movies. He knows that in the "good old days" people got along just fine without thinking about sexuality and without social emphasis on it.

He cannot imagine people in previous centuries even thinking about the topic, and now he is supposed to plan a convention because counselors want programs on sexuality. He says to you, "Why is it that there is so much more emphasis on sexuality today than there was in previous cultures?" He has done some historical reading, and rarely was the topic even brought up.

1. What can you tell him about the relative importance of sexuality in previous cultures?

2. Is the topic of sexuality more prevalent in today's society than in earlier societies? Give some examples.

3. Is it true that people got along fine without thinking about sexuality in previous times?

Case 6

Grappling with Group Gyrations: Handling the Activities of Groups

The principal of your school, Ms. Ima Pushover, calls you into her office one afternoon after classes and appears to be very concerned about something. Apparently some community members have heard that the school is planning to expand its sexuality education program so that it covers grades 7 to 12. Ms. Pushover tells you that community groups have already formed in opposition to any sexuality education in the school. These groups are demanding that no sexuality education be taught, and they are constantly calling and writing to Ms. Pushover to express their views. She indicates that she wants to do something about the situation but has no idea where to start. What should she do?

1. How should Ms. Pushover handle the groups?

2. What should she do about expanding the program?

3. What facts would be helpful to Ms. Pushover at this point?

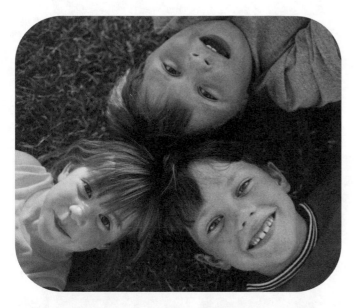

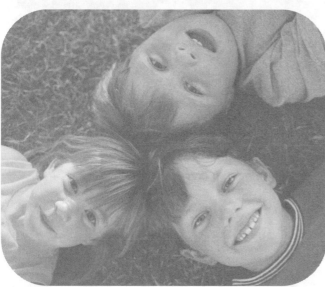

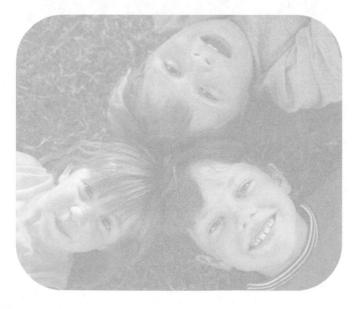

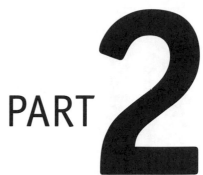

PART **2**

Biological, Psychological, and Sociological Aspects of Sexuality Education

Chapter 5

A View from the Inside

Chapter 6

The Cognitive and Psychological Side of Sexuality

Chapter 7

Family Life and Interpersonal Relationships

Chapter 8

The Sociological Side of Sexuality

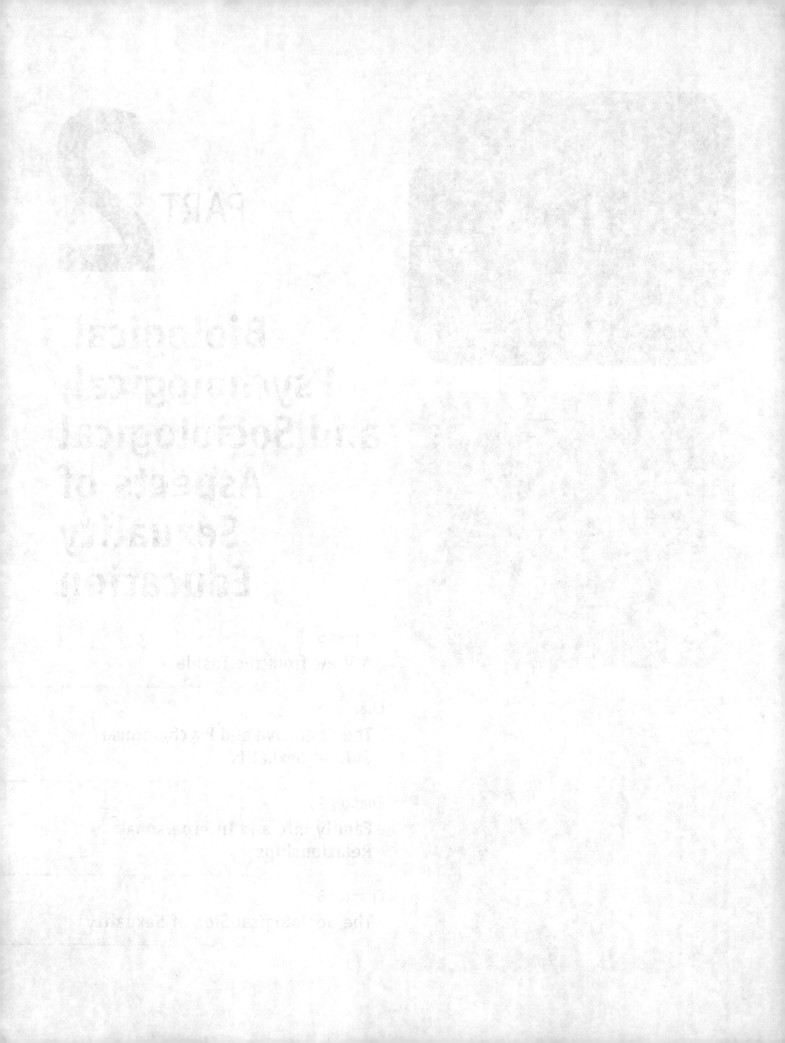

A View from the Inside

CHAPTER 5

Key Concepts

1. Male and female reproductive systems are well designed for their functions.

2. There are similarities and differences between male and female sexual responses.

3. Fertility control means intervention at some point in the reproductive process.

4. Pregnancy is a condition deserving serious attention and care.

This chapter is the only one in this book that focuses on the physical experience of human sexuality. We will look beneath our skins to determine what occurs during sexual stimulation and reproduction. Most important, we will find that although males and females certainly differ biologically, they are also quite similar and remarkably complementary.

Although this is not a human sexuality book, the information included in this chapter is vital to learners' understanding of their sexual selves, and the chapter demonstrates various ways of presenting this information.

Male and Female Reproductive Systems

Males

Some parts of the male reproductive system are external and some are internal. The external parts are the scrotum and the penis. The internal parts are depicted in Figure 5-1. The scrotum's function is to contain and protect the testes, which produce sperm and the male sex hormone, **testosterone.** Within the testes are the seminiferous tubules, the vasa efferentia, and the epididymis. The **seminiferous tubules** (approximately 1,000 in each testis) produce sperm. The average male produces about 150 million sperm each day.

Once sperm are produced in a testis, they travel via the vasa efferentia to the **epididymis,** where they are stored. The epididymis also provides nutrients to help the sperm develop. Some of the sperm leave the epididymis at this point and proceed to the ejaculatory duct via the vas deferens. These sperm are provided more nutrients from the seminal vesicles, which are located near the ejaculatory duct.

Just prior to ejaculation, the seminal vesicles empty and, with the sperm, their secretion (semen) enters the ejaculatory duct to make its way into the urethra. It is helpful that the urethra passes through the **prostate gland,** since the prostate secretes a substance that prolongs sperm life. In addition to the secretions already noted, preparation for ejaculation involves the lubrication of the urethra by a substance secreted into it by the **Cowper's gland.** This secretion from the Cowper's gland also neutralizes any acidity in the urethra that may remain from urine. (The preejaculatory fluid, which is observable, is really the Cowper's gland secretion with some sperm possibly included.) Semen (sperm and fluid) thus serves several purposes: it helps transport sperm, it serves as nutrition for the sperm (it has a fructose base), it helps neutralize the acidity in the vagina, and it helps to neutralize the acidity in the male urethra.

The semen in the urethra passes through the erect penis. Sexual stimulation causes the arterioles in the corpus cavernosum to become engorged with blood, which is what causes the penis to become erect.

---

scrotum　A sac that contains and protects the testes.

testosterone　Male sex hormone.

seminiferous tubules　The area in the testes that produces sperm.

epididymis　The place in the testes where sperm are stored and where nutrients help the sperm further develop.

prostate gland　A gland through which the urethra passes that secretes a substance that prolongs sperm life.

Cowper's gland　A small gland that secretes a lubricant and neutralizes any acidity in the urethra.

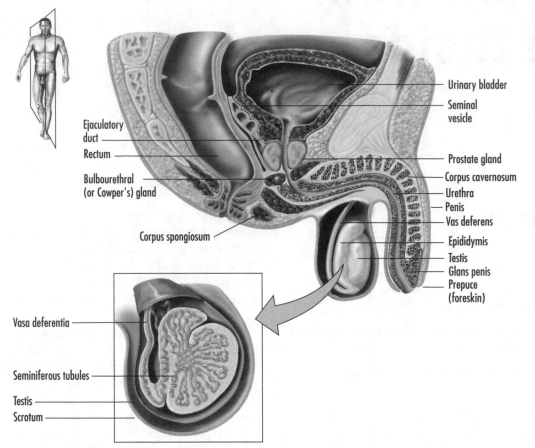

Ejaculatory
duct
Rectum
Bulbourethral
(or Cowper's) gland
Corpus spongiosum

Urinary bladder
Seminal
vesicle
Prostate gland
Corpus cavernosum
Urethra
Penis
Vas deferens
Epididymis
Testis
Glans penis
Prepuce
(foreskin)

Vasa deferentia
Seminiferous tubules
Testis
Scrotum

Figure 5-1   The Male Reproductive System. The external male sex organs include the penis and the scrotum.

Ejaculation can now occur (Figure 5-2). What happens at this point is a result of muscular contraction in the glands and ducts of the reproductive system. The ejaculatory duct and seminal vesicles contract. Also contracting is the bulbocavernosus muscle surrounding the corpus spongiosum

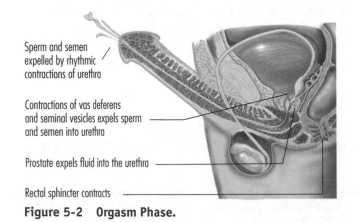

Sperm and semen
expelled by rhythmic
contractions of urethra

Contractions of vas deferens
and seminal vesicles expels sperm
and semen into urethra

Prostate expels fluid into the urethra

Rectal sphincter contracts

Figure 5-2   Orgasm Phase.

of the penis. The average ejaculate (semen) contains some 300 million sperm.

Females

The female reproductive system also contains external and internal structures. The external structures (called the vulva) are the labia majora, labia minora, clitoris, hymen, and vestibule (Figure 5-3). The two large folds of skin called the **labia majora** serve two main functions: protecting the external genitalia, and opening the vulva during sexual stimulation. The opening of the vulva occurs because of engorgement of blood in the labia majora.

The **labia minora** consist of two folds of skin lying inside the labia majora. Loaded with blood vessels and nerve receptors, the labia minora and particularly the clitoris are very sensitive to stimulation. Filling still further with blood during sexual excitement, the labia minora will spread, thereby providing access to the vagina.

ejaculation   The expulsion of semen from the penis as a result of muscular contractions.

labia majora   Outer folds of skin surrounding the labia minora.
labia minora   Inner folds of skin lying inside the labia majora.

Insight 5-1

Understanding the Male Reproductive System

To test your understanding of the male reproductive system, complete the matching quiz in Part A, and write in the name of the structures in the diagram in Part B.

Part A

Correct Letter	*Numbered Item*	*Lettered Item*
_____	1. Ejaculatory duct	a. Supports testes
_____	2. Scrotum	b. Surrounded by the bulbocavernosus muscle
_____	3. Corpus cavernosum	c. Stores sperm
_____	4. Epididymis	d. Stores sperm and contracts during ejaculation
_____	5. Corpus spongiosum	e. Produce sperm
_____	6. Seminiferous tubules	f. Its being engorged with blood results in erect penis
_____	7. Vasa efferentia	g. Carry sperm to the epididymis
_____	8. Vas deferens	h. Transports sperm from epididymis to ejaculatory duct

Part B

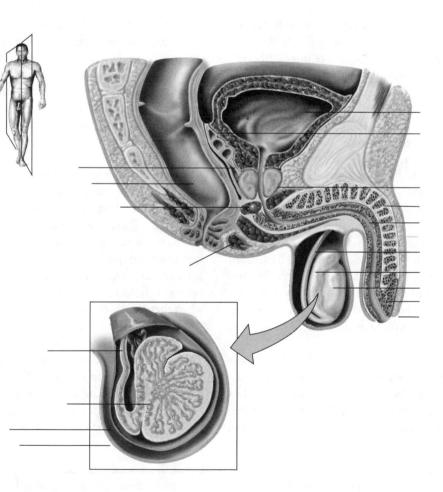

Check your answers with Figure 5-1.

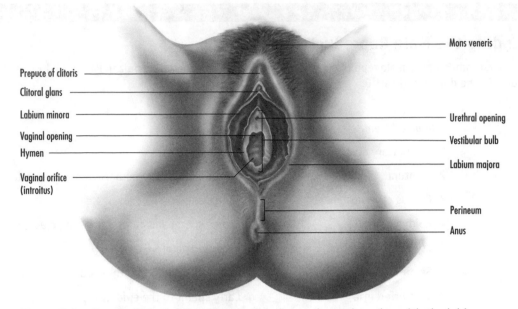

Prepuce of clitoris
Clitoral glans
Labium minora
Vaginal opening
Hymen
Vaginal orifice (introitus)

Mons veneris
Urethral opening
Vestibular bulb
Labium majora
Perineum
Anus

Figure 5-3   Female External Sex Organs. This figure shows the vulva with the labia opened to reveal the urethral and vaginal openings.

The **clitoris,** the most sensitive structure in the female body, is similar (homologous) to the male penis. As the penis contains a corpus cavernosum, so does the clitoris (although it does not also contain a corpus spongiosum). During sexual stimulation, the corpus cavernosum of the clitoris fills with blood and becomes erect. When the clitoris is erect and the labia minora are spread, the vestibule (vaginal and urethral openings) becomes visible.

The **hymen,** a thin connective tissue containing a relatively large number of blood vessels, separates the vestibule from the vagina. The hymen's function is to protect the vagina from infection. Blood is usually evident upon rupturing of the hymen, which may occur during the female's first sexual intercourse. Absence of the hymen does not necessarily mean that the female is not a virgin, however. The hymen varies widely in shape and thickness and in some women can be ruptured by accident, exercise, or, if need be, by a physician. In addition, the hymen has a small opening that allows for the insertion of a tampon, during a female's menstrual period.

Figure 5-4 depicts the internal structures of the female reproductive system. The **vagina** is a hollow, tunnellike structure, the function of which is to receive the penis and its ejaculate, to serve as the route of exit for the newborn, and to provide an exit for the menstrual flow (see the discussion of menstruation later in this chapter). The vaginal walls contain

muscular membranes that allow the vagina to expand so wide that a baby can pass through it. The vagina also serves to enhance coitus by secreting a lubricant from its walls during sexual stimulation. The secretion of this lubricant is the first physical sign of sexual excitement in the female. In this regard, the male and female differ. Although the clitoris is homologous to the penis, secretion of a lubricant from the walls of the vagina precedes the erection of the clitoris during sexual stimulation.

It should be noted that because of the muscular membranes in the vaginal walls, the vagina is capable of expanding and contracting so as to accommodate any size penis. It is incorrect, therefore, to assume that the size of the penis is related to the sexual satisfaction of the female. The vagina is capable of adapting to, and the female being satisfied by, any size penis. As a matter of fact, although the size of flaccid penises (unerect) may differ greatly, this difference lessens when they become erect.

The vagina's tunnellike structure opens outward to the labia minora, and at the opposite end, into the uterus. This end of the uterus connected to the vagina is called the cervix; the other end is termed the fundus. The uterus, like the vagina, is hollow and contains very muscular walls. Figure 5-5 depicts the vaginal change during orgasm. Notice that the shape of the vagina is transformed from tubelike to balloonlike.

---

clitoris   A highly sensitive structure of the external genitalia of females, which is homologous to the male penis.

hymen   A thin connective tissue that covers the vaginal opening to protect the vagina from infection.

vagina   A hollow, tunnellike structure of the female reproductive system that receives the penis during coitus.

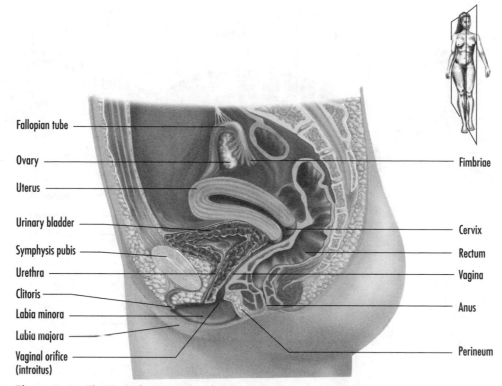

Fallopian tube

Ovary

Uterus

Urinary bladder

Symphysis pubis

Urethra

Clitoris

Labia minora

Labia majora

Vaginal orifice
(introitus)

Fimbriae

Cervix

Rectum

Vagina

Anus

Perineum

Figure 5-4   The Female Reproductive System. This cross-section locates many of the internal sex organs that compose the female reproductive system.

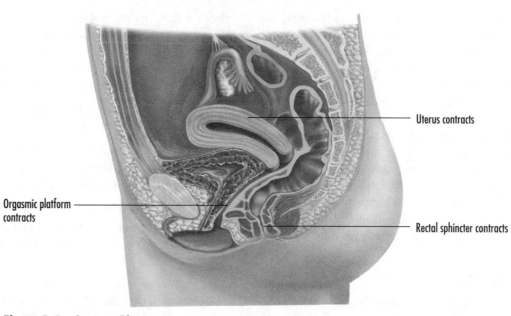

Orgasmic platform
contracts

Uterus contracts

Rectal sphincter contracts

Figure 5-5   Orgasm Phase.

The uterus is where a fertilized ovum is implanted and where the embryo and eventually the fetus will grow. Its three layers are most appropriate to its function. The perimetrium, the outermost layer, is elastic, thereby accommodating a fetus as it increases in size. The middle layer of the uterus, the myometrium, consists of smooth muscles, which aid in the pushing of the newborn through the cervix and into the birth canal (vagina). The innermost layer, the endometrium, is loaded with blood vessels that can provide nourishment for the embryo and fetus. It is this innermost layer that is partly discharged when fertilization does not occur and menstruation therefore begins.

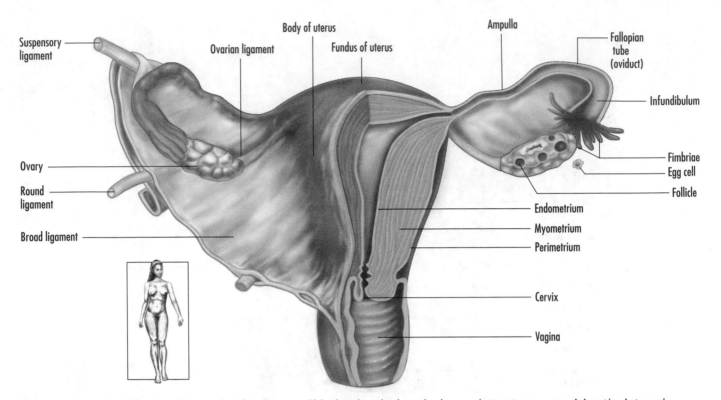

Figure 5-6   Female Internal Reproductive Organs. This drawing depicts the internal structures comprising the internal female reproductive organs.

The fallopian tubes lead from the uterus to the ovaries. The **fallopian tubes** (oviducts) serve as the route for an egg (ovum) to journey from an ovary to the uterus, and as the place where an egg can be fertilized by a sperm. These tubes are hollow and have muscular walls.

Ova are contained in the **ovaries.** The female has plenty of eggs to spare, since each ovary contains approximately 400,000 ova at birth. When an ovum is discharged by the ovary (usually alternating between ovaries in each cycle), the fimbriae at the end of the fallopian tube guide it into the tube (Figure 5-6). The ovaries are also responsible for the production of the hormones **estrogen** and **progesterone.** As will soon be described, these female hormones play a significant role in both the birth process and menstruation.

Male Hormones

Hormones help males develop certain characteristics termed secondary sex characteristics. These include hair on the chest, a deep voice, pubic hair, hair on the face, and a V-shaped chest. These secondary sex characteristics are influenced by hormones that, when secreted by glands, trigger various bodily responses. Examples of these hormones are as follows (Greenberg & Dintiman, 1992, 126):

1. *Thyroxin.* Secreted by the thyroid gland, it is related to growth differentiation.

2. *Dehydroepiandrosterone.* Secreted by the cortex of the adrenal gland, it stimulates the development of male sex characteristics (also called androgen).

3. *Follicle-stimulating hormone (FSH).* Secreted by the anterior portion of the adrenal gland, it stimulates growth of the seminiferous tubules in the testes.

4. *Luteinizing hormone (LH).* Secreted by the anterior portion of the adrenal gland, it controls the production and release of testosterone by the testes.

---

fallopian tubes   Tubes through which ova travel down, sperm travel up, and where fertilization takes place.

ova   Eggs that can be fertilized by sperm.

ovaries   The part of the female reproductive system in which ova are housed before traveling down the fallopian tubes.

estrogen   A female sex hormone.

progesterone   A female sex hormone.

5. *Testosterone.* Produced in the interstitial cells of the testes, it stimulates development and maintenance of male sex characteristics.

6. *Gonadotropic hormones.* A collective term for FSH and LH; FSH and LH (sometimes called ICSH, or interstitial cell stimulating hormone, in the male) are secreted by the anterior portion of the pituitary gland.

Female Hormones

Female hormones aid in the development of such secondary sex characteristics as rounded hips, pubic hair, and developed breasts. Female hormones also govern the menstrual cycle. Whereas male hormonal secretions affect the testes, female hormonal secretions affect the ovaries. In fact, many of the hormones secreted by females are the same as those secreted by males, such as LH and FSH. The difference is in their site of action.

The menstrual cycle commences with the secretion of FSH from the pituitary gland, signaling the ovary to ripen an egg. The anterior portion of the pituitary, in addition to secreting FSH, also secretes LH which further aids ovulation (the discharge of an ovum from an ovary). Following ovulation, the place in the ovary from which the egg is released (the graafian follicle) becomes a yellow body termed the corpus luteum. The **graafian follicle** secretes the hormone estrogen; the corpus luteum secretes the hormone progesterone. Progesterone's function is to signal the innermost layer of the uterus (the endometrium) to develop in preparation for a fertilized egg (**zygote**) that will be implanted within and nourished by the endometrium. If the ovum is not fertilized by a sperm, the corpus luteum degenerates and progesterone levels fall. This lack of progesterone alerts the body that an ovum has not been fertilized and that the developed endometrium, rich with blood and nutrients, is not needed. The discharge of the endometrium then begins (menstruation). **Menstruation,** from the Latin word *mensis,* meaning "month," has been called many names: "period," "curse," "monthly sickness," and many others.

Though the typical 28-day menstrual cycle does not really exist (it varies from woman to woman and may vary in any one woman from cycle to cycle), this length is used to show the relationship in time between events of the cycle. For example, during a 28-day menstrual cycle, ovulation will occur on the fourteenth day, progesterone will be secreted from day 14 until day 25, and menstruation will occur during days 1 through 5 (see Figures 5-7 and 5-8). Estrogen is produced throughout the menstrual cycle, although in varying amounts. The important point here is that ovulation is best determined by counting 14 days back from the first day of the menstrual flow. Unfortunately, having to wait for menstruation is too late to provide a basis for contraception. Thus, as we shall soon see, one of the problems with the rhythm method of contraception is determining the time of ovulation.

Menstruation does not occur throughout a woman's life. **Menopause,** sometimes termed the climacteric, is the end of a woman's menstruating or the end of her cyclical expulsion of a nourished endometrium. Commonly occurring somewhere between the ages of 40 and 55, menopause also is a function of hormonal activity. Just prior to menopause, FSH and LH secretions increase, thus disturbing the feedback mechanism of these hormones upon the pituitary gland (Masters, Johnson & Kolodny, 1992). The result is discontinuation of both ovulation and menstruation. This is a general rule, however, and there are exceptions. "Change-of-life" babies are evidence of this. These babies are born to women who have stopped menstruating yet who still periodically ovulate and have had an egg fertilized. Generally, though, menopause indicates the end of the childbearing years and, because of this, often results in increased enjoyment in sexual intercourse. One explanation of this fact is that since the fear of pregnancy is eliminated, coitus can be more fully enjoyed. In any case, menopause certainly does not mean the end of sexual activity nor of satisfaction derived from that activity. Neither does it mean that the woman has run out of eggs. Recall that thousands of ova are contained in each ovary at birth.

Still another myth associated with menopause is that women always experience upsetting symptoms during this time of life. Not so! Only about 25% of menopausal women experience any upsetting symptoms (McCary, 1982). This information is important for sexuality educators to know. When people expect something to happen, their expectations create a greater tendency for that event to occur. This tendency is termed a self-fulfilling prophecy. In other words, women who expect distressing symptoms as a result of menopause may experience these symptoms *just because* they expect them. It is the sexuality educator's role to provide accurate information and thereby help to prevent such symptoms.

---

graafian follicle   The area of the ovary from where an egg ruptures.

zygote   A fertilized egg.

menstruation   The cyclical sloughing off of blood from the vaginal opening.

menopause   The cessation of menstruation.

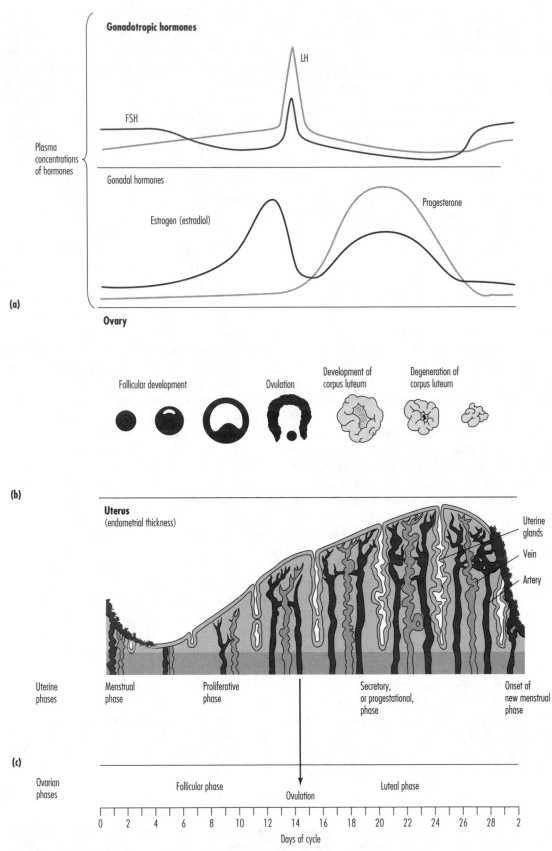

Figure 5-7   Changes occurring during the menstrual cycle.

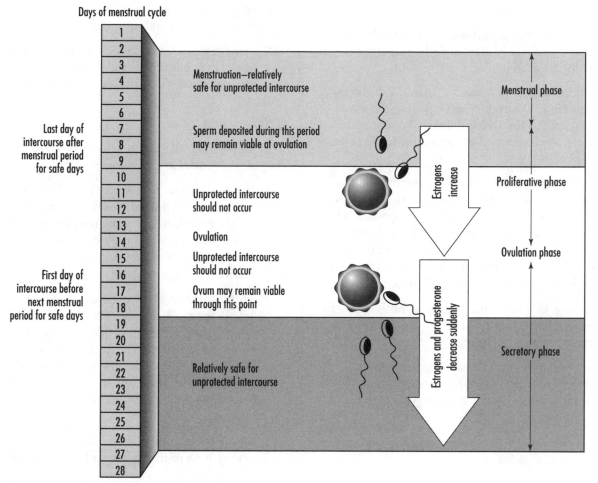

Figure 5-8   Occurrences during various phases of the fertility cycle.

Similarities and Differences Between Male and Female Sexual Responses

When one looks closely at males and females, one finds both startling differences and amazing similarities. This section will explore the differences and similarities between male and female sexual responses. It is important for sexuality educators to be able to present this information to learners for several reasons. In addition to emphasizing how much we have in common, it will help learners realize that their sexual responses can be understood, predicted, and studied, just as many of their other physiological processes can be. Sexual behavior, therefore, will more readily be viewed as a normal part of people's functioning.

Similarities

The most significant ongoing research relative to human sexual responses has been conducted by William Masters and

Virginia Johnson (1966). Masters and Johnson conclude that human sexual response, male and female, can be described and is consistent. They divide human sexual response into four phases:

1. *Excitement phase.* Sexual stimulation, which may be physical or psychological, begins.

2. *Plateau phase.* Sexual tension grows.

3. *Orgasmic phase.* The climax or orgasm occurs.

4. *Resolution phase.* Sexual tension is lost, and the person returns to preexcitement status.

Others have suggested adding a desire or appetite phase. This phase entails the desire for sexual activity. As we will see when we discuss sexual dysfunctions, it is at this phase that difficulty in the sexual response sometimes develops. Still others prefer to view the human sexual response as occurring in three phases, since the plateau phase is really an intensification of the conditions developed during the excitement phase.

During these phases, certain physiological reactions can be predicted. Those reactions that are similar for males and females include the following:

1. *Nipples.* Both males' and females' nipples become erect and increase in diameter when a person is sexually stimulated.

2. *Sex flush.* Males and females experience a darkening of the skin of the neck, face, forehead, or chest during sexual stimulation. This darkening of the skin is a result of blood accumulating in that area of the body.

3. *Muscle tension.* Commencing during the plateau phase and involving the legs, arms, abdomen, neck, and face, muscle tension (myotonia) appears in both sexes when they are sexually stimulated. Further, muscles of the abdomen, chest, and face are tensed during orgasm, after which (resolution phase) there is a release of muscular tension in both sexes.

4. *Breathing.* During sexual excitation, both sexes experience deep and rapid breathing. Such breathing is termed hyperventilation.

5. *Heart rate.* Increases of heart rate up to 180 or more beats per minute during orgasm are not unusual in either sex. Such an increase is termed tachycardia.

6. *Blood pressure.* There is an increase of blood pressure during sexual excitement.

7. *Perspiration.* Approximately one-third of males and females perspire following orgasm.

8. *Blood flow.* Increased blood flow to the pelvic area results in penile erection and vaginal lubrication. This increased blood flow is termed vasocongestion.

Differences

As noted earlier, differences do exist between the sexual responses of males and females:

1. *Nipples.* Whereas females are most likely to experience nipple erection during the excitement phase, males usually experience it during the plateau phase. Furthermore, female nipple erection disappears soon after orgasm, while male nipple erection often remains long after orgasm.

2. *Sex flush.* Whereas the male sex flush is experienced only in the plateau phase, the female sex flush can occur either late in the excitement phase or in the plateau phase. The neck, face, forehead, and chest of both males and females may show sex flush. In addition, the sex flush occurs over the lower abdomen, thighs, lower back, and buttocks of females.

3. *Muscle tension.* Muscular tension causes an increase in the length of the vagina and an expansion of the

---

Insight 5-2

Understanding Sexual Response

For each of the phases of sexual response, list three physiological occurrences for males and females.

	Males	Females
I. Excitement Phase		
II. Plateau Phase		
III. Orgasmic Phase		
IV. Resolution Phase		

diameter of the cervix in females; it causes elevation of the testes in males.

4. *Breathing.* After orgasm, males must wait for hyperventilation to diminish before being able to have another orgasm. Since the male is usually unable to achieve another erection at this point, this period of time is often referred to as a refractory period. Females, on the other hand, may have another orgasm prior to hyperventilation subsiding. Consequently, some females are capable of many orgasms in a short period of time. These women are described as multiorgasmic.

5. *Blood pressure.* In males, blood pressure has been found to increase 40 to 100 mm Hg systolic and 20 to 50 mm Hg diastolic during sexual stimulation. In females, the increase ranged from 30 to 80 mm Hg systolic to 20 to 40 mm Hg diastolic.

6. *Perspiration.* Sweating in males is usually limited to the soles of the feet and palms of the hands. Females are more likely to perspire over the back, thighs, chest, and sometimes the trunk, head, and neck.

7. *Orgasm.* As stated above, females can be multiorgasmic; males usually cannot. Further, orgasm for the females lasts longer than for males and does not involve ejaculation.

The next time you are sexually stimulated (either physically or through thoughts or fantasies), stop a moment and attempt to identify any of the responses described here.

It is our opinion that young people should be educated as to what to expect when they are sexually excited. Male erection and female vaginal lubrication are entirely natural occurrences. Whether it be photographs, films, thoughts, or another person that sexually excites young people, we believe that they will be less embarrassed, feel less guilt, and be more comfortable with their sexual responses if they know what to expect.

Fertility Control

To understand attempts to affect fertility, either enhancing or preventing it, students must recall their knowledge of the male and female reproductive systems. Since *preventing* conception is probably the major interest of those for whom you conduct sexuality education, we will limit our discussion to means of preventing conception.

Contraception

In many instances, the problem is not how to foster conception but rather how to prevent it. When one stops to analyze the consequences of sexual-behavior decisions such as pregnancy, abortion, adoption, and so on, **contraception** becomes an important consideration. This is not to say that sexuality educators should recommend that a form of contraception be employed. This area is fraught with controversy and religious and moral implications. We do know, however, that there are approximately three million unintended pregnancies each year in the United States. Of those unintended pregnancies, 43% result in induced abortions, 13% in spontaneous abortions (miscarriages), and 44% in births (*Fact sheet: Contraceptive use*, 1998). Unwanted children place a burden on parents; moreover, these children may suffer not only economically and socially, but physically as well.

Perhaps knowledge and proper use of a method of contraception would help prevent conception, thereby decreasing the number of low-birth-weight babies born. Since low birth weight is related to birth defects of many kinds, contraception might be expected to help decrease the incidence of birth defects.

What contraceptive methods are available, and how effective are they? It should be noted that effectiveness is difficult to determine exactly; consequently, the effectiveness rates cited in this chapter should be considered approximations. Furthermore, there is a difference between **theoretical effectiveness** (when used by researchers in

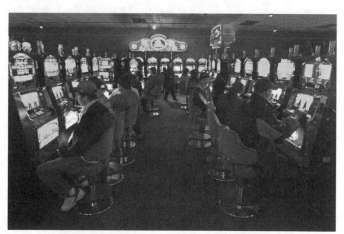

It is not unusual for people to gamble at racetracks or casinos for leisure. However, they usually gamble only what they have to lose. What are you gambling if you are sexually active and do not use a condom?

---

contraception   Methods designed to prevent conception (pregnancy).

theoretical effectiveness   The ability of a method of contraception to prevent conception when used under laboratory controlled circumstances

controlled laboratory settings) and **user effectiveness** (when used at home by people not being monitored). We will briefly discuss each of the available methods.

Abstinence.   One means of preventing the union of sperm and egg is refraining from coitus. This is the most effective means of birth control. Yet, there are people for whom sexual abstinence is not acceptable and others, for whom it is acceptable for long periods of time, but not indefinitely. The advantages of abstinence include preventing the contraction of a sexually transmitted infection as well as preventing conception.

Withdrawal.   Termed *coitus interruptus,* this method consists of the withdrawal of the penis from the vagina just prior to ejaculation. There are two basic problems with this method. First, it requires a great deal of control on the part of the male to interrupt a highly exciting moment to withdraw the penis. Second, the preejaculatory fluid may contain sperm and can itself be responsible for fertilizing the ovum.

Natural family planning.   There are basically three types of **natural family planning** methods: the calendar method, the ovulation method, and the sympto-thermal method. The **calendar method** involves recording the woman's reproductive cycles starting from day 1 (the first day of menstruation) to the last day (the day before the next menses). After accurately recording eight consecutive cycles, the shortest and the longest cycles are used to determine when the woman is ovulating. Recognizing that sperm can remain alive for up to 72 hours and that the ovum can be viable for as long as 48 hours, the objective is to refrain from sexual intercourse for 3 days before and after ovulation. Providing for some error, abstinence should be practiced from day 10 through day 17 of a 28-day menstrual cycle.

Ovulation methods involve charting the woman's basal body temperatures or cervical secretions. Using a basal body thermometer, a woman takes her temperature upon awakening each day and charts it on a monthly graph. Recognizing that body temperature rises approximately 0.4°F between 24 and 72 hours after ovulation, abstinence is practiced until after 3 days of elevated temperature.

Paying attention to cervical secretions is another form of the ovulation method. After menstruation there is little cervical secretion. However, as estrogen levels peak at mid-cycle, the secretions become clearer, stretchy, and slippery. After ovulation, the secretions become thick again. At that point, coitus is considered safe in terms of pregnancy (Greenberg, Bruess & Haffner, 2004).

The **sympto-thermal method** is a combination of the basal body temperature and cervical secretion methods. Both charting temperatures and paying attention to cervical secretions, and abstaining from coitus at the most fertile time of the menstrual cycle, add increased effectiveness in preventing conception.

The theoretical effectiveness of natural family planning methods of contraception is between 91% and 99%. However, when using the calendar method alone, that effectiveness rate decreases to 81% (Greenberg, Bruess & Haffner, 2004).

Condoms.   Termed *rubbers* in the vernacular, **condoms** cover the penis so as to prevent sperm from entering the vagina. Available in various shapes and colors, lubricated or not, condoms can be quite effective if used *correctly:* if the condom is placed on the penis before vaginal entry, with space provided between the condom and the tip of the penis to collect the semen and prevent its overflow into the vagina, and if the penis is removed from the vagina immediately after ejaculation, with the base of the condom held in place against the base of the penis (see Figure 5-9).

Some of the criticisms of condom use are that putting a condom on interrupts foreplay and that it decreases the sensations felt by the penis. However, condoms are relatively inexpensive, are easily obtained, and provide some protection from AIDS and other sexually transmitted infections (for example, vaginitis and nonspecific urethritis). Latex condoms provide this protection. Animal skin condoms' pores are too large to prevent organisms from passing through. Last but certainly not least, condom use eliminates the possible side effects associated with some of the other methods of contraception soon to be described.

One of the problems with condoms is the embarrassment that people may feel when purchasing them. If you are unsure of how purchasing a condom in a drugstore would affect you, why not try it and find out? You might also want

---

user effectiveness   The ability of a method of contraception to prevent conception when used by people in a real-life setting.

natural family planning   Methods of contraception that use "natural" means to prevent the sperm-egg union.

calendar method   A natural family planning method of contraception that entails recording the shortest and longest menstrual cycles over a period of time to determine a woman's infertile period.

ovulation method   A natural family planning method of contraception that entails determining a woman's infertile period by monitoring her temperature.

sympto-thermal method   A natural family planning method of contraception that entails monitoring temperature and cervical secretions to determine a woman's infertile period.

condom   A sheath that covers the penis, thereby preventing sperm from entering the vagina during sexual intercourse.

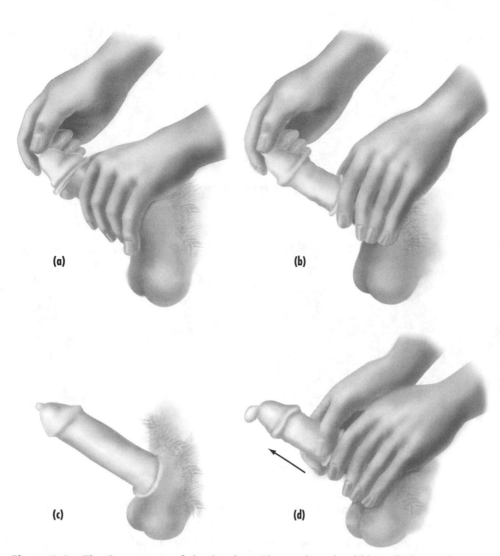

(a)

(b)

(c)

(d)

Figure 5-9   The Correct use of the Condom. The condom should be rolled over the erect penis, leaving a small space at its end to collect ejaculated semen. To do that, hold the tip of the condom as it is unrolled onto the shaft of the penis. When withdrawing the condom after coitus, hold its base to avoid spillage of semen.

to incorporate this as a learning activity when you are conducting sexuality education. However, be sure that such an exercise will be acceptable in the setting in which your program is conducted.

Given the interest in condoms that has developed as a result of the fear of AIDS and the desire to avoid the complications of the other methods of birth control, there have been recent noteworthy developments in the use of the condom. For example, a "woman's condom"—referred to in some quarters as an intravaginal or vaginal pouch—that is inserted within the vagina is available. Whereas the male condom is made of latex or animal skin, the female condom is made of polyurethane. It is believed that polyurethane makes the female condom stronger and more difficult for viruses and bacteria to penetrate. The female condom has a ring on each end. The ring on the closed end of the condom

is placed over the cervix (as a diaphragm might be placed). The ring at the open end extends outside the vagina and is designed to prevent any skin contact between sexual partners. Whereas the male condom has a theoretical effectiveness rate of 97% and a user effectiveness rate of 86%, the female condom's comparable rates are 95% and 79% (Hatcher, et al., 1998).

A condom has also been developed which only covers the glans penis thereby allowing the penile shaft to come in contact with the vagina. The intent is to enhance the pleasure of sexual intercourse while preventing pregnancy. It stands to reason that such a condom, however, will not provide the same degree of protection from AIDS and other sexually transmitted infections as the standard condom. Furthermore, to alleviate concern about the effectiveness of condoms that may have sat on the shelf for some time before being sold

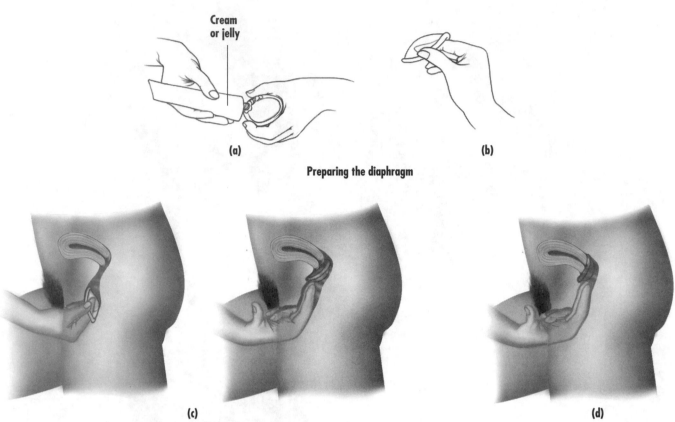

Figure 5-10   The proper use and placement of a diaphragm.

and eventually used, condom manufactures have agreed to put expiration dates on condom packages.

As you might expect, condom sales and usage have increased dramatically in recent years. The occurrence of AIDS has played the major part in this increase; although fear of the complications of other methods of birth control and the desire to prevent other STIs have played a role as well. Americans have purchased approximately 450 million condoms each year since the early 1990s (Hatcher, et al., 1998).

Diaphragm.   The **diaphragm** prevents the sperm from traveling through the uterus up the fallopian tubes and thus from fertilizing an egg. The diaphragm is a shallow rubber or synthetic rubber cap surrounding a collapsible metal ring that covers the cervix (see Figure 5-10). Since its purpose is to prevent sperm from going beyond the vagina, the fit of the diaphragm is very important. If the diaphragm does not fit just right, there is the chance that sperm can bypass this barrier. Consequently, diaphragms should be fitted by physicians and should be refitted after a woman gives birth or if she gains or loses a significant

amount of weight. The practice of using someone else's diaphragm is not recommended.

Some disadvantages of the diaphragm are that it has to be inserted prior to intercourse (one has to plan ahead) and that it must be inserted properly. Further, females must handle their own genitalia during its insertion, and this may make them uncomfortable. The diaphragm must remain in place at least 6 hours after intercourse. It should not be removed for each coitus during that time, and spermicide needs to be added for each repeated intercourse.

The two major advantages of using a diaphragm as a method of birth control are that it lacks harmful side effects and is effective in preventing conception. Inserted properly and used with a spermicidal cream or jelly, the diaphragm has a 94% theoretical effectiveness rate and an 80% user effectiveness rate (Hatcher, et al., 1998). The spermicide is used to kill any sperm that may bypass the mechanical barrier of the diaphragm.

A diaphragm may also be used in conjunction with a condom. This combination will provide two additional advantages: increased effectiveness in preventing conception and

diaphragm   A shallow cap that covers the cervix, thereby preventing sperm from entering the vagina during sexual intercourse.

shared responsibility for contraception. Shared responsibility is increasingly being sought by women who believe that the male should assume equal responsibility for contraception.

Cervical cap.   The **cervical cap** covers the cervix as does the diaphragm. However, it fits more snugly. The cervical cap is made of either rubber or plastic and is held in place by suction. The caps come in a limited number of sizes and shapes, so not all women can be fitted for one. Cervical caps can remain in place throughout the menstrual cycle except during menstruation and are, therefore, convenient.

The cap needs to be inserted prior to intercourse and remain in place for at least 6 to 8 hours afterward. It can be used with a spermicidal agent and is judged to be approximately as effective as the diaphragm (90% theoretical effectiveness and 80% user effectiveness). Although there are no serious side effects associated with the use of the cervical cap, they have been known to occasionally irritate the cervix, may cause an unpleasant odor or vaginal dryness, and may become dislodged.

Intrauterine devices.   These devices, often called **IUDs,** are small shapes of copper or synthetic materials designed to be inserted in the uterus. Originally, IUDs could only be used by women who had previously been pregnant. Today, however, all women having no contraindications can use them. In 1978 the National Center for Health Statistics reported that 20% of widowed, divorced, and separated women aged 14 to 44 who used some method of contraception used an IUD (National Center for Health Statistics, 1978a); and 12.5% of married women who used some method of contraception used an IUD (National Center for Health Statistics, 1978b). However, with reports of its potential side effects—pelvic inflammatory disease, perforated uterus, ectopic (tubal) pregnancy, pregnancy complications (stillbirths, birth defects, low birth weight), and infertility—the number of women who used IUDs in the 1980s dropped dramatically. By 1988, 1% to 2% of women aged 15 to 44 used an IUD (National Center for Health Statistics, 1990).

There are several theories as to how an IUD prevents pregnancy: that the IUD immobilizes sperm; that the IUD changes the chemical environment or the hormonal secretions required for a fertilized ovum to grow and develop; that the IUD makes eggs move faster through the fallopian tubes so that conception does not occur; and that the IUD

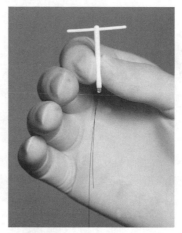

Once off the market due to concerns about health risks and resulting law suits, IUDs have made a comeback as they have been made safer.

causes more intense uterine contractions, thereby inhibiting implantation of the fertilized ovum. But no one knows for sure how the IUD works.

The major advantages of the IUD are that it is always there (planning before each coital experience is not necessary) and that it is effective. Since it contains a string that a woman can feel, its presence can usually be verified. The IUD is reported to be between 97% and 99% effective when studied in the laboratory setting, and 98% to 99% effective as actually used (Hatcher, et al., 1998).

Since no practical method of contraception is 100% effective, with the exception of abstinence, there is always the chance of conception occurring. If this should happen with an IUD still in the uterus, a woman who does not believe in abortion is presented with a dilemma. If the IUD is removed, there is a 25% chance of a spontaneous abortion. If it is kept in place, the result may be infection, blood poisoning, bleeding, or premature labor.

One type of IUD, the Dalkon Shield, proved to be linked to deaths from infection and other conditions. Consequently, lawsuits were filed against the manufacturers of that IUD. The fallout, though, affected other IUD manufacturers, so that in 1986 G. D. Searle & Co., protesting lawsuits against manufacturers as unwarranted, stopped selling its IUDs in the United States. They said that insurance and legal costs were too high. Today there are two types of IUDs available.

Spermicidal agents.   Spermicidal agents will kill or immobilize sperm on contact. A **spermicide** in foam,

---

cervical cap   A shallow cap that covers the cervix more snuggly than does the diaphragm, thereby preventing sperm from entering the vagina during sexual intercourse.

IUDs   Small devices that are placed within the uterus to prevent conception.

spermicide   A chemical that kills sperm on contact and is used as a method of contraception.

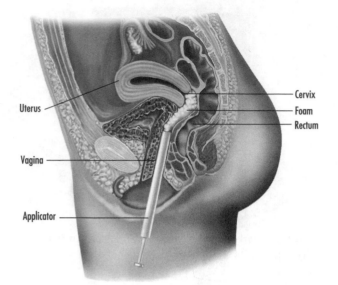

Uterus

Vagina

Applicator

Cervix

Foam

Rectum

Figure 5-11   Applying a spermicidal agent.

cream, or jelly form is usually placed against the cervix of the uterus with a syringe (see Figure 5-11) or can be placed directly on the top of the penis. A spermicidal agent may also be used with another method of contraception. For example, a spermicide may be placed directly on a condom or diaphragm and can be used in conjunction with an IUD. Using a spermicide with another method of contraception will increase the chances of preventing conception. Spermicidal agents have a 94% theoretical effectiveness rate but only a 76% user effectiveness rate (Hatcher, et al., 1998).

The disadvantages of using a spermicide include the need to interrupt foreplay to apply it or to plan ahead of time, the possibility (though unusual) of allergic reactions, and its unpleasant taste reported by couples engaging in oral–genital sexual activity.

Spermicidal sponge.   In April 1983, the U.S. Food and Drug Administration approved the marketing of a vaginal **contraceptive sponge** containing a spermicidal agent. (The brand name of this product is *Today* and it is manufactured by the VLI Corporation.) The sponge is moistened before it is inserted and then placed in front of the cervix. It can be inserted up to 24 hours prior to coitus and must remain in place for at least 6 hours, but no longer than 30 hours, after coitus. Some cases of toxic shock syndrome were suspected of being caused by the use of the sponge as a result of its being kept in the vagina too long or from fragmenting upon removal (Lundberg, 1984). The sponge works in several ways: its spermicide kills the sperm; the sponge itself absorbs the ejaculate, thereby preventing sperm from

entering the uterus; and it acts as a mechanical barrier to block the opening of the cervix. The sponge may cause vaginal itching or odor, may produce some vaginal discharge, and may dislodge (in particular during a bowel movement). However, these relatively minor side effects are a welcome relief to some women after hearing of the potential serious side effects of some other forms of contraception. Another advantage of the sponge is that it is relatively inexpensive.

The Pill.   Other than abstinence, sterilization, Depo-Provera, or hormonal implants, the birth control pill is the most effective means of preventing pregnancy. The Pill has been reported 96% effective as used, and 100% effective if used correctly all the time (Hatcher, et al., 1998). In addition to its effectiveness, the Pill is advantageous, because it does not necessitate an interruption of sexual activity, and because it helps to regulate the menstrual cycle. The disadvantages of the earlier birth control pills—those that contained larger doses of estrogen—were their side effects. Approximately 40% of users experienced some side effects, ranging from nausea, weight gain, headaches, and yeast infections to gallbladder disease, hypertension, and blood clots.

The pills of today can contain as little as 20 to 35 mcg of estrogen as compared to 150 mcg in many earlier versions. Consequently, the threat to the woman's health is lessened.

The Pill is really many pills. Some include estrogen and progestin, some just estrogen, and some just progestin (termed the mini-pill). Further, the amount of hormone varies from brand to brand. Consequently, those using oral contraceptives prescribed for someone else may be doing themselves a disservice and may be subjected to the side effects cited above.

The Pill is based on our knowledge of the menstrual cycle. The estrogen signals the brain's hypothalamus to prevent the pituitary gland from producing FSH or LH. This prevents ovulation. The body is tricked into believing that pregnancy has occurred and that, consequently, there is no need to ovulate. The progestin in birth control pills prepares the endometrium for implantation. It is also believed, though, that progestin used prior to ovulation inhibits implantation, and that it creates a cervical mucus resulting in decreased sperm transport and penetration.

One form of the Pill is taken for 21 days and not taken for the next 7. Another form is taken every day. Some companies used to produce sequential pills, which provided estrogen for 14 to 15 days and a combination of estrogen and progestin for the remaining days of the menstrual cycle. These pills are now banned by the federal government. They

---

contraceptive sponge (spermicidal sponge)   A sponge, filled with spermicides, that is placed in front of the cervix to prevent conception.

contained a greater amount of estrogen than combination-type pills (those with estrogen and progestin throughout), and estrogen has been implicated in many negative side effects of the Pill.

The mini-pill, which is taken every day (even during menstruation), contains only progestin. Since estrogen appears to be the culprit in side effects, the advantage of a pill containing no estrogen is obvious. However, the mini-pill is slightly less effective than the combined Pill and, therefore, relatively few women use the mini-pill.

One way in which oral contraceptives can be used is as an emergency contraceptive. **Emergency contraception** is used to prevent conception when coitus has occurred under conditions that place the woman at risk of pregnancy. For example, a couple might engage in unprotected intercourse as a result of being emotionally aroused, not planning, or the female's forgetting to take her oral contraceptive. Emergency contraception can also be used in cases of rape or incest. It entails administering two oral contraceptive pills within 72 hours of unprotected coitus; one pill taken immediately and the other taken 12 hours later. Over-the-counter emergency contraception kits are now available. Emergency contraception is 74% effective (Greenberg, Bruess & Haffner, 2004).

One other type of Pill contains diethylstilbestrol (DES) and is termed the morning-after pill. The morning-after pill functions after fertilization has occurred. Consequently this pill is considered by some to be a means of contraception, by others a means of abortion.

There are several conditions that indicate that a woman should not use the Pill as a method of contraception. These conditions include, but are not limited to, impaired liver function, hypertension, circulatory problems, sickle cell disease, asthma, varicose veins, epilepsy, and migraine headaches (Hatcher, et al., 1990). It is wise to use the Pill only after medical consultation.

Whether oral contraceptives increase the risk of contracting breast cancer has been a matter of debate for some time. An analysis of 54 studies on the issue concluded that use of the Pill slightly increased the risk (Collaborative Group on Hormonal Factors in Breast Cancer, 1996). The slight risk is eliminated as soon as use is discontinued. Studies continue to present contradictory studies regarding the relationship between breast cancer and the use of oral contraceptives.

Although the contraceptive pill's contraindications and potential unhealthy side effects have received widespread publicity, its positive side effects are not as widely known. Some researchers have found the use of the Pill to be related to a lowered incidence of noncancerous breast lumps, ovarian cysts, and rheumatoid arthritis; and a reduced risk of malignant endometrial and ovarian tumors, pelvic inflammatory disease, iron-deficiency anemia, and premenstrual symptoms (Harlap, Kost & Forrest, 1991).

Depo-Provera.   **Depo-Provera** is a form of progestin administered by injection every 12 weeks. Depo-Provera is very effective, with only 0.3% of users becoming pregnant during a year of use, and since it requires no action on the part of the user, its user effectiveness rate is the same as its theoretical effectiveness rate. In fact, its user effectiveness rate is even better than that of oral contraceptives. Depo-Provera use has several advantages. The user does not have to interrupt sexual activity to use it, it need not be readministered for 12 weeks, it is very effective, and it is reversible. However, some weight gain has been reported by some women, and there may be changes in a woman's period (either not menstruating, frequent bleeding, or spotting between periods). In addition, Depo-Provera provides no protection against sexually transmitted infections.

Hormonal implants.   In 1990, the Federal Drug Administration gave final approval for the marketing of **hormonal implants** as a means of contraception. Marketed under the brand name Norplant, these implants consisted of six matchstick-sized capsules containing levenorgestrol, a progesterone-like synthetic hormone. Levenorgestrol prevents ovulation. No egg means no fertilization. It also thickens the cervical mucus.

Norplant is surgically implanted by a physician in a simple procedure requiring a needle, by which the implants are inserted under the skin of the forearm. This procedure usually takes approximately 15 minutes. Once in place, the implants release a low, continuous dosage of levenorgestrol and remain effective up to 5 years. Studies of over half a million women in many countries have led researchers to conclude Norplant is 99.7% effective (user effectiveness) in preventing pregnancy. That makes it the most effective method of contraception to date, with the exception of sterilization, abstinence, or Depo-Provera.

The advantages of Norplant are many, not the least of which is its actual use effectiveness rate. In addition, once in place, it can be forgotten. There are no other actions needed

---

emergency contraception   The use of oral contraception in a prescribed manner after sexual intercourse has occurred to prevent pregnancy.

Depo-Provera   A synthetic chemical (a form of progestin) used to prevent conception.

hormonal implants   Matchstick-sized capsules containing hormones that release slowly over time to prevent conception.

to be taken by the user. Furthermore, should a woman want to become pregnant at a later date, the implants can be removed in a minor surgical procedure and fertility usually returns during the woman's next menstrual cycle. Lastly, although the initial cost for the implants may be higher than some other methods of contraception, over the 5 years that it remains effective, the total cost is less than the cost of oral contraceptives.

As with all means of contraception, implants also have their disadvantages. Some women may have difficulty affording the initial cost of insertion. Implants are also more effective in women who weigh less than 110 lb and significantly less effective in women weighing over 154 lb. Norplant can also lead to menstrual irregularities such as prolonged bleeding and more frequent bleeding (Keenan, 1991). Furthermore, although the safety of Norplant has been tested, and it does not contain any estrogen, the FDA still recommends that women with acute liver disease, unexplained vaginal bleeding, breast cancer, or blood clots refrain from using these implants. Lastly, anywhere from 2% to 7% of women using Norplant will experience side effects that lead them to have the implants removed. Among these side effects are menstrual irregularities and amenorrhea, ovarian cysts, headaches, acne, weight change, and hair growth. Given these advantages and disadvantages, one physician who is an expert on women's health recommends implants be considered if the following apply (Patterson, 1990):

a. You are interested in long-term contraception.

b. You are unable to use pills containing estrogen.

c. You have used barrier methods—for example, the diaphragm, spermicides, condom, cervical cap—and have become dissatisfied with them.

d. You are older than 35, since use of oral contraceptives after that age is becoming suspect.

Unfortunately, Norplant is no longer being marketed. In 2000, its manufacturer, Wyeth, became concerned that specified lots of Norplant might be ineffective due to a manufacturing error and, consequently, advised health care professionals to stop providing implants from those lots. In addition, Wyeth advised women who already had implants from those lots to use a barrier or hormonal contraceptive method to ensure protection from pregnancy. After conducting further tests, however, Wyeth concluded there was no problem with those lots and that women need no longer use a backup method of contraception. Unfortunately, the damage was already done to Norplant's reputation and, citing "limitation in product component supplies," Wyeth decided not to reintroduce Norplant to the market (Wyeth, 2002).

Sterilization.   To be sterilized is to be made biologically incapable of reproducing. Males or females may be sterilized. In males, **sterilization** entails intervention in the vas deferens. This intervention can be through cutting the vas deferens, plugging it up, or clipping it closed (see Figure 5-12). Either way, sperm are prevented from entering the ejaculate. Previously considered irreversible in 95% of cases, sterilization can now be reversed in many cases. Both removal of the plugs inserted in the vas deferens and microsurgery are means of reversing male sterilization. One word of caution: the male should consult his physician to verify sterility, since sperm may be present in the ejaculate for some time after a sterilization procedure.

Sadly, in the past, people who were institutionalized with disabilities were sometimes sterilized without their consent. It was believed that people with certain disabilities could not make responsible sexual decisions and that sterilization was in their best interests. Fortunately, this practice has virtually ceased, and people with disabilities have demonstrated sexual responsibility with appropriate support from their families and various supportive agencies when necessary.

The usual means of female sterilization are **tubal ligation,** electrocoagulation, and mechanical means of blocking the fallopian tubes. Tubal ligation involves cutting the fallopian tubes and tying them back. Electrocoagulation uses heat on or within the tubes to seal them closed. Mechanical means include clips, silicone rubber bands, or plugs to close the tubes. These procedures can be reversed in some cases, but the woman is advised that reversal is by no means guaranteed and, on the contrary, the procedures should be considered permanent. A tube (laparoscope) that contains a viewing scope is used during tubal ligation. The tube is inserted through one or two small incisions in the abdomen, and the fallopian tubes are then cut, tied, or cauterized. This procedure can be done under local anesthesia. Other methods of tubal ligation include making a larger abdominal incision (laparotomy) or reaching the fallopian tubes through the vagina (culpotomy). Still other means of female sterilization include surgical removal of the uterus (hysterectomy) or hormonal, irradiation, or chemical treatment.

---

sterilization   A means of contraception involving either cutting, plugging, or clipping the fallopian tubes or the vas deferens to prevent the union of egg and sperm.

tubal ligation   A means of female sterilization involving blocking the fallopian tubes.

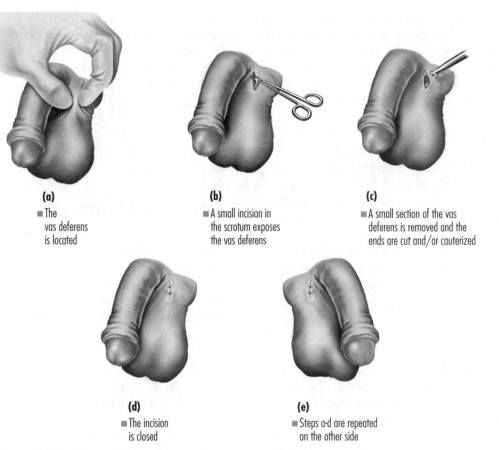

(a)
- The
vas deferens
is located

(b)
- A small incision in
the scrotum exposes
the vas deferens

(c)
- A small section of the vas
deferens is removed and the
ends are cut and/or cauterized

(d)
- The incision
is closed

(e)
- Steps a-d are repeated
on the other side

Figure 5-12   External view of a vasectomy.

Some newer methods of contraception. Methods of contraception that have been developed recently include the following:

NuvaRing. A vaginal ring that provides hormonal protection from pregnancy was approved by the U.S. Food and Drug Administration in 2001 and became available in 2002 (Organon, 2002). NuvaRing emits 0.015 mg of ethinyl estradiol (the estrogen component) and 0.120 mg of etono-gestrel (the progestin component) daily for 21 days. In contrast, low-dose estrogen contraceptive pills contain 0.005 mg more estrogen, and other contraceptive pills contain 0.015 mg more estrogen. Although the diaphragm and cervical cap need to be positioned correctly to provide maximum protection, NuvaRing need not. It cannot be inserted incorrectly, and it comes with a timer as a reminder for when it needs to be replaced. The hourglass-shaped timer shows the number of days the ring will remain effective, and beeps on day 21. Even if not removed immediately, protection remains for another week. NuvaRing costs approximately $40 in pharmacies and requires a prescription to be purchased.

NuvaRing is an effective hormonal contraceptive with many advantages. NuvaRing contains less estrogen than even the low-dose oral contraceptives, thereby decreasing the risks associated with synthetic estrogens. The ring does not require any daily action, as does taking a pill each day. All that is required is replacement of the ring after 21 days. Consequently, its user effectiveness rate is quite high. It has a theoretical and user effectiveness rate of 98% to 99%. Furthermore, the vast majority of women cannot feel the ring when it is in place, and report being satisfied with this method of contraception. In addition, NuvaRing's effects are reversible once removed.

As with all methods of contraception, there are also disadvantages associated with NuvaRing. The risk of synthetic estrogen is not eliminated, it is merely reduced. Therefore, as advised by the manufacturer, smokers, those with heart disease, and those susceptible to blood clots should not use the ring. Further, 14% of users experienced vaginitis (Redfearn, 2002), and 25% of men felt the ring during intercourse, although most reported they did not perceive that to be a problem. The manufacturer suggests removing the ring during intercourse if a partner finds it problematic. It can be removed for up to 3 hours without losing its effectiveness. Another disadvantage of the ring for women who are uncomfortable touching their genitalia is the need for the user to manually insert it through the vagina. In addition, NuvaRing does not offer any protection against sexually transmitted infections. Lastly, the monthly cost of the ring is slightly higher than the monthly cost for oral contraceptives and, at the time of this writing, is not covered by health insurance companies.

The contraceptive patch. In December 2000, Johnson & Johnson applied for approval to market the first contraceptive patch. In March 2003, the patch became available to women seeking a method of contraception that released a steady delivery of hormones over time. In a short time it became the second most popular form of nonoral birth control in prescriptions and sales (Long, 2002).

Similar to the nicotine patch, users wear it on their lower abdomen, buttocks, or upper arm. The patch is about the size of a matchbook and delivers a combination of estrogen and progesterone. Each patch is used for 7 days, then removed and discarded. Women wear successive patches for 3 weeks and then have a patch-free week while menstruation occurs. The primary side effects of the patch are headache, nausea, and site reactions, which were experienced by 20% of users in clinical trials (Contraception patch, 2001). The patch is approximately as effective as birth control pills. It is 99.7% effective when used perfectly, with typical use resulting in a 92% user effectiveness rate (Long, 2002).

The contraceptive methods now being researched include the following:

Male contraceptive implants. In 2001, clinical trials began on a male contraceptive implant. One hundred and twenty male volunteers in the United States and Europe received implants that contained the hormone etonogestral. This hormone is thought to prevent the production of sperm. If these trials prove safe and effective, it is possible that male contraceptive implants will be available as early as 2005 (Male contraceptive implant, 2001).

Implanon. Implanon is a single-rod progesterone implant, only about 4 cm long, that inhibits ovulation while impeding motility in the reproductive tract. A small dose of the same progesterone that is in the vaginal ring is released constantly. Implanon, designed to be used for 3 years, will include a device to allow women to insert and remove it easily. In clinical trials, no pregnancies were reported in over 53,000 menstrual cycles (Long, 2002).

Jadelle. Manufactured by Wyeth, the former manufacturer of Norplant, this two-rod implant system continually releases progesterone to inhibit ovulation. The rods are 4.3 cm long and must be inserted and removed by a trained clinician. Jadelle was determined to be as effective as Norplant in its first 3 years of use (Sivin, et al., 1998). Potential side effects are similar to those of Norplant and include periodic breakthrough bleeding.

Lea's Shield. Lea's Shield is a cervical cap that allows the release of cervical fluids and air. Elliptical in shape and made of silicone rubber, it is slightly larger in its posterior portion so as to allow for a good fit on the cervix. The shield acts as do other barrier methods. In spite of coming in only one size that fits all users, the shield requires a prescription. Reported to be comfortable and easy to use, the shield can be washed and used for up to 1 year. It is currently available in Germany, Austria, Switzerland, and Canada, although effectiveness data are limited (FDA approves Lea's Shield, 2002).

Essure. This method of birth control causes sterility without surgical anesthesia or incision and does not result in any visible scar. Passed through the vaginal canal and uterus, a small metal ring is inserted into the fallopian tubes. In 3 months an occlusion occurs, thereby blocking the union of sperm and egg. Essure has been 99.8% effective in clinical trials (Long, 2002).

Choosing a Contraceptive

One of the sexuality educator's functions is to discuss why people choose *not* to use a method of contraception. Obviously, both religious reasons and lack of knowledge are sometimes involved. Still others choose to conceive. However, studies of college students disclose that the majority do not use any means of contraception during intercourse.

In a study of 140 college female students who had previously experienced coitus, only 74 reported using any form of contraception the first time they had sexual intercourse (Sawyer & Beck, 1988). Reasons given by students who did not use birth control are summarized in Table 5-1. In another study of 569 female college students (Ogletree, 1990), it was found that 78% had experienced sexual intercourse but only 60% of these women reported using a method of contraception during their first coital experience. When these women's knowledge about contraception was studied, they scored fairly high. Consequently, it was concluded that knowledge is not sufficient to predict contraceptive usage. It was recommended that educational programs be conducted to teach college students interpersonal and social skills (for example, communication and assertiveness skills). Unfortunately, one study of contraceptive education reported too many high school students not receiving an in-depth sexuality education class (Taylor, et al., 1989). However, of those who did receive such a class, more had positive attitudes toward contraception than those who did not.

Other studies have validated the lack of consistent use of contraception for sexually active people. For example, in a national survey by Leigh and colleagues (1993), 13% of respondents reported engaging in sexual intercourse with more than one partner, but only 8% had used condoms consistently. Of the total population studied, 95% used condoms inconsistently, and of those respondents who reported engaging in sexual intercourse with a new partner, only 25% stated they had used a condom. In another study, of those who engaged in sexual intercourse over the previous 3 months, almost 36% did not use any method of contraception (Piccinino & Mosher, 1998). And, in a study of 15- to 19-year-olds, 27% of males who had engaged in sexual intercourse did not use a condom (Sonenstein, et al., 1998).

Table 5-1 Reasons Given for Not Using Any Form of Birth Control

Percent Who Said:	Yes	No	Maybe
Wanted to become pregnant	0.0	100	0.0
Didn't think I'd have sex at the time	56.3	39.1	4.7
I'm not really very sexually active	45.9	47.5	6.6
Didn't think I'd get pregnant	35.5	50.0	14.5
Partner didn't want to use a method	20.0	73.3	6.7
Partner didn't want *me* to use a method	10.2	83.1	6.8
Knew it was risky, but took a chance	62.3	18.0	19.7
Don't believe in birth control for moral or religious reasons	1.7	98.3	0.0
Think birth control is too messy and unromantic	6.9	86.2	6.9
Didn't know how birth control works	1.7	94.9	3.4
Didn't know where to get birth control	8.3	91.7	0.0
Didn't want to see a doctor to obtain birth control	19.7	78.7	1.6
Would seem like I was planning to have sex	10.3	86.2	3.4
I was too embarrassed to get birth control	6.8	88.1	5.1
I was drinking/using drugs at the time	15.0	83.3	1.7
I am concerned with the health risks of the methods	34.5	56.9	8.6
Was forced to have sex against my will	1.7	96.6	1.7
I cannot afford to use birth control regularly	5.2	89.7	5.2

From Robin Sawyer and Kenneth H. Beck, "Predicting Pregnancy and Contraceptive Usage Among College Women," in *Health Education* 19:42–47. Copyright © 1988 Journal of Health Education, Reston, VA. Reprinted by permission.

Some of the reasons most frequently given for not using contraception are reflected in the following statements:

1. It (pregnancy) couldn't happen to me.

2. I feel guilty (immoral) if I plan in advance.

3. I'm too embarrassed to buy contraceptives.

4. Someone (for example, parents) may find out I'm using contraceptives.

5. Once I use contraceptives, I couldn't stop myself from participating more.

6. It wasn't a planned experience.

7. It hasn't happened yet (pregnancy or coitus), so it won't.

8. It's not natural to use contraceptives.

9. It ruins the fun.

10. I'm too lazy.

11. I could not imagine myself having a child (it's beyond my comprehension).

12. I experience coitus too infrequently to be concerned with contraception.

Some people have gone so far as to suggest that contraception be mandated, especially now that we have so many effective contraceptive alternatives. In fact, a judge sentenced a child abuser—a woman convicted of abusing her children—to prison and ordered a contraceptive implant be inserted in her arm (Allstetter, 1991). The American Civil Liberties Union appealed this verdict on the grounds that it violated her procreative rights. What do you think is appropriate in this case?

Some research has suggested that many out-of-wedlock teenage pregnancies are not accidents but rather are intended. Whether to seek attention, to have someone to nurture, to punish parents, or for other reasons, many teenagers intend to conceive a child. Obviously, then, a study of this phenomenon needs to be included in sexuality education programs; a major focus of this study should be the consequences (both positive and negative) of out-of-wedlock pregnancy on the mother, father, and child.

The sexuality educator, as stated in Chapter 4, must be an advocate for responsible sexual behavior. One might appropriately question whether coitus without some acceptable means of contraception (even if a person's religion only allows natural family planning) is responsible sexual behavior. Such a consideration should be incorporated into sexuality education programs.

To select a contraceptive device, the following questions should be asked:

1. Is it safe? Are there any side effects? Will it interact with current medications?

2. Is it effective—both theoretically and as you would use it?

3. Is it affordable?

4. Is it convenient? Will it mean an interruption in sexual activity?

5. Is it consistent with your religious and moral values?

6. Is it compatible with your partner? (For example, some people may be allergic to some spermicides.)

7. Is it reversible? Will it affect any future decision to have children?

8. Is it available?

Recognizing that there is no "perfect contraceptive," one should select the method that "best" meets one's needs, and then attempt to minimize the imperfections in that method. For example, if one has selected a method that is accompanied by potential side effects, regular medical checkups should be scheduled so as to detect any side effects early enough to prevent them from causing serious injury.

Pregnancy, Childbirth, and Abortion

Pregnancy

Pregnancy begins when an egg is fertilized by a sperm and is successfully implanted on the endometrium to be nourished. Pregnancy can be determined through several means. The most frequent is to test the urine for the presence of **human chorionic gonadotropin (HCG),** a hormone produced by the placenta once implantation has occurred. Although conception can be chemically determined as early as 10 days after conception, most pregnancy tests are conducted around 6 to 8 weeks after the last menstruation. These tests are very reliable and are best conducted and analyzed by a physician or laboratory. Although pregnancy test kits can be purchased at drugstores for self-administration, they are not

recommended. Negative findings of such test kits are not reliable, the kits cost money, and using the kits properly is sometimes difficult.

Because the first trimester of pregnancy is the most important in the embryo's development, it is imperative that a pregnant woman seek prenatal care as soon as she determines that she is pregnant. This one piece of information is highly important to emphasize in sexuality education. First, pregnant women should be educated about the detrimental effects of drugs (alcohol, tobacco, and others) on the development of the unborn. Second, they should learn what kinds of physical activity pregnant women can engage in. Third, they should be told the kind of diet they should be following. They should also learn about the effects of radiation and communicable diseases on pregnancy. All of these topics can be discussed with a physician during prenatal care; the physician also monitors the pregnancy and the unborn's development. It is our belief that if sexuality education served no other purpose, it would be worthwhile if it resulted in pregnant women seeking prenatal care earlier and in greater numbers.

Sexuality educators should also inform people that the prepregnancy state of a mother is a factor in the development of the unborn. Women who prior to conception do not eat nutritionally sound diets may have deficiencies that will affect subsequent embryos and fetuses. Similarly, women who drink alcoholic beverages to excess, women who smoke tobacco, and women who abuse other drugs are developing their "inner environments" in such a way as to be harmful to subsequent pregnancies.

Some complications may arise for the fetus during pregnancy. These problems may stem from heredity or may be **congenital** (not transferable from generation to generation). One means of detecting fetal abnormalities is by testing the fluid (amniotic fluid) in which the fetus is developing. The process of extracting fluid for testing is called **amniocentesis** (not a routine procedure). The sex of the fetus can also be determined by analyzing fetal cells found in the amniotic fluid. Another means of detecting fetal abnormalities is **chorionic villi sampling** (sometimes called chorionic villi biopsy). This procedure involves extracting pieces of the villi (thin tissue) protruding from the chorion (outer layer of the amniotic sac) and analyzing it for birth defects. The advantage of this technique over amniocentesis is that it can be done 9 weeks after conception rather than the 16 weeks necessary for amniocentesis. Consequently, a decision to

---

human chorionic gonadotropin (HCG) A hormone produced by the placenta and whose presence in urine is tested to determine whether a woman is pregnant.

congenital A trait or condition that is not transferred from one generation to another.

amniocentesis Extraction of amniotic fluid to determine whether birth defects are present in a fetus.

chorionic villi sampling Extraction of pieces of the thin tissue protruding from the chorion to determine whether birth defects are present in a fetus.

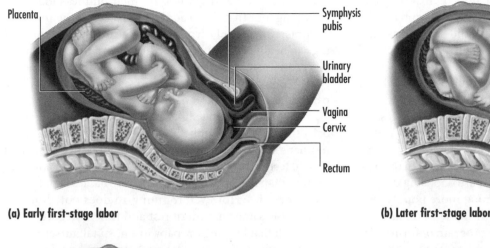

(a) Early first-stage labor

Placenta · Symphysis pubis · Urinary bladder · Vagina · Cervix · Rectum

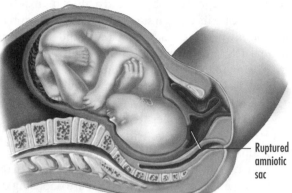

(b) Later first-stage labor: the transition

Ruptured amniotic sac

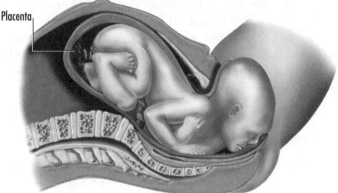

(c) Early second-stage labor

Placenta

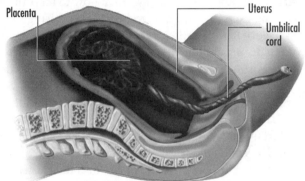

(d) Third-stage labor: delivery of afterbirth

Placenta · Uterus · Umbilical cord

Figure 5-13   Stages of the birth process.

abort the fetus or preparations to care for a baby born with a birth defect can be made all that much earlier.

After a normal pregnancy and birth, the mother may experience a period of depression. Such **postpartum depression** may be a result of fatigue, hormonal changes, the awesome responsibilities associated with parenthood, or a combination of these. In any case, sexuality education programs should inform people that such depression may occur and should discuss the interaction and understanding needed by women at this point in their lives.

Birth

The birth process is quite well defined. It consists of three stages of labor. The first stage lasts an average of 10.5 hours for the first pregnancy and 6.5 hours for other pregnancies. The purpose of this stage of pregnancy is to dilate the neck of the cervix wide enough (4 in.) for the fetus to exit.

The second stage of labor, lasting approximately 1 hour, results in the delivery of the fetus outside the mother's body. An involuntary contraction and pushing of the abdominal muscles aids this process. To prevent tearing of the vaginal tissue, physicians sometimes make an incision, called an episiotomy, in the vaginal opening. The final stage of labor delivers the placenta (afterbirth). See Figure 5-13.

Upon the baby's delivery, the umbilical cord that has served as the lifeline for the fetus, providing it with nourishment from the mother, is clamped and cut; the baby is checked for vital functions; and medicine in the form of drops (silver nitrate) is deposited in the baby's eyes to prevent blindness from a possible gonorrheal infection in the mother.

Routine childbirth can be anything but routine. In some instances the fetus may be positioned in the uterus with its buttocks where its head should be. This is termed a **breech birth** (it occurs in 4% of all births) and calls for specific physician involvement to successfully maneuver the fetus for birth. In

---

postpartum depression   Feelings of depression (sadness, fatigue) that occur after a woman has given birth.

breech birth   When a fetus is positioned with the buttocks, not the head, being the body part nearest the cervix during birth.

other cases the pressure on the head of the fetus may be so great as to decrease its oxygen supply. In these cases and in other situations where the mother or baby would be endangered by vaginal delivery, the best procedure for birth may be through an incision in the woman's abdomen. This surgical delivery is termed a Caesarean section; approximately 20% of births in the United States are delivered in this manner.

Other decisions regarding childbirth are necessary, and these should be considered in sexuality education programs. With the knowledge that anesthetics used during childbirth to decrease the mother's pain remain in the newborn long after birth, many women are choosing drugless births. Natural childbirth is becoming more popular. The Lamaze method of natural childbirth, named after its developer Fernand Lamaze, consists of a program of formal class instruction designed to teach women how to relax through breathing exercises and how to bear down during the second stage of labor. Further, partners are taught how to coach women during childbirth.

Choosing where to deliver is the next question needing attention. Although hospital delivery is still the predominant choice, some women are choosing home births, and hospitals are providing birthing rooms made to be more comfortable than typical delivery rooms. The advantages of home delivery include the familiar and comforting setting of the home, the important role given to the father, faster recovery than hospital births, and the ability to have the baby be an immediate part of the family (introduced to brothers and sisters right after birth). However, since medical resources available at hospitals are not available in homes, home births are recommended only in certain cases. These cases should involve low risk, meaning the following factors apply:

1. The mother should be between 20 and 30 years of age.

2. The mother should have had good nutrition.

3. The mother should have had one to three full-term births without complication.

4. No potential medical problems should be evident.

In any case, home birth should include the services of a qualified physician or nurse-midwife.

The next decision is how to treat the newborn immediately after birth. There seemed to be no question about this area until the ideas and practices of a French obstetrician, Frederick Leboyer, were publicized. Leboyer (1975) believed birth to be traumatic enough without our adding to it. He advised that newborns be delivered in dimly lit, quiet, warm rooms. Furthermore, he argued that babies should not be held by their feet and spanked on their buttocks to induce breathing, but that they should be placed on the mother's abdomen where her heartbeat can be heard and their breathing can begin gradually. Finally, he advised that the baby be placed in water at body temperature and bathed and rocked gently. Leboyer states that babies born in this manner will be psychologically better off in later life.

Another issue that should be considered is where the baby should be kept in the hospital—in a nursery or in the mother's room. Mothers who room-in with their first child tend to feel more competent and confident in their ability to mother than do those women who have babies kept in hospital nurseries. However, rooming-in does not allow the mother the same amount of rest and time to recover from childbirth that keeping the baby in a hospital nursery does.

It is obvious that many decisions need to be made regarding pregnancy and childbirth, and they must be made on the basis of as much and as accurate information as possible. The feelings and thoughts of mothers and fathers must also be explored. The role of the sexuality educator is to facilitate the decision-making process.

Abortion

The first decision that must be made once pregnancy is diagnosed is whether to let the pregnancy run its course. Sometimes the choice is made to foster the pregnancy, but something goes wrong and the unborn's development is terminated. Such a natural cessation of the unborn's growth and development is termed a **spontaneous abortion** (also called a *miscarriage*). On the other hand, some abortions are purposely initiated; these are called **induced abortions.** Some people believe that induced abortion is akin to murder, whereas others see it as just a medical intervention. The sexuality educator's role is not to recommend for or against induced abortions but rather to present the various religious, philosophical, sociological, medical, and scientific considerations that relate to this practice. The question of when life begins, for example, is central to the abortion debate. Some people argue that life begins at conception; others believe that life begins at the time the unborn can exist on its own; still others are convinced that life begins at birth. A decision for or against induced abortion depends not only on one's view of when life begins but also on one's perception of the magnitude of the population explosion, one's view on the importance of quality living as opposed to plain existing, and one's judgment about the degree of responsibility people should assume for their sexual behaviors.

---

spontaneous abortion   A natural cessation of pregnancy, also called a miscarriage.

induced abortion   The forced termination of a pregnancy.

The important question for you as a sexuality educator is whether you can objectively facilitate consideration of abortion without imposing your own view. Can you?

In 1973, in the Roe versus Wade case, the U.S. Supreme Court ruled that abortion should be available for women during the first trimester of pregnancy and that the decision to use this option is one that should be made by the pregnant woman and her physician. Regarding abortions scheduled during the second trimester, the Supreme Court ruled that individual states can develop regulations they deem necessary to maintain maternal health. The court has ruled that the states can prohibit abortions after the second trimester as long as the mother's health is not in jeopardy.

The medical techniques used for abortion include the following (Greenberg & Dintiman, 1992):

1. *Vacuum aspiration.* Pressure vacuums out the products of conception.

2. *Dilatation and curettage.* The cervix is dilated and an instrument is inserted to scrape out the products of conception.

3. *Evacuation and curettage.* When the products of conception are too large to be sucked out through the vacuum tube, they need to be scraped into smaller parts by a curette. Once small enough, they are then sucked out with the vacuum.

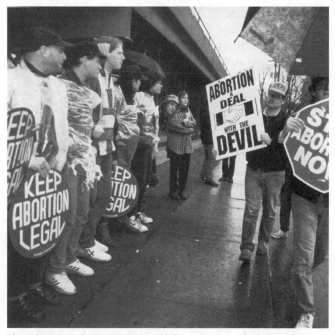

Abortion remains a controversial topic. Pro-choice and pro-life views both need consideration in sexuality education programs.

4. *Induced labor.* Labor is induced by injection of saline solution into the amniotic fluid. Sometimes prostaglandins (synthetic hormones) are used instead of saline solution.

5. *Hysterotomy.* An abdominal incision is made and the products of conception are removed through the incision. This method is only rarely used.

6. *Chemicals.* Either diethylstilbestrol (DES) or RU 486 are used to create a spontaneous abortion.

Since abortion is an issue debated by citizens, ruled on by the judiciary, and legislated by elected representatives, it is a topic that needs the fullest possible study. Sexuality education can contribute to an informed citizenry by offering educational experiences that will objectively explore the ramifications of the practice of abortion. Sexuality educators must be prepared to conduct such experiences and to be able to justify their inclusion in sexuality education.

RU 486: A Method of Nonsurgical Abortion

A drug that has been dubbed the "morning after pill" has been used extensively in Europe in place of surgical abortion. Called **RU 486,** it was discovered in 1978 by research scientists at Roussel Uclaf, a French pharmaceutical company. RU 486 blocks the action of progesterone when taken within 49 days of a woman's last menstrual flow. Given that it works after conception occurs, RU 486 is considered an abortifacient; that is, it "aborts" a fertilized egg by preventing its implantation on the endometrial lining of the uterus, precipitating uterine contractions, and sloughing off the egg in the menstrual flow.

Research indicates RU 486 is a safe, economical, medical alternative to surgical abortion procedures (Allukian, 1990). In addition, RU 486 is thought to have potential for treating breast cancer, endometriosis, meningioma (a form of brain cancer), Cushing's syndrome (an adrenal gland disorder), and other hormonal-related maladies (Suplee, 1990).

RU 486 is effective in only 60% of cases in which it is administered alone. However, when the woman returns 36 to 48 hours after taking RU 486 and receives an injection of a prostaglandin (misoprostol), the effectiveness rate increases to about 95%. Treatment with RU 486 usually involves four visits to a physician. The first is for an examination, the second is for the administration of RU 486, the third is to receive the prostaglandin, and the fourth is to verify the abortion is complete and to identify any side effects (such as bleeding). Misoprostol can result in mild cramps, nausea, vomiting, and diarrhea. Further refining the use of RU 486 to make it

RU 486   A chemical that can terminate a pregnancy.

as safe as possible, in 1991 the French government banned its use in women over 35 years of age or women who have smoked more than 10 cigarettes a day for more than 2 years (Herman, 1991). This was a result of the fear that heart attacks could be induced if such women were to be administered RU 486. This fear is not unfounded, since several heart attacks have actually occurred in otherwise healthy women as a result of prostaglandin injections following the use of RU 486.

Summary

The male and female reproductive systems are well designed for their functions. The male system is designed to produce sperm and to implant these sperm within the female system. The female system is designed to produce ova and to provide an environment for growth of the developing organism. Males and females produce similar hormones; the male hormones influence secondary sexual characteristics and the production of sperm, while the female hormones regulate the menstrual cycle as well as produce secondary sexual characteristics.

There are both similarities and differences between the sexual responses of males and females. Masters and Johnson describe four phases of the human sexual response cycle: the excitement phase, the plateau phase, the orgasmic phase, and the resolution phase.

Fertility control means intervention at some point in the reproductive process. Those who wish to prevent conception may choose from a variety of methods, each of which has particular advantages and disadvantages. Some methods provide a mechanical barrier between sperm and egg (condoms, diaphragms, sponge, cap), some kill or immobilize the sperm (spermicides), and some prevent the egg from implanting in the uterus (IUD). Methods that do not require expense or mechanical aids include abstinence, withdrawal, and the ovulation method. The most effective approach of all is sterilization. The role of the sexuality educator is one of education, not of advocacy. Since religious and moral considerations must be a part of decisions regarding the use or nonuse of contraception, the educator's role is to facilitate discussion and knowledge of the consequences of coitus without contraception, rather than to argue for the use of birth control methods.

With regard to pregnancy and the normal growth and development of the fetus, the educator's role is to emphasize the importance of early parental care. The sexuality educator must also discuss the normal course of pregnancy and childbirth, as well as the possible complications that can arise for both mother and child. Couples expecting a child have many decisions to make, including whether to use natural childbirth, where to give birth, whether to use the Leboyer approach, and whether to room-in with the baby after it is born. If a couple prefers not to have a child, the couple must consider the moral, emotional, legal, and medical aspects of abortion. The role of the sexuality educator relative to abortion is to develop a citizenry with sufficient understanding of the issue and to encourage individuals to make informed decisions for themselves.

References

Allstetter, B. Compulsory contraception: Does the punishment fit the crime? *American Health* (May 1991), 32–34.

Allukian, M. Where in the world RU 486? *The Nation's Health*, 20 (1990), 2.

Collaborative Group on Hormonal Factors in Breast Cancer. Breast cancer and hormonal contraceptives, *Lancet*, 347 (1996), 405–11.

Contraceptive patch, *The Contraception Report*, 12, no. 4 (2001), 12–14.

Fact sheet: Contraceptive use. New York: Alan Guttmacher Institute, 1998.

FDA approves Lea's Shield, *The Contraception Report*, 13, no. 2 (2002). Available: http://www.contraceptiononline.org/contrareport.issue.cfm.

Greenberg, J. S., Bruess, C. & Haffner, D. *Exploring the dimensions of human sexuality* 2nd ed. Boston: Jones and Bartlett, 2004.

_____ & Dintiman, G. B. *Exploring health: Expanding the boundaries of wellness.* Englewood Cliffs, NJ: Prentice Hall, 1992.

Harlap, S., Kost, K. & Forrest, J. D. *Preventing pregnancy, protecting health: A new look at birth control choices in the United States.* New York: The Alan Guttmacher Institute, 1991.

Hatcher, R. A., et al. *Contraceptive technology, 1990–1992.* 15th rev. ed. Manchester, NH: Irvington Publishers, 1990.

Hatcher, R. A., Trussell, J., Stewart, F., Cates, W., Stewart, G. K., Guestr, F. & Kowal, D. *Contraceptive Technology.* 17th rev. ed. New York: Advent Media, 1998.

Herman, R. French ban use of RU 486 by smokers, women over 35, *Washington Post Health* (April 30, 1991), 5.

Keenan, F. Imperfect implant, *American Health* (March 1991), 9.

Leboyer, F. *Birth without violence.* New York: Alfred A. Knopf, 1975.

Leigh, B. C., Temple, M. T. & Trocki, K. F. The sexual behavior of United States adults: Results from a national survey, *American Journal of Public Health*, 83 (1993), 1400–08.

Long, V. E. Contraceptive choices: New options in the U.S. market, *SIECUS Report*, 31 (2002), 13–18.

Lundberg, G. TSS and the Sponge, *Journal of the American Medical Association*, 251 (1984), 1015–16.

Male contraceptive implants. Sexhealth.com (July 11, 2001). Available: http://www.sexhealth.com.

Masters, W. H. & Johnson, V. E. *Human sexual response.* Boston: Little, Brown, 1966.

_____ & Kolodny, R. C. *Human sexuality.* 4th ed. New York: Harper Collins, 1992.

McCary, J. L. *Human sexuality.* 4th ed. Belmont, CA: Wadsworth Publishing, 1982.

National Center for Health Statistics. Contraceptive use in the United States, 1973–88, *Advance Data,* 181 (March 20, 1990).

_____. Contraceptive utilization among widowed, divorced, and separated women in the United States, *Advance Data,* 40 (September 22, 1978a), 3.

———. Contraceptive utilization in the United States, *Advance Data,* 36 (August 18, 1978b), 6.

Ogletree, R. J. Contraceptive use at first intercourse as reported by college women in personal health classes, *The Eta Sigma Gamma Monograph Series,* 8 (1990), 19–23.

Organon. NuvaRing, world's first vaginal birth control ring, now available in U.S. news release, July 16, 2002.

Patterson, J. Have you switched to low-dose oral contraceptives yet? *Shape* (June 1986), 30–32.

Patterson, J. The contraceptive implant, *Shape* (August 1990), 30–31.

Piccinino, L. J. & Mosher, W. D. Trends in contraceptive use in the United States: 1982–1995, *Family Planning Perspectives,* 30 (1998), 4–10, 46.

Redfearn, S. A new ring cycle: Contraceptive woos the way, *Washington Post* (August 6, 2002), F1, F4.

Sawyer, R. & Beck, K. H. Predicting pregnancy and contraceptive usage among college women, *Health Education,* 19 (1988), 42–47.

Sivin, I., Lahteenmaki, P., Mishell, D. R., Alvarez, F., Diaz, S., Ranta, S., Grozinger, C., Lacarra, M., Brache, V., Pavez, M., Nash, H. & Stern, J. The performance of levonorgestrel rod and Norplant contraceptive implants: Year randomized study, *Human Reproduction,* 13 (1998), 3371–78.

Sonenstein, F. L., Ku, L., Lindberg, L. D., Turner, C. F. & Pleck, J. H. Changes in sexual behavior and condom use among teenaged males: 1988–1995, *American Journal of Public Health,* 88 (1998), 956–59.

Suplee, C. Hill holds heated hearing on RU 486, *Washington Post* (November 20, 1990), A21.

Taylor, M. E., Wang, M. Q., Leonard, J. Jr. & Adame, D. D. Effects of contraceptive education on adolescent male contraceptive behavior and attitudes, *Health Education* (1989), 12–117.

Wyeth. Back-up contraception no longer required for women using Norplant system. News release, July 26, 2002.

Suggested Readings

Boston Women's Health Book Collective. *Our bodies, our selves for the new century: A book by and for women.* New York: Simon and Schuster, 1998.

Byer, C. O. & Shainberg, L. W. *Dimensions of human sexuality.* Dubuque, IA: William C. Brown Communications, 1997.

Crooks, R. & Baur, K. *Our sexuality.* Pacific Grove, CA: Brooks/Cole, 1999.

Kaschak, L. & Tiefer L., eds. *A new view of women's sexual problems.* Binghampton, NY: Haworth Press, 2002.

Rathus, S. A., Nevid, J. S. & Fichner-Rathus, L. *Human sexuality in a diverse world.* Boston: Allyn and Bacon, 2000.

The Cognitive and Psychological Side of Sexuality

CHAPTER 6

Key Concepts

1. Psychosexual development has been explained by various theories.

2. Self-esteem is the key to sexual maturity.

3. Attitudes are not always converted into behavior.

4. Having children should be more a matter of choice than of chance.

5. Sex-role stereotyping is not to the advantage of males or females.

6. Society contributes to sex-role stereotyping.

The psychological aspects of human sexuality are far less understood than its biological aspects. It is important, however, for the sexuality educator to include knowledge of the stages of psychosexual development, the importance of self-esteem to sexual maturity, the relationship between sexual attitudes and behavior, and the limits of traditional sexual roles on healthy sexuality as components of the psychological side of education for sexuality.

Theories of Psychosexual Development

Theories have been proposed and research has been conducted to attempt to explain the psychological components in the development of people's sexual attitudes and behaviors.

Freud

Although all people develop differently, theorists look for common threads. Freud, for instance, believed that personality and sexuality developed together. He described this development as occurring in a series of stages.

1. *Self-love.* Lasting from infancy to about 4 or 5 years of age, this stage is characterized by concentration on oneself. Attitudes about oneself are formed during this stage of development, attitudes such as self-concern, tenderness, and involvement. A child needs to experience loving physical contact in order for these attitudes to develop adequately. If love is expressed to the child and the child feels secure, the child will develop positive attitudes regarding himself or herself. These attitudes will then allow the child, as an adult, to feel and express love and concern for others.

2. *Parental identification.* Sexual roles are learned during this stage, which starts at age 5 or 6 and lasts for about 1 year. Close contact with an adult of the same sex is important during this time. This adult serves as a model for the child, demonstrating the appropriate sexual role for a man or woman in the child's society. Some theorists believe that homosexuality is a result of a failure to successfully accomplish the task of this stage of psychosexual development.

3. *Gang.* Lasting through the elementary school years, this stage is easily recognized: each sex tends to avoid the other. Although Freud termed this stage the **latency period** because he believed that little occurred sexually during this time of life, we now know that during these years children engage in much sexual experimentation. They play "doctor" and "show and tell," and there is a good deal of bickering between the sexes. The gang stage also helps the child learn cooperative behavior and strengthen masculine and feminine roles.

---

latency period   A time described by Freud that lasts through the elementary school years during which it was thought little sexual development occurred, although we now know much development does occur at this time.

4. *Heterosexual adult.* Beginning with the onset of puberty, children turn their attention to the opposite sex. Dating occurs at this time.

According to Freud, each of these stages of sexual development provides a foundation for the next stage. People with trouble at any one stage are said to be fixated or stuck at that stage. These people may proceed through other stages but will not completely and satisfactorily meet the tasks of the stage at which they are fixated. If, for example, a person is not given tenderness, physical comfort, and security during the self-love stage, that person may not develop the ability to be tender and caring. The person may not love himself or herself well enough to be able to love, or show love, to others.

Erikson

Erik Erikson (1963) divided life into eight stages, each of which requires the achievement of some task. This task is presented in the form of a crisis with which individuals must cope. These stages and their crises are as follows:

1. *Birth to age 1.* The crisis for an infant is of trust versus mistrust. Will he or she find that the world can be trusted, that parents will meet his or her needs, and so on?

2. *Ages 1 to 3.* The crisis is autonomy versus shame. The child discovers a mind and will of his or her own. A balance between autonomy and cooperation must be learned.

3. *Ages 3 to 5.* The crisis is initiative versus guilt. The child must be able to experiment while developing an emerging conscience.

4. *Ages 5 to 12.* The crisis is between industry and inferiority. Knowledge and skills are developing rapidly, and the child loves recognition but is sensitive to criticism. Too much criticism or difficulty in acquiring knowledge and skills could result in a feeling of inferiority.

5. *Ages 12 to 17.* The crisis during the adolescent years is between identity and confusion. This is the period of time when a sense of identity is developed. The person develops this sense of identity or feels confusion (termed **identity diffusion** by Erikson).

6. *Ages 17 to 22.* The crisis is intimacy versus isolation. Intimacy pertains to closeness with friends as well as with the opposite sex. A failure to develop intimate relationships can result in isolation and alienation.

Insight 6-1

Stages of Sexual Development

To consider your own present stage of sexual development, take a moment to answer the following questions:

1. At which one of Erikson's stages are you?

2. How is the crisis of this stage manifesting itself?

3. How do you expect this crisis to be resolved?

4. What form do you expect the crisis of the next stage to take?

---

7. *Middle adult years.* The crisis is generativity versus self-absorption. Will one develop a concern beyond oneself (such as parenthood or a cause)? Or will one seek satisfaction of one's selfish needs?

8. *Older adult years.* The crisis is integrity versus despair. One who successfully copes with this crisis develops a feeling of continuity with those who have come before and those who will come after. He or she identifies with all of humanity. A failure to resolve this conflict successfully may result in a sense of despair, a feeling that life has been useless.

The sexuality educator should recognize the particular stage of psychosexual development at which the learners are at the time of instruction. In this way, the educational process can be geared to the needs of the learners.

Social Learning Theory

Another explanation of the development of sexual attitudes and behaviors may be found in the **Social Learning Theory.** Based on the work of Kurt Lewin (1935) and Julian Rotter (1954), and more recently Albert Bandura (1977, 1986), Social Learning Theory states that reinforcements that occur in society shape attitudes and behaviors. If you behave in a loving way and receive love in return, you are likely to continue behaving lovingly toward people. However, if you behave lovingly but receive ridicule from friends, it is less likely that you will soon behave that way again.

Social learning goes on to suggest that as children, and even as adults, we learn by modeling our behavior on other people. If our parents demonstrate affection for one another

---

identity diffusion   The state of confusion when one does not have a clear sense of one's strengths, values, and other important components of one's makeup.

Social Learning Theory   A theory of human behavior that states societal rewards and punishments shape attitudes and behaviors.

and if they openly kiss and hug, we learn to behave similarly—especially if we observe positive consequences for their behavior. However, if one parent demonstrates affection and the other rejects it, we might learn to avoid rejection by withholding expressions of affection. Adults, too, experience "vicarious learning" in this manner by observing the consequences of various sex-related behaviors and expressions of attitudes.

Self-Esteem and Sexual Maturity

Theorists and researchers who study psychosexual development generally agree that **self-esteem** is the most significant variable in sexual maturation.

How is self-esteem related to sexual maturity? If you have high self-esteem, you feel good about your assets and limitations; you accept who you are. If, during your early years, you do not or cannot deal satisfactorily with the stages of psychosexual development, you may develop a negative image of yourself. For example, if you do not receive tender love, you may conclude that you are not worthy of love. If you receive too much criticism during what Erikson calls the industry versus inferiority stage, you may develop the belief that you are inferior.

Guilt may also affect sexual behavior. McCary (1982, 107) went so far as to state that "the more guilt a young person feels about his sexual behavior, the more restricted is his level of intimacy in premarital sexual experiences." Erikson referred to guilt as interfering with the tasks of a major stage of human development, and Freud regarded guilt feelings as the cause of many psychological difficulties. Masturbatory behavior has been said to be harmless *except* for the psychological harm from guilt that may be associated with it.

In an article written for physicians, Burchell (1975), a physician himself, described the relationship between self-esteem and sexuality. He stated that low self-esteem weakens relationships, whereas high self-esteem "provides a foundation for risk taking and growth that is nurturing to any relationship." Burchell believed that much sexual malfunction is a result of low self-esteem. Freedom to *receive* pleasure, to *acknowledge* individual sexual tastes and pleasures, to *search* for individual sexual tastes and desires, and to help *satisfy* one's sexual tastes and desires requires, according to Burchell, high self-esteem.

Self-esteem affects women in our society somewhat differently than it affects men. Our culture values attractiveness and the "ideal" body shape. The vast majority of women cannot match up to this image and develop less confidence in themselves as a result. Self-esteem has been described as "intimately related to what others think of us, and if we fail

to impress others, we lose esteem in our own eyes" (Sabini, 1992, 251). One unfortunate consequence of low self-esteem in young women is the development of eating disorders (Pettijohn, 1992). Disorders such as bulimia and anorexia nervosa are caused by various attitudes. Among these is the attempt by women to control their body shapes and mold them into their perception of the ideal.

It follows that the sexuality educator's responsibility is to provide a learning environment conducive to the development of high self-esteem. There have been books written to help you do this (Greenberg, 1998), and specific instructional strategies are discussed in Chapter 12 of this book. For now, we hope you recognize the importance of this variable in sexual maturation. Self-esteem is the master key that can unlock psychosexual maturation, thereby opening the door to the actualization of one's human sexuality potential.

Sexual Attitudes and Behavior

Sexual attitudes are developed throughout life through experimentation and reinforcement. Newborns are dressed in colors denoting their gender (blue for males, pink for females), children play "I'll show you mine if you'll show me yours" games and engage in autoerotic genital play, while teenagers engage in group masturbation. Attitudes are formed as a result of experiences like these as well as from knowledge. Cognitive knowledge and facts lead us to believe, for example, that loving someone can be demonstrated through physical contact such as hugging, kissing, and hand-holding. We might try this knowledge out in the real world by demonstrating our love for someone in these ways. We choose a loved one, hold and kiss that person, and the good feelings of acceptance, caring, and love we experience reinforce the attitude that physical contact between loved ones is appropriate. As a consequence, we are apt to demonstrate our love in these ways again.

Unfortunately, the relationship between attitudes and behaviors is not always so well defined. Although an attitude is a predisposition to behave in a particular way, we often behave differently. For example, people who risked showing affection in infancy but were rejected, or those who as infants explored their genitalia and were scolded for it, might hesitate to express affection physically as adults. Think of all those who have the attitude that conception should be a planned event and yet do not use some method of contraception during coitus. Or consider those men who believe that there should be equality of the sexes but who require their wives to stay home, clean house, and raise the children. The problem appears to be that we have many, many attitudes and that some of them contradict others. When our attitudes are in

---

self-esteem How highly or positively you regard yourself.

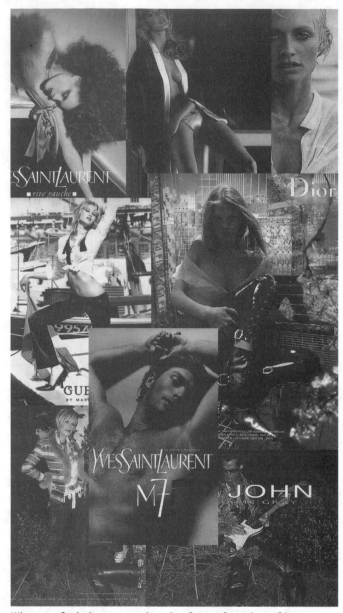

What we feel about ourselves is often a function of how advertisers depict the ideal person. Do these ads reflect your ideal man or woman, or do you depict the ideal to be more multidimensional?

conflict, we choose the most important attitude to manifest in behavior. The husband who believes in equality of the sexes, for example, might also believe that children need a full-time mother with whom to interact in order to grow up emotionally healthy.

The sexuality educator's role is to help learners identify their attitudes and values. With their attitudes and values clarified, people are more likely to make sexual decisions that are suited to their needs and interests than otherwise might be the case. Attitudes and values can be clarified through large-group, small-group, and introspective learning strategies, which are described in Chapter 12. The purpose of such

educational experiences is to help learners clarify *their* attitudes and values so that they may choose sexual behaviors consistent with those attitudes and values; the purpose is not to instill a particular predetermined attitudinal or value structure in learners.

There are several influences on attitudinal development. Parents play a major role by serving as role models to emulate. Females identify with mothers, males with fathers (or other same-sex role models) and develop attitudes accordingly. Parental influence is particularly important in one's early years, since contact with societal institutions and other people is limited at that time. Schools socialize students and play a major role in attitudinal development as well. Siblings and peers are significant to the development of attitudes by serving, like parents, as role models. Attitudes and even behaviors of peers are adopted throughout one's life. However, as parental influence wanes sometime during adolescence, peer influence takes on added significance. Effective sexuality educators will aid learners in sorting through and making sense of these influences on attitudinal development so that their sexual decisions can be more sensibly arrived at.

Sex-Role Stereotyping

Years ago (Centers, 1971), college students were asked which abilities and aptitudes were desirable for males and which for females. They listed the following as desirable for males:

- Athletic ability
- Mechanical ability
- Leadership
- Economic ability
- Observational ability
- Intellectual ability
- Scientific understanding
- Theoretical ability
- Common sense
- Achievement and mastery
- Occupational ability

They cited the following for females:

- Social ability
- Interpersonal understanding
- Art appreciation
- Art-creative ability

- Moral-spiritual understanding
- Domestic ability
- Affectional ability
- Sartorial ability (dress nicely)
- Physical attractiveness

According to these students, males and females ought to possess very different kinds of abilities. Traditionally, these abilities have defined male and female sex roles in Western culture. Categorizing men and women according to these traditional roles is called **sex-role stereotyping.** Do you think college students of today would respond similarly? Before proceeding further, complete the exercise in Insight 6-2.

Archer, Kimes, and Barrios (1978) found that subjects asked to draw pictures of men and women tend to draw men with faces that are almost twice as prominent as women's faces. These researchers also studied magazine photographs from stories and advertisements and found that publications emphasize the faces of men and the bodies of women. These researchers drew the following conclusions:

If the unique qualities of men are associated with the face, with its lively features and nearness to the brain, these qualities are likely to be conceptualized in terms of personality or intellect. If the unique qualities of women are associated with the body, these qualities are likely to be conceptualized in more physical terms, such as weight, physique, and general attractiveness.

Did your drawings indicate any sex-role stereotyping on your part? Would you describe the abilities and aptitudes desirable for males and females as those above? Do not be surprised if you answered yes to these questions, since sex-role stereotyping is quite pervasive.

There are some significant disadvantages of sex-role stereotyping. One obvious disadvantage is that people are limited in their lifestyle options. Males are expected to be mechanics, females nurses. Male nurses and female mechanics, though they exist, are rare and might be viewed with suspicion. Sex-role stereotyping limits other options as well. For example, men are not supposed to cry and women are not supposed to be independent. Women must be nurturing, emotional, passive; men must be dominant, aggressive, competitive, and rational.

Women have experienced significant changes within the past 40 years. For example, more and more women are working outside the home. In 1998, there were 52.4 million women in the workforce (U.S. Census Bureau, 1999). In addition, more women today are in powerful positions at work. For example, 49% of the professional, managerial, and administrative workforce are women (Greenberg, Bruess & Haffner, 2004, 207). Furthermore, 86% of Fortune 500 companies have at least one woman board member (Wellington, 1998).

In general, though, women have not faired well economically. The attitude that women work just for "pin" money, that they will get pregnant and leave, and that women are weak and get sick often (such as each month during menstruation) has worked against occupational equality for women. Of course, these allegations are all untrue, but they persist, and they influence female hiring, paying, and promotion practices.

The government keeps statistics on the workforce and has reported the following (U.S. Census Bureau, 1999):

1. The female workforce has risen from 27.5 million in 1970 to almost double that amount (52.4 million) in 1998, with an estimate of 57.6 million in 2006. Almost 60% of adult women were in the workforce in 1998.

Insight 6-2

Men/Women Drawings

In the space provided, draw a man on the left and a woman on the right.

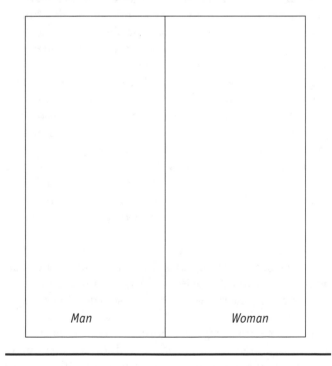

Man   Woman

---

sex-role stereotyping   Categorizing men and women according to highly defined traits and abilities.

2. Whereas 37% of women with children under 6 years of age were in the workforce in 1975, by 1998 that amount increased to 64%.

3. In 1998, of married couples with children under 6 years of age, 61% of mothers were employed. As children get older, more mothers join the workforce. Of married couples with children between the ages of 6 and 17, 74% of mothers were employed.

Causes of Sex-Role Stereotyping

There is agreement that society contributes to sex-role stereotyping. Girls are taught to be ladylike; boys are supposed to be rough and tough. Girls are supposed to be clean and neat; boys' play is expected to result in dirty clothes, faces, and hands. Girls may help mother set the dinner table; boys remain outside playing. Boys can call girls for dates; girls

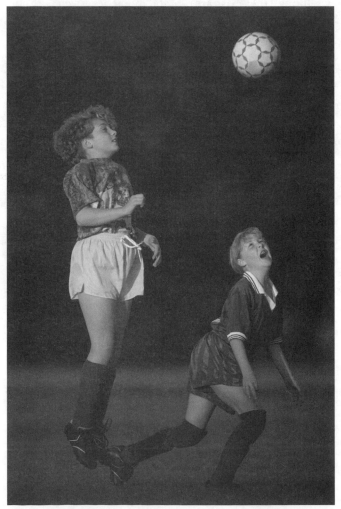

Legislation and government interpretation of that legislation have led to schools and colleges paying more attention to equal opportunity in sports. The results are intended to lead to more women whose talents are recognized and used.

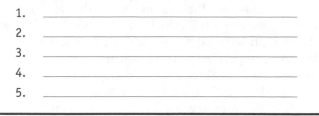

Schools and Sex-Role Stereotyping

Schools have been accused of contributing to sex-role stereotyping. List below ways in which you think schools are guilty, based on your own experiences or that of someone else you know.

1. _____
2. _____
3. _____
4. _____
5. _____

must wait by the telephone. Although this division between boy and girl behaviors is less prevalent today than in the past, it persists nonetheless.

The Decision to Engage in Sexual Intercourse

Many sexual decisions are a function of psychological considerations and needs. One of these is the decision of whether to engage in sexual intercourse. Some people seek coital connections *because they feel unloved* and want to have someone hold them, kiss them, and be close physically. These needs can be met in other ways, but sexual intercourse is often seen as the most physical demonstration of being loved. Others engage in coitus because of the *pleasant sensations* that sexual intercourse evokes. Still others are *attempting to be mature* and "adult" and see coitus as one form of adult expression. *Peer pressure* is certainly operative in many people's decisions to experience sexual intercourse. In a diary that one of your authors requires students to keep, several students have described the immense pressure they experienced from dormmates and friends to be "sexually active"—a euphemism for sexual intercourse. And *curiosity* motivates others to engage in coitus.

Whatever one's motivations, several other variables should be considered before the decision is made to be coitally active. For example, the age of the person is important. There is quite a difference between a 50-year-old deciding to experience sexual intercourse and an 11-year-old deciding the same. Related to age is the emotional maturity of the person. In addition, one's motivations and alternative means of satisfying those motivations are important. Other factors that need to be considered when deciding whether to engage in sexual intercourse include marital status, previous coital experience, morals, religious teachings, and (not the least of considerations) the chance of conception and the desire for the same. It is the sexuality educator's responsibility to help those enrolled in the program to recognize these factors and to process them in order to make a rational decision and one that will meet their needs.

Teenage Out-of-Wedlock Pregnancy

A word must be mentioned here of the high rate of pregnancies in unmarried teenage women. Although the rate of teenage pregnancies is alarming, it actually has been decreasing. In 1998, the birth rate for U.S. teenagers aged 15 to 19 was 51.1 births per 1,000 women, which was 2% lower than the rate in 1997. However, the actual number of births to teenage women increased from 483,220 in 1997 to 484,895 in 1998 due to the increase in the number of teenagers. Of these births to teenage women, 79% were to unmarried women. The percentage of teenage out-of-wedlock birth rates has steadily increased from 1950 (National Center for Health Statistics, 2000). Partially explaining this phenomenon are data that show that from the early 1970s to the early 1990s, teenagers became two-thirds less likely to marry before birth of a premaritally conceived child (Bachu, 1999). The U.S. teenage out-of-wedlock pregnancy rate is higher than other developed countries. The Alan Guttmacher Institute concluded that teenagers in these other countries do not engage in sexual intercourse later or less frequently than do American teenagers. Rather, the cause of the difference in rates, the Guttmacher staff concluded, is a result of the lack of sexual information (in particular about contraception) and a lack of emphasis on the importance of avoiding pregnancy. The Guttmacher researchers advised as follows:

> *Although the specific approaches vary from country to country, those approaches that increase the legitimacy and availability of contraception and sex education have been effective in reducing teenage pregnancy rates in other developed countries, and there is no reason to believe that such an approach would not be successful in the United States. (Yates, 1986, 46)*

Given that 54% of students in grades 9 to 12 report having experienced sexual intercourse, with almost 40% having had sexual intercourse in the month prior to the survey (Sexual behavior among high school students—United States, 1990; 1992), the risk of pregnancy among teens is understandably high. To compound this risk are data that indicate only 36% of teenagers can correctly identify the period during the menstrual cycle when women are most fertile (Reschovsky & Gerner, 1991). The Alan Guttmacher Institute conclusions are given greater weight when these data are considered.

The Decision to Marry

Another important decision is whether to marry. There are many attractions of marriage. *Marriage provides companionship.* It is nice to have someone committed to spending time with you and sharing important occasions in your life. *Marriage provides emotional security.* The intimate nature of the marital relationship can help alleviate the anxieties, fears, and insecurities people experience in today's society. *Marriage provides for a sexual outlet.* The knowledge that your sexual needs will be satisfied in a loving, caring relationship can be quite appealing. *Marriage can improve self-esteem.* Just knowing that you are worthy enough for someone else to marry can make you believe that you are an attractive, appealing, valuable person. *Marriage can provide financial security.* The addition of another wage earner, or someone who can earn money while you both contribute to the partnership by doing chores that would cost money to pay someone else to do, can make you more financially able to live the life you desire. *Marriage can legitimize reproduction.* If you want children and you believe that they will do best in a societally sanctioned family—a marriage—you might want to be married.

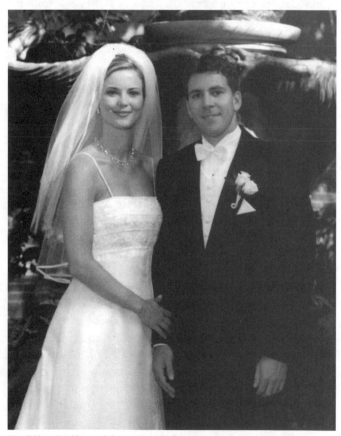

Deciding to live with someone for the rest of one's life should not be made emotionally or without considerable thought. Students should be helped to appreciate the level of commitment marriage entails.

Recognizing that marriage has many attractions, we should also recognize that not all marriages actualize these expectations. The high divorce rate evidences this fact. Furthermore, the single life also has many attractions. For example, singlehood provides for greater flexibility in career choices and goals, since moving from one city to another or working late may not affect other people as much. Singlehood may also allow for variety in sexual partners, psychological and social autonomy, more time to spend with friends and outside groups (such as social or political organizations), and may prevent disappointment from a potentially unsatisfying and legally bound relationship—marriage.

The decision to marry should take these attractions into consideration—those of marriage and those of singlehood. The sexuality educator's role in this regard is to aid the program's participants to be aware of the factors that should enter into a sensible, rational decision regarding marriage.

The Decision to Have Children

Another important psychological aspect of sexuality education concerns the decision of whether to have children. Obviously, parenthood entails an important responsibility. Yet some enter parenthood without much thought as to what is actually involved. Children can serve many psychological needs. Recall that Erikson saw generativity as the major task of the middle adult years. One way to perpetuate oneself is through one's progeny. Parenthood can therefore serve this need of the middle adult years. For people who equate the ability to make a baby with their manhood or womanhood, parenthood might serve to verify their masculinity or femininity.

Those entering parenthood to perpetuate themselves or to prove their manhood or womanhood, or those who enter parenthood unintentionally, are in for a shock. The responsibilities of parenthood, like its joys, are immense. Consider the economic challenge. The amount of time and energy involved in parenting is also extensive and may involve an interruption of promising careers in order to attend to pregnancy and childrearing.

Table 6-1 presents some questions that the sexuality educator can employ to explore the impact of parenthood. Since it is reasonable to assume that those who conceive unwanted children will, as a rule, not be as prepared for parenthood (psychologically, physically, or financially) as those who plan pregnancies, sexuality educators need to incorporate the implications and consequences of unplanned pregnancy into sexuality education programs. It is unfortunate when children suffer for the mistakes or lack of foresight of parents. It would be nice if all pregnancies were planned and wanted—if people not wanting to be parents would abstain from coitus or use some method of contraception that they can accept. This practice might be expected

to result in fewer birth defects, less child abuse, fewer emotional problems for parents and children alike, and greater happiness in general.

The role of the sexuality educator is not to discourage parenthood but rather to encourage well-thought-out decisions as to whether to parent. One part of sexuality education programs, therefore, must be concerned with the responsibilities and benefits of parenthood *and* an exploration of the non-parenthood option. Should one choose parenthood, one must be willing to pay attention to that task. It is sad to become a parent and realize, too late, that one has not provided one's children with the attention they needed. Witness one parent's regrets (Anonymous, 1977):

My hands were busy through the day;
I didn't have much time to play
The little games you asked me to.
I didn't have much time for you.
I'd wash your clothes, I'd sew and cook,
But when you'd bring your picture book
And ask me please to share your fun
I'd say: "A little later, son."
I'd tuck you in all safe at night
And hear your prayers, turn out the light,
Then tip-toe softly to the door . . .
I'd wish I'd stayed a minute more.
For life is short, the years rush past . . .
A little boy grows up so fast.

No longer is he at your side
His precious secrets to confide.
The picture books are put away,
There are no longer games to play,
No good-night kiss, no prayers to hear . . .

That all belongs to yesteryear.
My hands, once busy, now are still.
The days are long and hard to fill.
I wish I could go back and do
The little things you asked me to.

Summary

In this chapter we began by describing three theories of psychosexual development. Freud's four stages of psychosexual development are self-love, parental identification, gang, and heterosexual adult. Erik Erikson defined eight life stages and particular crises to be met at each stage that are related to psychosexual development. Lewin, Rotter, and Bandura viewed attitudes and behavior dependent on social reinforcement—either directly or vicariously. They called their theory Social Learning Theory.

Self-esteem is the most important factor in a person's sexual maturity. The sexuality educator's role is to provide a learning environment conducive to the development of

Table 6-1 Are You Parent Material?

Does having and raising a child fit the lifestyle I want?

1. What do I want out of life for myself? What do I think is important?

2. Could I handle a child and a job at the same time? Would I have time and energy for both?

3. Would I be ready to give up the freedom to do what I want to do, when I want to do it?

4. Would I be willing to cut back my social life and spend more time at home? Would I miss my free time and privacy?

5. Can I afford to support a child? Do I know how much it takes to raise a child?

6. Do I want to raise a child in the neighborhood where I live now? Would I be willing and able to move?

7. How would a child interfere with my growth and development?

8. Would a child change my educational plans? Do I have the energy to go to school and raise a child at the same time?

9. Am I willing to give a great part of my life—AT LEAST 18 YEARS—to being responsible for a child? And spend a large portion of my life being concerned about my child's well being?

What's in it for me?

1. Do I like doing things with children? Do I enjoy activities that children can do?

2. Would I want a child to be "like me"?

3. Would I try to pass on to my child my ideas and values? What if my child's ideas and values turn out to be different from mine?

4. Would I want my child to achieve things that I wish I had, but didn't?

5. Would I expect my child to keep me from being lonely in my old age? Do I do that for my parents? Do my parents do that for my grandparents?

6. Do I want a boy or a girl child? What if I don't get what I want?

7. Would having a child show others how mature I am?

8. Will I prove I am a man or a woman by having a child?

9. Do I expect my child to make my life happy?

Raising a child? What's there to know?

1. Do I like children? When I'm around children for a while, what do I think or feel about having one around all of the time?

2. Do I enjoy teaching others?

3. Is it easy for me to tell other people what I want, or need, or what I expect of them?

4. Do I want to give a child the love (s)he needs? Is loving easy for me?

5. Am I patient enough to deal with the noise and the confusion and the 24-hour-a-day responsibility? What kind of time and space do I need for myself?

6. What do I do when I get angry or upset? Would I take things out on a child if I lost my temper?

7. What does discipline mean to me? What does freedom, or setting limits, or giving space mean? What is being too strict, or not strict enough? Would I want a perfect child?

8. How do I get along with my parents? What will I do to avoid the mistakes my parents made?

9. How would I take care of my child's health and safety? How do I take care of my own?

10. What if I have a child and find out I made a wrong decision?

Have my partner and I really talked about becoming parents?

1. Does my partner want to have a child? Have we talked about our reasons?

2. Could we give a child a good home? Is our relationship a happy and strong one?

3. Are we both ready to give our time and energy to raising a child?

4. Could we share our love with a child without jealousy?

5. What would happen if we separated after having a child, or if one of us should die?

6. Do my partner and I understand each other's feelings about religion, work, family, child raising, future goals? Do we feel pretty much the same way? Will children fit into these feelings, hopes, and plans?

7. Suppose one of us wants a child and the other doesn't? Who decides?

8. Which of the questions listed here do we need to really discuss before making a decision?

Source: Are You Parent Material? Copyright © National Alliance for Optional Parenthood Washington, DC.

positive self-worth. The exploration of feelings of guilt and their relationship to self-esteem should also be a part of sexuality education.

The development of sexual attitudes is an important topic in sexuality education. Attitudes are developed as a result of cognition and experience. The relationship between attitudes and behavior, however, is inconsistent. Some attitudes are not expressed behaviorally; when contradictory attitudes are present in the same person, some attitudes are given priority and the person acts on the most important ones. The sexuality educator's role is to help learners clarify their sexual attitudes and values and determine which have priority.

Both evidence and causes of sex-role stereotyping should be explored in sexuality education. Sex-role stereotyping limits options (occupational and otherwise) for women and is also disadvantageous for men. Sexuality educators should help learners explore the consequences, both positive and negative, of sex-role stereotyping. Such exploration should result in sex-role stereotyping that is only employed for beneficial purposes (if it is useful at all), rather than remaining merely because of tradition and habit.

Finally, the significance of parenthood should be recognized in sexuality education. Sexuality education should include the study of the financial, psychological, physical, and sociological implications of parenthood, as well as the study of nonparenthood as an alternative lifestyle.

Sexuality depends to a very large extent on psychological factors. Experts in the field may disagree on how much of our sexuality is learned and how much is innate. However, they will agree that a good deal of sexuality is actually learned behavior. The theories of psychosexual development described in this chapter help explain the relationship between psychological factors and sexuality, as do the concepts of self-esteem, attitude development, and sex-role stereotyping.

References

Anonymous. To My Grown-up Son. Appeared in Ann Landers' column, *Buffalo Evening News* (August 6, 1977). Copyright News America Syndicate. Used by permission.

Archer, D., Kimes, D. D. & Barrios, M. Face-ism, *Psychology Today* (September 1978), 65–66.

Bachu, A. Trends in premarital childbearing: 1930 to 1994, *Current Population Reports*, ser. P-23, no. 197 (1999).

Bandura, A. Human agency in social cognitive theory, *American Psychologist*, 37 (1986), 1175–82.

———. *Social learning theory*. Englewood Cliffs, NJ: Prentice Hall, 1977.

Burchell, R. C. Self-esteem and sexuality, *Medical Aspects of Human Sexuality*, 9 (1975), 74–90.

Centers, R. Evaluating the loved one, *Journal of Personality*, 39 (1971), 311.

Erikson, E. *Childhood and society*. New York: W. W. Norton, 1963.

Greenberg, J. S. *Health education: Learner-centered instructional strategies*. Boston: WCB/McGraw-Hill, 1998.

Greenberg, J. S., Bruess, C. E. & Haffner, D. W. *Exploring the dimensions of human sexuality*. 2nd ed. Boston: Jones and Bartlett, 2004.

Lewin, K. *A dynamic theory of personality*. New York: McGraw Hill, 1935.

McCary, J. L. *Human sexuality*. 4th ed. Belmont, CA: Wadsworth Publishing, 1982.

National Center for Health Statistics. Variations in teenage birth rates, 1991–98: National and state trends, *National Vital Statistics Report*, 48 (2000), 1–2.

Pettijohn, T. F. *Psychology: A concise introduction*. 3rd ed. Guilford, CT: The Dushkin Publishing Group, 1992.

Reschovsky, J. & Gerner, J. Contraceptive choice among teenagers: A multivariate analysis, *Lifestyles: Family and Economic Issues*, 12 (1991), 171–91.

Rotter, J. B. *Social learning and clinical psychology*. Englewood Cliffs, NJ: Prentice Hall, 1954.

Sabini, J. *Social psychology*. New York: W. W. Norton, 1992.

Sexual behavior among high school students—United States, 1990, *Morbidity and Mortality Weekly Report*, 40 (January 3, 1992), 885–87.

U. S. Census Bureau. *Statistical abstracts of the United States, 1999*. Washington, DC: U.S. Government Printing Office, 1999.

Wellington, S. Cracking the ceiling, *Time*, 152 (1998), 187.

Yates, S. U.S. far exceeds other nations in teen pregnancy, *Health Link*, 2 (1986), 45–46.

Suggested Readings

Francoeur, R. T. *The international encyclopedia of sexuality*. Herndon, VA: Continuum Publishing Company, 1999.

Gibbs, N. The war against feminism, *Time* (March 9, 1992), 5–55.

The impact of adolescent pregnancy and parenthood on educational achievement: A blueprint for education policymakers' involvement in prevention efforts. Washington, DC: National Association of State Boards of Education, 2000.

Johnson, D. R. & Booth, A. Marital quality: A product of the dyadic environment or individual factors? *Social Forces*, 76 (1998), 883–904.

Luker, K. *Dubious conceptions: The politics of teenage pregnancy*. Cambridge, MA: Harvard University Press, 1997.

Pollock, K. *Statistics on safe haven laws*. New York: Child Welfare League of America, 2001.

Schone, B. & Weinick, R. Health-related behaviors and the benefits of marriage for elderly persons, *The Gerontologist*, 38 (1998), 618–627.

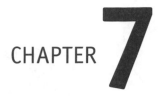

CHAPTER 7

Family Life and Interpersonal Relationships

Key Concepts

1. Sexuality education and family-life education are inseparable.

2. Dating serves many purposes.

3. Cohabitation is increasing.

4. Marriage is staying the same, yet changing.

5. The family is evolving.

6. Parenting is a skill that can be learned.

Sexuality Education and Family-Life Education

Once again we return to the theme of this book: sexuality refers to who and what one *is* rather than to what one *does*. Consequently, sexuality education must include a study of one's roles as a family member and of the intimacies these roles require. Notice that the word *roles* is pluralized. Consider your own family roles. Sometimes you act as a brother or sister, other times as a son or daughter; you may be a parent, a grandchild, and so forth. Before reading further, complete Insight 7-1.

Family roles are only one type of role that you play. Some of you are students, some of you are girlfriends or boyfriends, some are workers (waiters, resident advisors, and so forth), and still others may be athletes or student-government representatives; some may even be leaders in the community. You can probably add many more roles to this list. Let us now, though, concentrate on the family roles you listed in Insight 7-1. As with other roles in your life, you are very good at some, while you recognize the need for improvement in others. Choose one family role on your list that you would like to perform better. Let us now demonstrate how family-life education, an integral component of sexuality education, can help *you* improve *your functioning* as a family member for the role you judge needs improvement.

Insight 7-1

Family Roles

List as many of the family roles as you can think of that you play:

_____

_____

_____

_____

_____

_____

Did you include cousin in your list? Some very close relationships can develop between cousins; they can even become marriages, as was the case with Franklin and Eleanor Roosevelt. Did you include aunt, uncle, nephew, or niece? Did you include *close friend* in your listing? How many times have we heard "They're like sisters to one another" or "He spends so much time at our house, he's like one of the family"? The relationship between close friends often includes the degree of intimacy expected in family relationships. In fact, in some families in which intimacy and communication are at a minimum, close friends are the only ones who can provide the support one needs.

Conflict Resolution

We are willing to bet that most if not all of you have chosen a role for which a better ability to resolve conflicts would be a valuable asset. There are several problems that arise when people try to settle arguments: lack of listening, insistence on winning, inability to demonstrate understanding of the other person, and rigidity that prevents consideration of alternative solutions. Consider the following conversation:

Paul:　　*Well, Barbara, as you know, Thanksgiving vacation is coming soon, and I'd like you to come home with me and spend it with my family.*

Barbara: Now you ask! I've already told my folks to expect us for Thanksgiving dinner!

Paul: You've got some nerve! You didn't even ask me if I wanted to go to your house for Thanksgiving.

Barbara: Ask you? You've been studying so much lately that I've hardly seen you long enough to say hello, much less ask you to Thanksgiving dinner.

Paul: What would you rather I do, fail my courses? You're pretty selfish, aren't you?

Barbara: I've had it! Either we're going to my house for Thanksgiving, or you can say good-bye right now.

Paul: In that case, good-bye!

Here is a situation in which both Paul and Barbara are trying to win. That is, they are both trying to get the other to spend Thanksgiving vacation with their own families. However, neither Paul nor Barbara can win in this example. You see, they have three choices presented to them, either overtly or implied: (1) spend the vacation at Paul's house, (2) spend the vacation at Barbara's house, or (3) break up their relationship.

If they decide to spend the vacation at Paul's, Barbara will have to cancel her plans with her family and put up with the inconvenience that would entail. Further, she might feel that her wishes are not very important in her and Paul's relationship. The bottom line is that she will resent being at Paul's for Thanksgiving. On the other hand, if they spend the vacation at Barbara's house, Paul will resent having to be there. He might feel that since he asked first, they should be at his house. Further, he might object to Barbara's assuming that she can make plans that include him without even bothering to consult him.

It becomes evident, then, that regardless of where they spend the vacation, one of them will be resentful. This resentment will probably result in a Thanksgiving vacation that is uncomfortable and unenjoyable for all concerned. In other words, no matter who wins, both really lose. They both wind up with a miserable vacation. The third possibility, dissolving the relationship, is obviously a no-win solution as well.

How might the decision as to where to spend Thanksgiving vacation have been better determined? Consider the following dialogue:

Paul: Well, Barbara, as you know, Thanksgiving vacation is coming soon, and I'd like you to come home with me and spend it with my family.

Barbara: Now you ask! I've already told my folks to expect us for Thanksgiving dinner!

Paul: You thought we would go to your house for Thanksgiving vacation?

Barbara: Yes, and my parents have already made preparations.

Paul: Your parents would be upset if we canceled Thanksgiving dinner with them?

Barbara: You bet! And I wouldn't want to be the one to have to tell them either!

Paul: You think that your parents would really hassle you if you didn't spend Thanksgiving with them?

Barbara: Yes.

Paul: Would you also feel embarrassed if you had to change plans that your parents thought were definite?

Barbara: Yes, I guess I would.

Paul: It sounds like you were really looking forward to our being together at your house and with your family this vacation.

Barbara: Yes, I really was.

Paul: I'm glad that you included me in your Thanksgiving plans, but I was really looking forward to spending this vacation together with you and with my family. I haven't seen my family for a while, and I know that they would really like you. Also, I'm a little bothered that you didn't consult me before making plans for the vacation.

Barbara: Gee, I guess you have some rights too. I'm sorry.

Paul: Well, let's see if there are some possibilities that we haven't considered.

Barbara: Maybe we could spend half the vacation at my house and half at yours.

Paul: Or perhaps we could invite your family to my house.

Barbara: How about staying here and not spending Thanksgiving with either of our families?

Paul: It seems like we have several possibilities. We could spend half of the vacation at each of our houses, but that would mean wasting a good part of the vacation in travel.

Barbara: It's not very realistic either to expect that my whole family would cancel their plans and go to your house.

Paul: At the same time, if we stayed here, both families would be disappointed. That would be cutting off our noses to spite our faces.

Barbara: Would it make sense to agree to spend this Thanksgiving vacation at one of our houses and the next vacation at the other's?

Paul: That seems sensible, and since you've already made plans, let's spend Thanksgiving at your house.

Barbara: OK. Remember, though, the next vacation will be at your house.

In this example, Paul followed a simple procedure for resolving interpersonal conflict. He began by using a technique called **active listening** or reflective listening. This technique requires the listener to paraphrase the words of the speaker so that the speaker knows that his or her meaning has been received. Further, it requires the listener to go beyond the words of the speaker and to paraphrase the feelings left unspoken. Note that Paul understood that Barbara would be embarrassed to have to cancel Thanksgiving vacation with her family even though she never explicitly stated that she would. The effect of the listener's reflecting back the speaker's words and thoughts is that the speaker becomes aware that the listener cares enough to really understand the speaker's views. Once the speaker appreciates this fact, he or she is likely to be more receptive to listening and understanding the listener's viewpoint. The net result is that both people not only understand each other's point of view better but are less insistent that their way is the only way.

The next step is to use brainstorming to explore alternative solutions; that is, to list all possible solutions prior to evaluating their appropriateness. Once all possible solutions are listed, each proposed solution can then be evaluated until one is decided upon. With this technique, it initially appears that no one wins. In fact, however, everyone wins. In our example, Paul will accompany Barbara to her house for Thanksgiving without being resentful. He will know that she now understands his need to be involved in their planning and that the next vacation is going to be spent with his family. Consequently, he will be better able to enjoy being with Barbara and her family. The vacation will be fun, and everyone will win.

The steps of this communication process, then, are as follows:

1. *Active listening.* Reflecting back to the other person his or her words and feelings.

2. *Identifying one's position.* Stating one's thoughts and feelings about the situation.

3. *Exploring alternative solutions.* Brainstorming other possibilities.

4. *Evaluating alternatives.* Deciding which work and which do not.

Communication

In addition to learning to resolve conflicts well, other communication skills will help you be a better family member—as well as improve your relationships in general.

Clarify Nonverbal Communication

When you participate in group activities, such as a class, notice the body posture of group members. During an interesting lecture or activity, most people will probably be leaning or

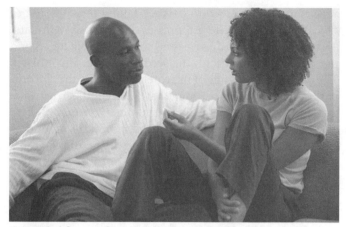

Nonverbal forms of communication, such as body postures and facial gestures, can convey thoughts. What do this couple's nonverbal signals communicate?

looking toward the lecturer or the center of the group, indicating that they are involved in what is going on. During a boring class, they will probably be leaning away from the lecturer or group. We call this physical behavior body language. Communicating by the posture of the body often says as much as the spoken word, and when people feel uncomfortable about expressing their thoughts or feelings verbally, body language is sometimes the only form of communication they participate in.

We all recognize the importance of communicating nonverbally, since we smile when we say hello, scratch our heads when perplexed, and hug a friend to show affection. (We also have an array of body terms to describe our nonverbal behavior: "Keep a stiff upper lip," "I can't stomach him," "She has no backbone," "I'm tongue-tied," "He caught her eye," "I have two left feet," "That was spine-tingling.") We show appreciation and affection, revulsion and indifference with expressions and gestures. We tell people we are interested in them merely by making eye contact and, like the male peacock displaying his feathers, we display our sexuality by the ways we dress and walk and even by how we stand.

Unfortunately, the nonverbal expression of feelings and thoughts is easy to misinterpret. Consequently, depending on nonverbal communication alone to express yourself is to risk being misunderstood. Furthermore, if another person is depending on nonverbal communication to express feelings to you, it is up to you to ask—verbally—whether you are getting the right message. Without such a reality check, the other person, while totally failing to connect, might assume that he or she is communicating effectively. For example, imagine that a couple on their first date begin hugging, kissing, and caressing each other after a movie. One partner's breathing

active listening Listening to a communication and then paraphrasing it when responding, also called reflective listening.

speeds up and the second partner, taking this as a sign of sexual arousal and interest, presses onward. When the first partner suddenly pushes free and complains that the second partner is too impatient, the second partner is confused. The problem here is one of interpretation rather than incompatibility: the rapid breathing that the second partner took as a sign of arousal was really a sign of nervousness. If these people had been more effective verbal communicators, they would have been able to clarify the situation in the beginning. Instead, they reached a silent impasse, with one confused and the other resentful. Check out your impressions of someone's nonverbal communication, and improve your communication by making your nonverbal and verbal messages as consistent as you can.

Plan Time to Talk

One common barrier to communication is the television set. We are often so busy watching it that we do not take the time to talk with those around us. In order to improve your communication with others, you may need to plan time for discussions. In setting up such times it is wise to follow some guidelines (Greenberg, Bruess & Mullen, 1993):

1. Make sure that you allow sufficient time to have a meaningful discussion.

2. Don't allow interruptions. Disconnect the phone and don't allow other people to barge in on you.

3. Accept all feelings and the right for the verbal expression of these feelings. For example, it is just as appropriate to say, "I feel angry when . . ." as it is to say, "I feel terrific when . . ."

4. Take a risk and really describe your thoughts and feelings. Don't expect the other person to guess what they are.

5. Approach your discussions with both of you understanding that the goal is to improve your relationship.

Listen

This aspect of communication seems obvious and yet, as was demonstrated when we discussed conflict resolution, it is often ignored. The listening and paraphrasing approach (active or reflective listening) is effective in regular conversation as well as during conflict. All of us can do a better job at listening. Try to pay more attention to this aspect of your communications.

Begin with Agreement

You would be surprised at how much better you can communicate with someone with whom you disagree if you start your message with a point on which you do agree. Of course,

this requires you to listen carefully, so that you can identify something with which you can agree. For example, if you are disagreeing about who should do the dishes, you might begin by saying "I agree that it is important that the dishes be cleaned. . . ." If you look and listen intently, you can always find a point of agreement.

Use "And," Not "But"

The word "but" is like an eraser; it erases everything that precedes it. When someone says, "Yes, your needs are important but . . ." they are saying, "Your needs may be important but let's forget about them because I'm about to tell you what's *really* important." In other words, the importance of your needs are being erased and now we can focus on the real issue. Listen to how people use the word "but" and you will get real insight into how people communicate. Listen to how *you* use "but"!

Substituting the word "and" for "but" is so simple and yet so significant. "And" leaves what preceded it on the table and *adds* something to it. "Your needs are important and . . ." means that we will not discount (erase) your needs; we will just consider them in addition to considering what will be presented next.

Use more "ands" and fewer "buts."

Use "I" Statements

Too often we try to get other people to behave or believe as we do. Others naturally resent that, as we do when others do it to us. Part of this problem relates to the words we use when communicating. Consider the example of a worker whose boss expects her to work on Saturdays. If she wanted to talk with her boss about this, she should not say, "When *you* expect me to work on Saturdays, I feel I'm being treated unfairly." Instead, she should use a statement such as, "When *I'm* expected to work on Saturdays . . ." In this manner she does not place the focus on the boss's behavior but on the situation and her feelings regarding that situation. Consequently, the boss need not get defensive, and they can better discuss and resolve the situation. When we say "you" we are making the other person feel that he or she is being criticized and needs to defend himself or herself. When we say "I" we are focusing on our feelings, beliefs, and interpretations. Feeling less defensive, the other person is more likely to listen to us and the result is more effective communication (Greenberg, Bruess & Haffner, 2000).

Avoid "Why" Questions

As with statements that include "you" instead of "I," questions that begin with "why" make the other person defensive. "Why did you leave so early?" makes the other person have to justify leaving early. In addition, "why" questions are often veiled criticisms. "Why don't you spend more time with me?" may be asked to get an answer but, more often than not, is a critical statement ("You don't spend enough time with me!") rather than a question. Avoid "why" questions.

Now you can use these techniques to improve your communication pattern so that you can better perform the family role you have identified as needing improvement. If you had been taught and had had the opportunity to practice these communication skills, wouldn't you be better at that family role?

The point is that if sexuality is who and what you are, and if part of what you are is a member of a family, sexuality education should give you learning experiences related to family life. There are many techniques for improving family interaction (see Chapter 12, Learning Strategies for Sexuality Education); this is but one such technique. These techniques should be practiced to be effective. One of the purposes of dating, for example, is to allow for trying out such things as conflict resolution skills and ways of improving communication.

Dating

Although sexuality educators may instruct both married and unmarried students as well as heterosexual and homosexual students, it is wise to include dating as a topic of study in sexuality education programs.

What purposes does dating usually serve in our society? First, dating is usually for fun. Dating occurs during recreational or leisure time and, therefore, is supposed to be enjoyed. In fact, all other things being equal, people do not usually date each other more than once if they do not enjoy being with each other.

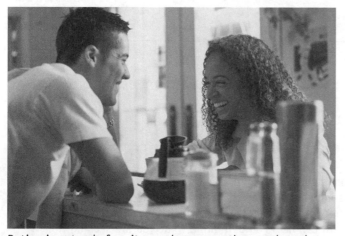

Dating is not only fun, it can also serve other needs such as providing recognition and enhancing self-esteem.

The question may then be asked, why *do* people who *do not* enjoy themselves on their first date sometimes date each other again? Recognizing that this situation occurs leads us to conclude that dating is designed for needs other than pure enjoyment. For example, people date for companionship. It is much more pleasant to be with someone during dinner than to be alone.

People also date for recognition and esteem. "I'll be the envy of all my friends," they think, "when they see me out with her/him."

People also date for sexual activity. They may believe that, since sexual activity is enjoyable, it is a good way to spend their recreational time.

People also date for love. Some seek love from another, and some seek to give love to another. Dating provides an opportunity intimate enough to allow for the practicing of these love responses.

Dating also provides the opportunity for intimacy in general. This intimacy may subsume many of the other reasons for dating. Physical intimacy, the intimacy present in love relationships, and the intimacy fostered through companionship all have closeness at their core. There are other reasons for dating (for example, to relieve boredom or because everyone else is doing it), but its major societal purpose is probably to provide people with the opportunity to practice seeking, nurturing, and improving intimate relationships.

It is important to note that some of these intimate relationships will result in marriages, whereas others will not. Dating, therefore, is not necessarily used as a preparation for marriage. Although this is a common belief, marriage is not always the goal people have in mind—effective relationship is. There are those who would argue that intimacy may be possible in a marriage relationship, but that it is lacking in many marriages. Conversely, they point to nonmarriage relationships that include a great deal of intimacy. Dating is useful for practicing a *relationship*, and that relationship may take varied forms, as we will see.

Cohabitation

Between 1970 and 1976, the number of people living together with someone of the opposite sex without marrying had doubled to 1.3 million people. In fact, until around 1970, **cohabitation** was illegal in all 50 states (Greenberg, Bruess & Haffner, 2004, 468). By 1997 it was reported that there were 4.1 million Americans cohabiting with someone of the opposite sex (National Center for Health Statistics, 1997) and another 1.5 million cohabiting with someone of the same sex (Miller & Solot, 1999). Women between the ages of

---

cohabitation   Living together with someone with whom a romantic involvement exists.

Insight 7-2

Dating Analysis

Complete the chart below for up to six people you have dated. List the names of your dates in the first column and then complete the rest of the information requested.

Name of Date	Where You Went	What You Enjoyed about the Place	What You Did Not Enjoy about the Place	What You Liked about the Person You Dated	What You Did Not Like about the Person You Dated

Now analyze your dating chart by attempting to generalize from the information included. For example, did you like dates who had a good sense of humor, or dates who could carry on an interesting conversation? Did you like to be with people at a place where talking was encouraged (such as over dinner), or did you prefer places where you and your date did not converse as easily (such as a noisy rock concert)? Your pattern can help you determine what you are seeking from a relationship. Are you seeking companionship, sexual activity, status (dating the most popular people), a possible marriage partner, or something else?

20 and 24 (112,000) are most likely to be currently cohabiting, with women between the ages of 25 and 29 (98,000) being the next most likely (U.S. Census Bureau, 1999, 59).

Cohabitation serves several useful purposes. Cohabitation is usually not viewed as a screening device for a future marriage. It is often considered something between a marriage and a dating relationship. Yet, as we have seen, large numbers of cohabitations result in marriage. It affords people the opportunity to have a "trial" marriage without the commitment a real marriage might entail. For older cohabitants, living together might provide companionship without a legal and financial commitment. In addition, it might provide them the companionship often sought when one's spouse dies and the grown children have busy lives of their own.

Cohabitation also provides an avenue to meet sexual needs and desires. In a classical study of cohabiting couples, Blumstein and Schwartz (1983) found that these couples had more frequent coitus than married couples, and that cohabiting women initiated sexual activity more often than did married women. These researchers also found only one-third of these cohabitants have sex with someone outside their relationship.

The increasing prevalence of cohabitation makes it a topic to which sexuality education programs and sexuality educators must address themselves. Such considerations as the religious and moral issues related to cohabitation, financial concerns, role definitions within such a relationship, problems arising from friends' and families' perceptions of living together, and what is involved in the breakup of these relationships should be incorporated into sexuality education curricula.

As you can see, living with someone may require a good deal of adjustment. The sexuality educator should help students to appreciate this fact of life.

Marriage

There are many aspects of marriage that have remained unchanged for centuries, and many others that have changed radically. June marriages are still the most popular, more adults still get married rather than remain single, marriage is still a legal entity requiring a marriage license and a marriage ceremony (either civil or religious), and more women still take their husbands' last names than do not.

On the other hand, marriage has changed considerably over the years. Although people of the same sex still cannot be legally married, some states recognize homosexual unions as a form of common-law marriage. In 1998, 110.6 million adults (56% of the adult population) were married and living with a spouse. Yet, a large number of adults are not married. Among people 25 to 35 years of age, over one-third (34.7%) have never been married. Marriage does not always work out. In 1998, 19.4 million people were currently divorced, representing almost 10% of the adult population. (U.S. Census Bureau, 1998).

How do you decide who to marry? And how can this decision be made so as to decrease the chance of divorce? These questions can be answered based on the research on marriage. However, this research is valid as it regards *groups* of people; so if you are looking for a formula a person can use to select a mate, there really is none. We do know, though, that marriages between people of similar characteristics and backgrounds are more likely to be successful. That is, people who are of the same religion, ethnic background, intelligence, physical attractiveness, and socioeconomic class are more likely to have a successful marriage than are people who differ on these variables. It stands to reason that the more people are alike, the less they will find to argue about; although being similar to a prospective mate does not guarantee that the relationship will be a good one. In any case, prospective mates should discuss their values, aspirations, sexual preferences, desire for children, who will be responsible for contraception, who will work outside the home, and numerous other important issues to determine how similar and compatible they are.

The Evolving Family

Today's family is somewhat different from the family of the past, and many of these differences can probably be attributed to our developing technological society. Think, for example, of the increased mobility of families today. In the past, people usually grew up in a city or town, probably married someone who grew up nearby, and settled down to live in that town for the remainder of their years. Nowadays, however, many adults are living far from where they grew up and from where their **extended families** (aunts, uncles, grandparents, and so on) are living. The **nuclear family** (a married couple and their children) may still be together (although the divorce rate leads one to question even this assumption), but the extended family is not. Family mobility can be partially attributed to the ease of travel and communication. By means of short airplane trips and relatively inexpensive long-distance telephone calls and e-mail, nuclear and extended families

---

extended family Family members other than a married couple and their children.

nuclear family A married couple and their children.

can still maintain communications. What is missing, however, is the day-to-day interaction that characterized the past. Where grandparents used to visit at least on the weekends, they now may visit only during some select holiday season.

There are those who have accused technology of doing *within* the nuclear family what it has done between the nuclear and extended families. These people would argue that, because of television, VCRs, and video and computer games, there is less communication among family members than in the past, and that, because of the automobile, there is a greater tendency for family members to engage in activities away from each other and the home. Even the changing role of women in society and the use of technological wizardry to release them from household chores, some suggest, has had a significant negative impact on family life.

Other changes have occurred in family life. The declining birthrate reflects the fact that families tend to be having fewer children. Similarly, the increasing life span has increased the number of elderly family members. Fewer children might result in less of parents' lives being devoted to childrearing and, consequently, in greater freedom to do other things. The increase in the number of elderly family members might mean just the opposite: less freedom because of the need to care for aged parents. This creates an interesting paradox, which some adults are solving by delegating care for elderly relatives to nursing-care facilities or homes for the aged. Others are choosing to care for the elderly at home.

New forms of family structure have emerged in response to societal, technological, and philosophical trends. First, many people are choosing not to marry and not to establish a nuclear family. Others who are marrying are choosing a childless lifestyle. They are making a conscious decision never to have children. Those choosing not to marry but to cohabit may be viewed as similar to those choosing to marry but to remain childless. However, there are some important distinctions between these two lifestyles; those marrying are making a greater commitment financially, legally, and familially than are those who are cohabiting.

Other family lifestyles have been tried. Over 30 years ago, Vance Packard described some of them in his book *The Sexual Wilderness* (1968). He wrote of **serial monogamy** as taking the place of traditional monogamy (marriage to only one person at any particular time) for many people. In serial monogamy, a person is married to only one person at one time, but divorces and marries several people in sequence. A glance at remarriage statistics shows that serial monogamy is not a far-fetched idea.

In many families, called dual-career families, both husband and wife work outside of the home, and both share household and childrearing responsibilities. Other families, as a result of divorce, separation, death of a spouse, or out-of-wedlock pregnancies are single-parent families. Such families are increasing in number and are becoming more feasible than in the past. Because the stigma of divorce has lessened and more jobs have been made available to women, single mothers are finding greater psychological and financial sets within which to function as a single parent.

Societal changes have led to new forms of families, or, at least, new versions of the old form. For example, many divorces occur in the United States, and many of these divorced people remarry. This often results in children from divorced families forming new families together with their remarried parents. These "blended families" bring with them various challenges. Sometimes there is jealousy for the affections of the parents. Squabbling sometimes occurs among the children, with some feeling disadvantaged. Further, the necessity to accommodate previous family rules and regulations into ones with which the new family feels comfortable requires special care.

Still another phenomenon occurring in today's families is the return of adult children to living with their parents after having lived on their own for a time. This is often the result of divorce or difficult economic times in which the children cannot be self-sufficient and live the lifestyle desired. These "boomerang" children also create challenges for the family. Having become accustomed to the freedom associated with living on their own, boomerang children usually must accept less privacy and assume more family responsibilities around the house.

Group families have also been attempted. Some of these experimental communities have taken the form of one large family, with household chores, financial responsibility, sexual behavior, childrearing, and so forth being shared. Others have taken on more of an extended family nature, with separate and distinct nuclear families sharing one roof and some duties and responsibilities. The latter type of group living arrangement has been termed a "cluster family."

In a contractual marriage, the partners agree to periodically renew their marriage contract. At the time for renewal, they renegotiate the contract or simply renew it for another time period. These contractual arrangements are legally binding as long as they do not contradict existing laws. Another type of contractual marriage is one in which the prospective marital partners agree to certain conditions upon which the marriage will be based. For example, the woman may agree to do the housecleaning and cooking, while the man may agree to work and help with the laundry and childrearing chores.

---

serial monogamy   The practice of marriage to one partner at any one time, but repeated divorces and remarriages.

In any case, experimentation with varied male-female liaisons is occurring. This experimentation appears to be the result of a growing number of people's dissatisfaction with presently existing family structures.

Parenting

Sexuality educators also need to direct students' attention toward parenting.

It is amazing to realize that one of the most significant roles some of us will ever play, that of parent, is one for which we receive so little preparation. True, we have all observed many parents—our own as well as others. It would be nice to think that such observation and experience would lead to our being better parents, that we would not repeat the mistakes of our parents, and therefore that each succeeding generation of parents would be better than their predecessors. Unfortunately, the evidence does not support this conclusion. Psychologists tell us that we identify with our parent of the same sex, modeling on his or her behavior. Parenting behavior is no exception to such identification. For example, parents who have been found to physically abuse their children tend to come from families in which they themselves were physically abused. And children from homes in which at least one parent was an alcoholic have a greater chance of becoming alcoholics themselves.

Lest there be confusion at this point, it should be noted that we are not destined to repeat the mistakes of our parents. It just seems that there is a tendency for this to happen. But there are also attempts being made to train parents to parent better. Organizations and individuals involved in parenthood education believe that people can be taught how to be better parents—that they need not repeat the mistakes of their parents but rather can learn from them.

Several organizations have developed parenthood education programs. The National Parent-Teachers Association (PTA) and the National Foundation/March of Dimes have joined to lobby for the inclusion of parenthood education as an integral part of the curriculum in public schools. As envisioned by these two organizations, a comprehensive parenthood education program, although needing to be custom-tailored to local needs, should include the following basic items:

1. Biological factors of reproduction
2. Genetics
3. Pregnancy, fetal development, and childbirth
4. Nutrition
5. Environmental hazards, including alcohol, cigarettes, and other drugs
6. Prenatal and postnatal care of mothers
7. Infant care
8. Child growth and development
9. Family structure and function
10. Parental roles and responsibilities
11. Family planning and population control
12. Community resources to aid in parenting

The Sexuality Information and Education Council of the United States formed a national task force to develop guidelines for comprehensive sexuality education. Among these guidelines are the following concepts to be presented during a sexuality education program (National Guidelines Task Force, 1991):

- Parenting children can be one of life's most rewarding responsibilities.

- People who have or adopt children are responsible for taking care of them.

- Parenting is an adult job.

- Parenting is a lot of work.

- People who decide to have children need to provide for them.

- People need information and skills to be good parents.

- Parents may not be able to do a good job of parenting because they have difficulties in their own lives.

- It can be a difficult job balancing job and parenting responsibilities.

- It is rewarding to raise a happy child.

- Parenting methods vary among cultures, but all parents must provide for their children's development.

- It is extremely difficult to be a teenage parent.

- For a teenager, parenting responsibilities can interrupt schooling, employment plans, social and family life.

- Deciding not to be a parent may be difficult because of societal pressure to have and raise children.

- As children grow, the nature of the parent/child relationship changes.

The communication and conflict resolution skills presented earlier can be used to improve the relationship between parent and child.

Most of the parenthood training programs have common goals: improved communication between parent and child, better recognition of each other's needs, and better ways of determining appropriate behavior for parent and child. In any case, parents can be taught to parent. They need not be

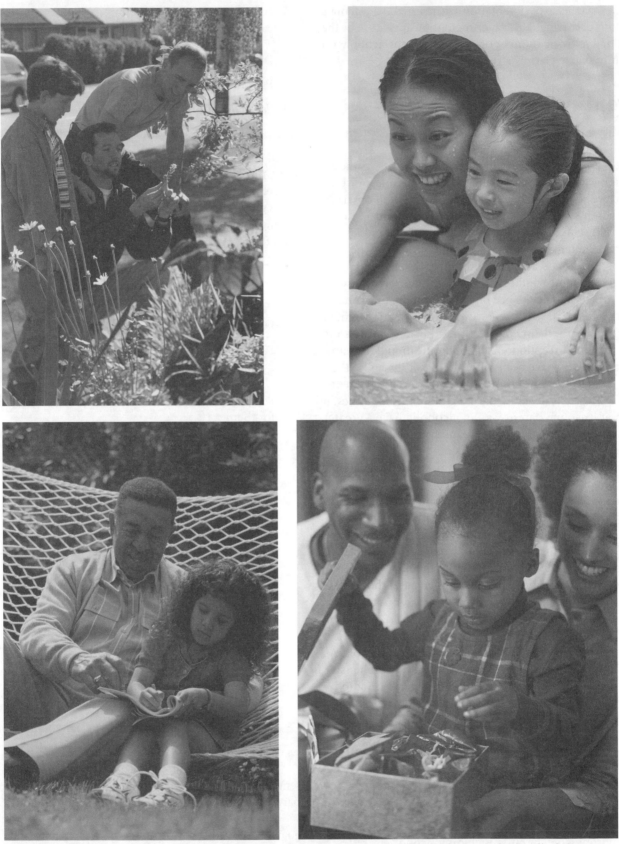

In today's society, one person's idea and experience of family can be very different from another's. All of these families have a positive role to play in shaping children's attitudes toward sexuality.

limited to the parenting style they learned from their parents. Individuals and organizations, both for-profit and non-profit, are mobilizing to respond to the need for parenthood education. Certainly, sexuality educators should be at the forefront of this movement.

Single-Parent Families*

Families with a single parent are becoming increasingly prevalent. According to the U.S. Census Bureau, the number of single-parent families doubled between 1970 and 1990, from 6% to 12% of all families. Between 1990 and 1999 it increased another percentage point. Almost 29% of children under age 18 live with a single parent. Among African-Americans 64% of children under age 18 live with a single parent (U.S. Census Bureau, 2000). More than 7.8 million children with a single parent live with their mother, and just over 1.7 million live with their father (Schmid, 1998). Most of the increase in single-parent families is as a result of marital separation, divorce, and out-of-wedlock pregnancies—rather than the death of one parent (Family composition begins to stabilize in the 1990s, Census Bureau reports, 1998).

Usually when we think of single-parent families, we think of them as being headed by women. Although this is generally true—about 82% of single-parent families are headed by women—the number of men heading such families is rising dramatically. For example, in 1990, 14% of single-parent families were headed by a man; in 1999, the comparable figure was 19%. Father-headed, single-parent families often place the father in a new role. We say often because nowadays more and more men in two-parent families are helping with what were previously considered to be the wife's household chores and responsibilities. For these husbands the adjustment to heading a single-parent family will be less difficult. They are used to cooking, cleaning, nurturing, and changing diapers. For the more traditional husband, the adoption of these necessary chores and responsibilities, added to the financial and emotional burdens of divorce, means that a more significant adjustment is required.

Life in a single-parent family can be stressful for the adult and the children. Members may unrealistically expect that the family can function as a two-parent family does and may feel that something is wrong if it cannot. The single parent may feel overwhelmed by the responsibility of caring for the children, maintaining a job, and keeping up with the bills and household chores. Typically, the family's finances and resources are drastically reduced following the parents' breakup.

Single-parent families deal with pressures and potential problem areas that the nuclear family does not have to face

(Single parenting and today's family, 1998):

- Visitation and custody problems

- The negative effects of continuing conflict between the parents

- Fewer opportunities for parents and children to spend time together

- Negative effects of the breakup on children's school performance and peer relations

- Disruptions of extended family relationships

- Problems caused by the parents' dating and entering new relationships

The demand for social services to meet the special needs of single-parent families is growing. Because single-parent families often have financial, psychological, custodial, and other needs that are more acute than those of conventional, two-parent families, they often need counseling or support groups. Many single parents have the added responsibility of providing role models for their children of the opposite sex. Day care, a virtual necessity (as it also is for many two-parent households) solves some problems, yet it may also be a source of anxiety, or at least concern, for financial, educational, psychological, or other reasons.

Although some of these research findings might seem discouraging—or they might seem wrong to readers who come from single-parent families—it is important to remember that these findings refer to trends in groups and have no bearing on particular individuals. Children from single-parent families are often very successful. Our intention here is to suggest that single parenthood does require special care and consideration. Perhaps most of all, the special needs of single-parent families should be understood both by family members themselves and by teachers, employers, and others with whom they interact. To meet this need for understanding, a group called Parents without Partners serves as a sounding board and a source of counsel for single parents.

The need for good parenting skills remains constant regardless of the parent's marital status. However, the situation can be more demanding for both the parents and children in single-parent households. The following are some suggested guidelines:

1. Be honest with your children about the situation that caused you to become a single parent.

2. In case of a separation or divorce, assure children that they are not responsible for the breakup of the relationship.

---

*Jerrold S. Greenberg, Clint E. Bruess, and Debra W. Haffner. *Exploring the Dimensions of Human Sexuality.* 2nd ed. (Boston: Jones and Bartlett, 2004), 484–87.

3. Try to maintain as much of the same routine as possible.

4. Do not try to be both mother and father to the children. Establish a family atmosphere of teamwork.

5. In the case of divorce, acknowledge that the relationship between you and your former partner is over, and do not encourage your children to hope for reconciliation.

6. Reassure children that they will continue to be loved and cared for (by both parents, if true).

7. Do not use children to gain bargaining power with a separated or divorced spouse.

8. Encourage relatives to help children maintain a sense of belonging to a continuing family.

Summary

Sexuality education and family-life education are inseparable. Because sexuality involves who and what you are, it definitely includes your role as a family member. You can improve your family life by improving communications. For example, you can try to solve conflicts by actively listening, presenting your point of view, identifying possible solutions, and then choosing one of the solutions to be implemented. When this method of problem solving is used, both people feel satisfied with the solution—a result not usually found in such conflict situations.

Family members can also learn to communicate better with each other. Paying attention to nonverbal communication, planning time to talk, listening well, beginning with points of agreement, using "and" instead of "but," using "I" statements, and avoiding "why" questions will all help improve communication among family members.

Dating meets many needs, including needs for fun, sex, love, intimacy, recognition, and self-esteem. Of these, the need for intimacy probably predominates, since it is a part of many of the other needs. In addition, dating helps in the practice of and improvement of relationship skills.

A practice becoming more frequent is cohabitation—two unrelated people of the opposite sex living together without being married. Cohabitation is practiced by the elderly as well as by young adults and college students. Sexuality educators should include in their programs consideration of the religious and moral issues, practical issues, and psychological issues relevant to cohabitation.

Marriage and divorce are changing. It is still true that more adults marry than do not, homosexuals still cannot be legally married, and a marriage license must be issued by the state for a marriage to be legal. On the other hand, approximately one-third of 25- to 35-year-olds have never been married, some states recognized unions between homosexuals as a form of common-law marriage, and at last count, only 56% of adults were living with a spouse. In 1998, 19.4 million Americans were currently divorced, and these divorces involved a large number of children. In 2000, almost 29% of children under 18 years of age were living with one parent.

Alternative family lifestyles have developed in recent years. There has been a change from a focus on the extended family to a focus on the nuclear family. This change has been a result of our technological society. Dual-career families, cluster families, blended families, contractual marriages, serial monogamy, and single-parent lifestyles are among current experiments in family life.

There are now parenthood education programs that teach parenting skills, with emphasis on improving communication between parent and child and developing better ways of determining appropriate behavior for parents and children. Parenthood education programs of nonprofit organizations as well as for-profit programs are proliferating.

Family life, then, is an integral part of sexuality education and should include, though not be limited to, such topics as dating, cohabitation, marriage, divorce, roles of family members, and parenting.

References

Blumstein, P. W. & Schwartz, P. *American couples.* New York: William Morrow, 1983.

Greenberg, J. S., Bruess, C. E. & Haffner, D.W. *Exploring the dimensions of human sexuality.* 2nd ed. Boston: Jones and Bartlett, 2004.

———, Bruess, C. E. & Mullen, K. D. *Sexuality: Insights and issues.* Dubuque, IA: William C. Brown Communications, 1993.

Miller, M. & Solot, D. *Organization for unmarried people condemns cohabitation report.* February 8, 1999.

National Center for Health Statistics. Fertility, family planning, and women's health: New data from the 1995 National Survey of Family Growth, *Vital and Health Statistics*, 23, no. 19 (1997).

National Guidelines Task Force. *Guidelines for comprehensive sexuality education.* New York: Sexuality Information and Education Council of the United States, 1991.

Packard, V. *The sexual wilderness.* New York: David McKay, 1968.

Schmid, R. E. Unmarried couples top 4 million, AP/AOL (July 27, 1998).

Single parenting and today's family, American Psychological Association, 1998.

U.S. Census Bureau. Family composition begins to stabilize in the 1990s, 1998.

U.S. Census Bureau. Marital status and living arrangements: March 1998 (update), *Current Population Reports*, ser. P20, no. 514 (1998).

U.S. Census Bureau. *Statistical abstracts of the United States, 1999.* Washington, DC: U.S. Government Printing Office, 1999.

U.S. Census Bureau. *Statistical abstracts of the United States, 2000,* p. 58. Washington, DC: U.S. Government Printing Office, 2000.

Suggested Readings

Dornbusch, S. M., Herman, M. R. & Lin, I. Single parenthood, *Society,* 33 (1996), 30–32.

Howell, S. H., Portes, P. R. & Brown, J. H. Gender and age differences in child adjustment to parental separation, *Journal of Divorce and Remarriage,* 27 (1997), 141–58.

Hoyt, C. 22 minutes to a better marriage, *McCalls,* 124 (1997), 124ff.

Morrow-Kondos, D., Weber, J. A., Cooper, K. & Hesser, J. L. Becoming parents again: Grandparents raising children, *Journal of Gerontological Social Work,* 28 (1997), 35–46.

Popenoe, D. & Whitehead, B. D. The state of the Union 2000: The social health of marriage in America. Rutgers, NJ: The National Marriage Project, 2001.

Treas, J. & Giesen, D. Sexual infidelity among married and cohabiting Americans, *Journal of Marriage and the Family,* 62 (2000), 48–60.

The Sociological Side of Sexuality

CHAPTER 8

Key Concepts

1. People of all ages, types, and conditions are sexual beings.

2. There are now a wide variety of lifestyle possibilities related to sexuality.

3. Sexuality and the law are related in several ways.

In this chapter we briefly examine the relationship between sexuality and a number of social topics. The person working in a sexuality education program needs an awareness of the relationship between sexuality and various social issues, since they have numerous educational implications. For example, it has traditionally been thought that sexuality education should begin when young people reach the stage of puberty, neglecting the fact that people are sexual beings from the day of birth. Is it not logical that society address the educational needs of younger sexual beings?

As we will soon see, the educational needs of other groups—older people, those of different races, physically disabled, individuals with cognitive defects, and ill people—have also been neglected. In addition, there has been in our society a lack of understanding of various sexual lifestyles and many confusions about the relationship between sexuality and legality. These are all social issues of which those working with sexuality education programs need greater awareness. We hope to increase awareness with our discussion of the sociological side of sexuality.

The sociological side of sexuality offers excellent examples of how cultural diversity can impact sexuality. For example, country of origin and familial practices influence sexual values, attitudes, and behavior. You do not even have to compare people from various countries to see examples of cultural diversity. People with urban backgrounds may differ from people with suburban or rural backgrounds. Those from higher socioeconomic classes may differ from those from lower socioeconomic classes, etc. Even peer groups, the media, and other social institutions affect our sexuality.

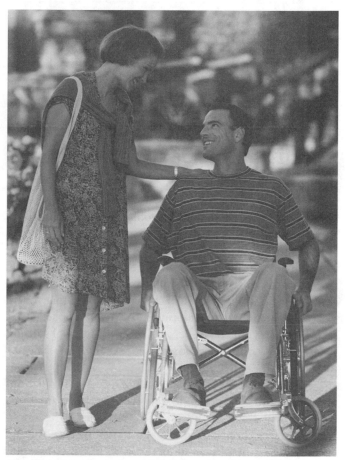

All people have sexual needs, although some are often ignored.

Consistent with our handling of the preceding three chapters, this chapter will approach the sociological side of sexuality mainly from the standpoint of basic factual material. Since the overall theme of this book is on handling the topic of human sexuality, however, we will discuss how to treat some of the specific sociological material in Chapter 14.

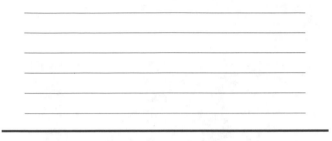

As has often been stated, it is not a choice whether to have sexuality education, since sexuality education for young people occurs every day in many social ways. The choice, instead, is what type of sexuality education young people should have.

Older People

At the other end of the spectrum of life are people of older ages. There are many myths about sexuality and the aged. In our society, as young people grow up, they learn that older people are supposed to be asexual beings. This sometimes results in a self-fulfilling prophecy whereby as these young people grow old, they become asexual beings themselves.

Many people have never even considered that older people are sexual beings. Keep in mind what our total concept of sexuality involves—feelings, relationships, and self-concepts, as well as sexual activity. If we are honest with ourselves, how could anyone be asexual?

To check yourself, fill out Insight 8-2 to help determine your knowledge about sexuality and aging. Then we will proceed with a little more information.

People of All Ages, Types, and Conditions as Sexual Beings

Young People

As we established in Chapter 1, people are sexual beings from birth to death. In practice, society has not been prepared to deal with—and perhaps is even opposed to dealing with—the sexuality of people near the ends of the age spectrum. From the moment a baby is born, many people treat it in certain ways, depending on its sex. As a child grows older, many social forces influence the development of his or her sexuality. Television, cartoons, commercials, movies, and books are just a few sources of information about sexuality and expected behavior.

Recognizing that these sources of sexual "stimulation" are all around us, we need to help young people, and those working with them, to understand some basics. For example, very young children are curious about their own and others' bodies. It is natural for children to play games such as "show me yours and I'll show you mine." Adults often react emotionally when young people play at sexual activity; in fact, there is no need to react at all unless some explanation is deemed necessary. We need to remember that the primary motivation of such play is experimentation and that the play is not the same as adult sexual activity.

We have not done a very good job of providing sound sexual facts for young people. In addition to reading, their major source of information is their peers, which results in a pooling of ignorance. We ought to be able to provide better sources of information. We need to help young people realize that erotic thoughts and fantasies are natural and that they are not evil people if they have such thoughts. Curiosity, as well, needs to be treated in a natural, matter-of-fact way.

Insight 8-2

Facts about Sexuality and Aging

Consider each of the following statements about sexuality and aging, then briefly jot down your response or reaction to each of the statements:

1. Older people are asexual beings. _____
   _____

2. Older people rarely participate in sexual acts.
   _____

3. Menopause causes serious physical difficulties for all women. _____

4. Sexual performance problems are a result of using oneself up in earlier years. _____
   _____

5. A hysterectomy means the end of a couple's sexual activity. _____

6. Certain foods or vitamins have sexually stimulating or aphrodisiac qualities that help sexual response.
   _____

7. Prostatic surgery for men means the end of their sexual activity. _____
   _____

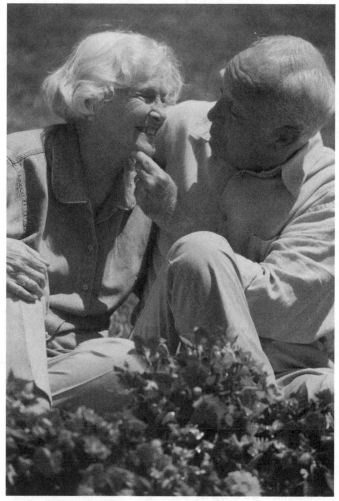

The sexuality of older people has too often been neglected.

We hope you realized that all of the statements in Insight 8-2 are myths. As mentioned earlier, our total concept of human sexuality recognizes that there are no asexual beings. Although physiological response may tend to become a little slower and possibly less intense with age, it is still essentially the same as in earlier years. For the average person in good health, sexual interest, desire, and activity continue throughout life.

Older people *do* participate in sexual acts. The major hindrance to sexuality in older people seems to be that part of the anatomy that lies between the ears. It is known that such things as monotony, preoccupation with career, mental or physical fatigue, overindulgence in food or drink, physical or mental infirmities, or fear of unsatisfactory sexual performance can hinder sexual activity; however, most of these factors relate to attitudes rather than to physical problems.

Regarding menopause, only a small percentage of females need medical help at this time, and many have few, if any, symptoms. Most women do not report a loss of sexual satisfaction as long as their attitudes do not get in the way.

There are many myths about hysterectomies, but the fact is that, generally, whatever the level of the woman's sexual response was before the surgery, it will continue unchanged provided that she has been assured that this will be so. In many cases a hysterectomy does not in any way interfere with basic hormonal production, and it is the hormones that influence feelings and drives—not the presence or absence of a uterus.

Unfortunately, with all the other myths about sexuality and aging, older people are more likely to wish to search for some nutritional element that will help sexual performance. No food or chemical has ever been proven to improve sexual performance—any apparent effects are typically psychological.

Although a number of men at some time in their lives will experience some prostatic problems, even in cases in which surgery is needed, sexual activity does not usually end. Those men who functioned well before surgery will usually continue to do so following surgery. Of course, there are exceptions, but medical personnel and counselors can greatly help by encouraging positive attitudes as they discuss this matter with their patients or clients.

Cross (1989) felt that the health of the elderly would be significantly improved if people would remember and apply the following six, simple rules:

1. **All older people are sexual.** They all have sexual beliefs, values, memories, and feelings. Many, if not most, also participate in sexual activity.

2. **Older people have a particular need for a good sexual relationship.** Many older people experience many physical, mental, and social changes. Perhaps they cannot easily do the enjoyable things they used to do. An excellent antidote for some of their problems is the warmth, intimacy, and security of a good sexual relationship.

3. **Sexual physiology changes.** In general, physiological changes are gradual and can be compensated for. For men, erections may take longer to achieve. Ejaculation might take longer, be less forceful, and is smaller in amount. This slowing down can easily be compensated for by taking more time. Women may experience atrophy and drying of the vagina, but estrogen administration or use of lubricants can help.

4. **Social attitudes are often frustrating.** Since society tends to deny the sexuality of the aging, laws, regulations, and customs tend to restrict the sexual behavior of older people. For example, those living in nursing homes or retirement homes often experience a lack of privacy.

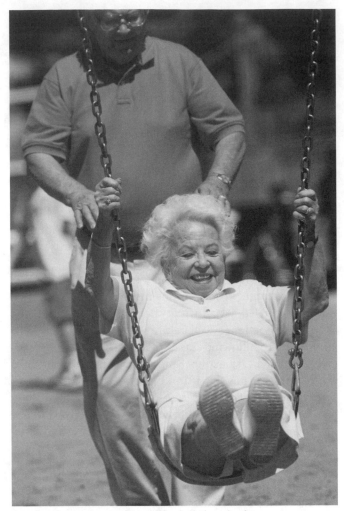

Age is often more a matter of mind than body.

5. **Use it or lose it.** Sexual activity cannot be stored and saved for a rainy day. Instead, it is a physiological function that tends to deteriorate if not used.

6. **Older folks do it better.** While the young would win out if "better" means a harder penis or a more moist vagina, the elderly have some advantages. They usually have lots of experience, they have more time, and attitudes can improve with aging. Some old folks have mellowed and learned to roll with the punches. Also, they no longer need to prove themselves.

It can easily be seen that there are many educational implications related to sexuality and aging. Educators have an obligation to help those who are aging (which includes everyone) to have adequate knowledge and healthy attitudes about sexuality. This can even pay off in a greater likelihood of sexual activity in later years. For example, men seem to remain sexually active because of the value that sexual behavior has in their lives, the frequency and range of past sexual behaviors, their motivation and ability to experiment

and develop compensatory strategies, and the supportive attitude of their partners (Schiavi, 1990).

For older women as well, past experience related to the importance of sexual behavior and more positive personal attitudes about sexuality, based on formal education, are influential determinants of sexual motivation. In addition, cultural attitudes that discourage sexual behavior in older people are likely to act as effective discouragers of sexual motivation (Sherwin, 1991).

There is still a lack of information about sexual health issues related to older Americans. There are at least several sexual health issues that educators and health care providers need to discuss with older people (Kreinin, 2002). First, there is a need to help some older people negotiate new relationships. Many widowed or divorced older people find themselves experiencing intimacy under unfamiliar circumstances. Second, there is a need to help older adults learn about sexual health issues. Older people must be educated about protecting themselves from some of the negative consequences of sexual behavior. While young people have hopefully learned to protect themselves through educational programs, for many older adults the current sexual health landscape is filled with terms like STI, HIV, and AIDS, to which they do not personally relate. Third, older adults need help coping with the physical effects of aging on intimacy and sexuality. As people's bodies age, for example, they need to know about the effects of such change. Fourth, older people have a need to become "askable" adults. Many older adults are serving as caregivers to grandchildren. Many others play important roles in the lives of relatives, friends, and neighbors. They are in a unique position to serve as role models and resources for younger people.

It is the mind and not the body, then, that tends to get in the way of understanding sexuality and aging. Parents, teachers, administrators, counselors, and medical personnel need to be aware of this, since each of us can do a great deal to help prevent and deal with problems associated with sexual attitudes and behaviors of older people. This problem ought to be relatively easy to deal with if each of us accepts a little of the responsibility.

People of Different Races

What does race have to do with sexuality? Recall that in Chapter 2 we talked about a double standard that became prevalent during the time of the Southern colonists in the United States. Part of this double standard had to do with "protecting" white women from black males while allowing white men to have sexual activity with black females.

Consequently, there was a need to develop a supportive structure of myth to justify this inconsistent behavior. Myths developed about supposed differences among races regarding sexual desires, sexual abilities, and even anatomical structure. In fact, there are no inherent racial differences

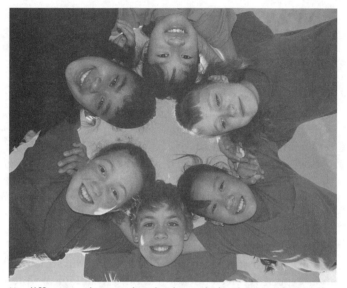

No differences in sexual attitudes or behaviors can be attributed only to racial differences.

that have significance in terms of human sexuality. But those working in sexuality education programs need to be aware of the emotional potential of this topic. Efforts are needed to help people put sexuality and racism into perspective.

Since people still believe myths about different races that have implications for human sexuality, sexuality education programs need to include opportunities for the myths to be dispelled. Although it is certainly true that cultural differences can have a real impact on sexual attitudes and behavior, it is not true that any of these differences can be attributed to race.

More recent considerations related to race and sexuality education are the increasing numbers of interracial relationships and the issue of adoption of a child by a parent of a different race. Both of these issues lend themselves to interesting discussion in sexuality education.

Physically Disabled People

For the purposes of this discussion, "physically disabled people" are people with any type of physical difficulties including damage or deterioration of the central nervous system (for example, cerebral palsy, seizure disorder, traumatic head injury, or spina bifida); musculoskeletal conditions (for example, muscular dystrophy, juvenile rheumatoid arthritis, scoliosis, or osteomyelitis); congenital malformations (for example, rubella, fetal alcohol syndrome, asthma, cystic fibrosis, diabetes, sickle cell anemia, hemophilia, cancer, or tuberculosis); and incapacities resulting from accidents and other physical conditions (for example, AIDS, child abuse and neglect, or children born of substance abusing mothers).

The fact that physically disabled people are sexual beings has been neglected in society's haste to see that the basic physical and security needs of physically disabled people are met. Concerns related to sexuality are often basic for physically disabled people and need to be addressed.

Depending on the type of disability, a variety of possible feelings may need attention, including feelings of loss of control over one's bodily functions, an inability to care for all of one's personal needs, a fear of being less of a person, and feelings of unacceptability. Almost always, the general issue of a physically disabled person's body image is important and ideally should involve the partners of the physically disabled too.

Individuals with Cognitive Deficits

As with the physically disabled, in our society people have generally tended to neglect the sexuality of individuals with cognitive deficits. When attention has been given to the sexual behavior of these individuals, it has generally been to restrict that behavior on the assumption that individuals with cognitive deficits are not interested or cannot manage sexual feelings or behaviors. As families, educators, and other professionals have become more aware of the lifelong needs of these individuals, sexuality has surfaced as an area that needs specific consideration. Cognitive disabilities do not change a human being into an asexual entity. Individuals with cognitive deficits need sexuality education and counseling designed to meet their individual needs, just like people without disabilities. The content, issues and teaching methodology must be tailored to reflect the effect of the disability on an individual's ability to learn and use information as well as the effect of the particular disability on an individual's psychosocial development and personal quality of life.

Our society has been reluctant to support the use of materials and methods that are sexually explicit, citing their use as pornographic and suggestive. There has been some progress made in this area as a result of the concerted efforts of disability advocates, parents, and individuals with disabilities (Bernstein, 1990).

More recently there has been increased attention given to the possibility of individuals with cognitive challenges getting married and having children. As an example, the 1999 movie *The Other Sister* tells the story of the families and lives of two young people with disabilities who marry.

Ensuring that sexuality education meets the needs of individuals with cognitive disabilities is part of the total responsibility of sexuality educators. More information about this topic is presented later in this text.

Ill People

People may have little experience with the very young, the aged, the physically challenged, or the mentally challenged. However, almost all of us know ill people, and we become ill

---

Insight 8-3

Sexuality and Illness

Before we answer them for you, jot down your responses to the following questions:

1. What types of medical problems are likely to result in disturbances of sexual function? _____

    _____

2. Why do you think people with physical medical problems often develop sexual problems? _____

    _____

3. How can we all help reduce sexual problems associated with illness? _____

    _____

---

ourselves on occasion. The ill are another group whose sexuality has largely been ignored.

In the past, most discussions between medical personnel and clients or patients excluded any mention of sexual topics. This was, no doubt, because both the patient and the medical person were too embarrassed to mention the word "sex." Now, questions about sexual history as well as other aspects of medical history are more likely to be considered routinely in the medical setting.

People with physical medical problems often develop sexual problems unnecessarily. Some people feel a sense of guilt when they get sick and try to determine where their guilt lies. Since the topic of sexuality is a leading producer of guilt, they may consciously or unconsciously avoid sexual activity. For others, illness can restrict sexual activity, not because restriction is necessary, but because medical personnel fail to let patients know that restriction is not necessary. The implications for sexuality education should be obvious.

Medical personnel need to help people feel that sexuality is appropriate to discuss and that guilt feelings are common. In addition, in all cases of illness, sexual activity should be resumed at the earliest possible time, consistent with the person's health, in order to avoid other detrimental effects on interpersonal relationships as well as on the self-concept of the ill person. Medical personnel also need to realize that sexual problems might be expressed through physical symptoms, such as in the case of a person who asks for an examination of the genital area because of a supposed concern about cancer or some other more "acceptable" difficulty than a sexual one.

There can also be concerns related to surgery—particularly for women (Rothenberg, 1991). In cases of breast surgery, hysterectomy, cesarean delivery, or other reproductive surgery, women may focus on an altered appearance,

a concern about an incision opening during sexual activity, or a concern about whether they can still function sexually. Educational programs can do wonders to ease the adjustment.

The cardiac patient may also be concerned about returning to sexual activity (Papadopoulos, 1991). Fears that sexual activity will bring on a heart attack or that it is no longer possible to participate in sexual activity can lead to a drastic reduction or elimination of sexual activity. Patients, their partners, and physicians need education to be able to ease the adjustment back to "normal" sexual activity. In most instances, a full life, including sexual activity, is possible after the development of cardiovascular disease.

Unfortunately, it is still true that many medical personnel are not well educated when it comes to sexuality. The situation is improving, but many medical people who are looked to as experts receive education about physiological functioning and disease, but not the many other important aspects of total sexuality.

Although it may appear that the issue of the relationship between illness and sexuality needs attention only in medical settings, this point of view would overlook basic educational prevention possibilities. Educators, parents, administrators, and community leaders need to see that such topics are addressed through sexuality education to help reduce the incidence of problems in medical settings.

Sexual Lifestyles

In Chapter 7 we described a number of lifestyle possibilities reflected in marriage and divorce statistics, changes in the nuclear family, cohabitation, serial monogamy, single parenthood, group family arrangements, and contractual marriages. At this point we want to consider additional related information.

Marriage

Consider first the subject of marriage in Insight 8-4.

Insight 8-4

What Should Marriage Vows Be Like?

Try the following exercise alone or with others: Take 15 minutes to contemplate what marriage should be all about. Then compose marriage vows you would like for your own marriage. These vows should reflect your feelings about appropriate arrangements within a marriage.

Examples of marriage vows that have resulted from this exercise include the following (Greenberg, 1992):

1. Together we will walk through life
   Known either as husband or wife.
   If we both grow tired of this affair,
   We'll split and never again care.

2. Let us consider these two people joined together at this point in time knowing full well that this relationship can and will be terminated at the request of one or both parties. If termination occurs, property acquired before the relationship will go to the individual owners, property acquired after will be divided equally. Both individuals have consented not to bear children. If a child is born, it then becomes the property of the state unless one of the parties consents to care for it, with the other's approval.

3. A recipe for a happy and successful marriage includes many ingredients and this I will give unto you:

   3 cups of love
   2 cups of understanding
   1 1/2 cups of patience
   3/4 cup of joy
   1/2 cup of good sense of humor
   Sprinkle with sunshine and serve daily with care.

How do you feel about these three marriage vows? How are they similar to or different from your own composition?

Nonparenthood

It is obvious that many married couples are choosing not to have children. Before going further, complete Insight 8-5 about reasons *to* have children.

Are you convinced by your reasons? Did you realize that some studies indicate that childless couples report being happier and more satisfied than couples with children?

Insight 8-5

Reasons for Having Children

Before we consider nonparenthood, take a moment to list the reasons why people *should* have children if they so decide.

1. _____
2. _____
3. _____
4. _____
5. _____

While at one time it was probably assumed that a married couple would have children, changes in attitudes have been occurring for at least three reasons: (1) In earlier, rural settings children were economically valuable and needed for their labor. Today they can be a painfully expensive proposition. (2) Children are no longer considered a necessary and inevitable part of marriage. (3) Due to feminism, and because of economic need, more women than ever are working.

It is not the role of sexuality educators to talk anyone into or out of having children. But sexuality educators must be prepared to raise levels of awareness and provide opportunities to consider alternatives on this issue. Strong arguments can be made for having children and against having children. People need to be aware that there are choices and to be prepared to make intelligent and informed decisions.

Living Together

Living together before marriage is a significant family trend. It is defined as couples who are sexual partners, unmarried, and sharing a household. By 1997 the total number of unmarried couples living together in the United States was over 4 million, up from less than half a million in 1960. Over half of all first marriages are now preceded by cohabitation (Poponoe & Whitehead, 2000).

Not only is cohabitation common, but it is widely accepted by young people. For example, 60% of high school seniors agree that it is usually a good idea for couples to live together before getting married to find out whether they really get along. Other reasons commonly given for living together are to share expenses, to learn more about each other, and to find out if a partner has what it takes to be married. Further, if things do not work out, breaking up is relatively easy to do. Interestingly, research indicates that living together before marriage increases the risk of breaking up after marriage, increases the risk of domestic violence for women, and increases the risk of physical and sexual abuse for children. Unmarried couples also report lower levels of happiness and well-being than married couples (Poponoe & Whitehead, 2000).

Insight 8-6

Living Together Before Marriage

To clarify your feelings on this topic, take a moment to list any reasons you can think of why people should *not* live together before marriage:

_____

_____

_____

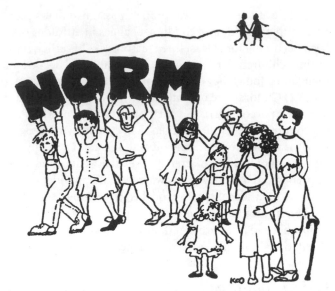

Some people choose not to go along with the norm.

Clusters, Groups, and Communes

For many years people have attempted to unite groups of families in order to get the benefits of an extended family. Several examples of this lifestyle are cluster marriages, group marriages, and communes.

In **cluster marriages** there is a cooperative relationship among a cluster of individual families of many types and ages. There is no common economic base, and possessions are generally privately owned. The clustered families live in close proximity and meet periodically to discuss values and share secrets. Services to each other can be provided to extend the boundaries of the intimate family.

In **group marriages** there are several people married to each other. This includes a communal living arrangement, but not all communal arrangements are group marriages. Most group marriages are small; if more than six partners are involved, the arrangement becomes more like a commune. In a group marriage, the mechanics of daily living can become complex, because more people are involved in basic decisions. There are both advantages and disadvantages to forming intimate relationships with three or four partners as part of an overall relationship.

In **communes** larger numbers of people unite around a common idea or objective, such as shared religious principles, a desire to withdraw from traditional society, or a desire to experience closer community with people with similar goals.

There have been so many different types of communes that it is impossible to generalize about the kinds of people who choose to become involved in this lifestyle. In order to escape more completely from traditional society, people in communes have commonly developed means for considerable economic self-sufficiency. Leadership in communes is assumed rather than bestowed. All members are expected to contribute to the well-being of the commune. In some communes there is sexual freedom, whereas in others there is not. Children are often treated as belonging to the total commune and not to a specific family. Most communes emphasize the idea of a nuclear family, but the nuclear units may shift from time to time.

Contract Marriages

To some people, the idea of having a written contract for a marriage is unthinkable. Such people feel that the institution of marriage is too sacred and personal to be treated as a mere legal arrangement. Other people feel that a contract is a good idea, because the strong emotions generated in such an important relationship might hamper rational thinking.

Insight 8-7

Contract Marriages

To clarify your own attitudes, take some time to think about how you would write a marriage contract. For this exercise, it does not matter whether you are already married or not, or whether you ever wish to get married. Thinking about what might be in a marriage contract is a way of thinking about what needs to be considered in a marriage. To simplify matters, consider the situation as if you were leasing an apartment—only in this case you are "leasing" a partner. What are the major sections of the contract you would wish to include? For example, maybe you want to spell out household responsibilities, financial matters, whether you to wish to have children, what you will do if you decide to terminate the relationship, and so on. On a separate piece of paper, list the major headings of your marriage contract.

Do you think contracts should be required before people can get married? Should the contracts be renewed periodically?

---

cluster marriage   Cooperative relationship among a group of individual families. There is no common economic base, possessions are generally privately owned, and the families meet periodically.

group marriage   Several people are married to each other and there is a communal living arrangement.

commune   Larger numbers of people unite around a common idea or objective (such as a shared religious principle). There are many types of communes.

One form of a **contract marriage** is defined with respect to the overall relationship. For example, a couple may decide that every 3 years they will either renew their commitment or go their separate ways. Another form of contract involves the spelling out of many details within the relationship as well as what the partners will do if they decide to change or sever the relationship. Some contracts cover both periodic renewals and details of the relationship.

While not really a contract marriage, increased use has been made of a written document called a *prenuptial agreement* (a written agreement drawn up and agreed to prior to marriage). Obviously, anything that is legal could be agreed to in a prenuptial agreement. Generally, however, this agreement has become more common in situations where one or both parties have been previously married. There might be such matters as previously earned assets, property owned by each party, obligations for child care, and preferences for an inheritance that might be worked out prior to a marriage. Prenuptial agreements can be as simple or as complicated as desired by the participants.

It is essential for sexuality educators to provide a format for discussing and learning about different lifestyle possibilities from an educational viewpoint. The personal values of sexuality educators should not be imposed on students; rather, the sexuality educator's role is to help students be aware of possibilities and be more secure in their own decisions.

Sexuality and Legality

The relationship between sexuality and legality is broader than many people think, for it encompasses more than the legal regulation of sexual behavior. It also includes the legal situation with respect to access to treatment and services related to sexuality, the legality of sexual discrimination, and the legality of educational activities related to sexuality.

Legal Regulation of Sexual Behavior

There are many laws that restrict sexual behavior between consenting adults in our society. These differ from state to state, are rarely enforced, date back to Old England and Puritan New England, and are very slow to change. There has been a trend throughout the years to leave these laws alone rather than risk a possible controversy in attempting to change them.

In some states people have seen fit to legalize (or not legislate against) any sexual behavior between consenting adults. This is a growing trend.

Perhaps the best example of a sexual behavior receiving legal attention in recent years is homosexuality. At different times legal rulings have been made for and against the right to participate in homosexual behavior. For example, in 1985 a federal appeals court in Texas upheld a Texas state law banning homosexual acts. The nine judges in the majority said the law is constitutional "in view of the strong objection to homosexual conduct which has prevailed in western culture for the past seven centuries." A dissenting judge, however, said, "If ever there was a constitutional right to privacy, Texas has violated it by blatantly intruding into the private sex lives of fully consenting adults" (Law ban of homosexuals upheld, 1985).

Then, in 1986 the U.S. Supreme Court ruled (5 to 4) that a state may outlaw sodomy among homosexuals, even if it is practiced in the privacy of a home. While one justice suggested that actually imprisoning homosexuals for their sexual conduct might violate the Eighth Amendment's ban against "cruel and unusual punishment," the majority rejected as "unsupportable" the idea that "any kind of private sexual conduct between consenting adults is constitutionally insulated" (Knocking on the bedroom door, 1986).

Although some cities and localities across the country have passed antidiscrimination legislation, as of 1992 only 5 states (Connecticut, Hawaii, Massachusetts, New Jersey, and Wisconsin) had passed legislation banning discrimination on the basis of sexual orientation. Seven states had legislation prohibiting sexual behaviors between people of the same sex, and 16 other states and the District of Columbia had laws either labeling certain sexual activities as "deviate sexual intercourse" and/or criminalizing their practice by either heterosexual or homosexual couples. Several other states had struck down such laws as violating the civil rights of people in the state (Haffner, 1992).

This controversy continues. In 2000, the governor of Vermont signed a bill making Vermont the first state to legally

---

The Law and Sexual Behavior

Do you believe that people should be free to participate in any sexual behavior they choose with another consenting adult? Why or why not?

_____

_____

_____

_____

_____

---

contract marriage   A written agreement spelling out aspects of a marriage. It may relate to details of the relationship, what happens if the marriage is severed, or periodic renewals of the contractual relationship.

recognize relationships between gay and lesbian couples. Although the measure did not allow for gay or lesbian marriages, it did enable such couples to form "civil unions" and entitle them to all rights and benefits enjoyed by married couples under state law, including the ability to make medical decisions on behalf of their partners and qualification for certain tax breaks (Vermont backs gay civil union bill, 2000).

After this bill existed for about a year, about 80% of the 3,000 gay-union licenses in Vermont were issued to nonresidents. In other states, gay and lesbian couples have filed lawsuits for the right to marry (Drummond, 2001).

Even in 2003, 24 states had sodomy laws prohibiting certain sexual behaviors (often oral–genital contact and anal intercourse) between consenting adults, even in the privacy of their own homes. However, in June 2003, the U.S. Supreme Court ruled that sodomy laws are unconstitutional. Many people felt that the decision would have far-reaching implications for discussions about gay rights—specifically related to such issues as marriages among homosexuals, partner benefits, adoption, and parental rights (Murphy, 2003).

Legality and Access to Treatment and Services

The idea that minors have the right to make important decisions about health care has been well established in federal and state policy. Many states specifically authorize minors to consent to contraceptive services, testing and treatment for HIV or other sexually transmitted infections, prenatal care and delivery services, treatment for alcohol and drug abuse, and outpatient mental health care. With the exception of abortion, lawmakers have generally resisted attempts to impose a parental consent or notification requirement on minors' access to reproductive health care and other sensitive services. Nevertheless, the movement to "restore" parental rights and to legislate parental control over minors' reproductive health care decisions is still active (Minors and the right to consent to health care, 2000).

One big controversy surrounding the rights of minors to access treatment and services related to sexuality arose in

---

Insight 8-9

Minors' Rights to Health Care Services

If you were going to present arguments for legislators on why minors should have the right to consent to their own treatment in areas related to sexuality, what would you tell them? Could you also argue the other side of the coin? For what reasons should the consent of parents or guardians be required in order for minors to get treatment?

1982 (Kenney, Forrest & Torres, 1982). At that time, the U.S. Department of Health and Human Services proposed a regulation requiring family-planning clinics funded under Title X of the Public Health Service Act to notify parents or the legal guardian of patients under the age of 18 within 10 days after the adolescent receives prescription drugs or services from a clinic.

This Parent Notification Proposal, or "Squeal Rule" as it was often called, was tested immediately in the courts and not upheld. Since that time, however, there have been additional attempts at the state and federal levels to implement such a rule.

For example, during the 1980s the Adolescent Family Life Act allowed religious and charitable organizations to receive funding for sexuality education. At the same time, it prohibited agencies who "advocate, promote, or encourage abortion" from receiving government funding. This meant agencies receiving federal funding could not provide abortion counseling, make abortion referrals, or provide information about abortions. A legal ruling in Connecticut indicated this provision violated the First Amendment protection for freedom of speech, since speech informing a woman about her health and a privacy-related activity (abortion) was a constitutionally protected right. However, an opposite decision was reached in New York (Bullis, 1991).

In May of 1991, the U.S. Supreme Court upheld the administration's "Gag Rule" restrictions on federally funded clinics. A pregnant woman who asked about abortion could only be told that the clinic does not consider abortion to be a method of family planning. Clinicians could not refer women, even if there were a medical emergency, to a facility that performed abortions (Haffner, 1991). Even though President Clinton reversed the "Gag Rule" in 1993, at the time you are reading this it is likely that a related debate is going on in some state or at the national level.

For example, following up on a successful 1998 ballot initiative in Colorado requiring parental notification in a minor's abortion, antiabortion lawmakers in 1999 succeeded in enacting such requirements in 3 more states. At the beginning of 2000, 38 states had laws on the books mandating some kind of parental involvement in abortion. Newer bills are designed to make an existing law even more restrictive, by switching from parental notification to parental consent (Sonfield, Dalal & Nash, 2000).

The advertisement and sales of contraceptives have become less restricted. Laws in some states that previously prevented the sales of contraceptives to minors, the sales of contraceptives by stores other than pharmacies, the sales of contraceptives to unmarried people, and the advertisement of services related to sexuality have been overturned.

The abortion issue has been a major part of the controversy surrounding the right of people to receive sexual-related services. In the early 1970s, it became illegal for states to

Feelings about the Legal Aspects of Abortions

In 1992, the United States Supreme Court ruling on a Pennsylvania abortion law set the stage for states to consider abortion laws that would sharply restrict, but not ban abortions. The Court approved most of the restrictions on abortion in Pennsylvania, but also said that the more permissive legislation of the early 1970s (Roe vs. Wade) must be upheld. The main points of the 1992 ruling are listed below. After each one, indicate how you feel about it.

1. Women have a constitutional right to an abortion.

   _____

2. Prior to an abortion, doctors must tell women about abortion alternatives and fetal development. _____

   _____

3. Women must wait 24 hours after hearing the information mentioned in number 2 before having an abortion. _____

   _____

4. A female under 18 must get permission from one parent or a judge before having an abortion.

   _____

5. Married women do not have to tell their husbands before getting an abortion. _____

   _____

Share your feelings about each point with several classmates and discuss similarities and differences among your feelings.

---

prohibit abortions in the early months of pregnancy, and many people considered abortion to be a right of females. Then a controversy developed over whether medical facilities had to provide abortion services. Some legal opinions indicated that a medical facility had to provide abortion services, since it was the female's right to receive the service; other opinions indicated this was not the case if medical personnel were morally opposed to abortions.

In recent years there has been a great deal of legislative activity related to abortion. Related issues involve circumstances under which an abortion can be performed, a waiting period (usually 24 hours) for an abortion, required counseling before an abortion can be performed, parental consent (or parental notification) requirements for minors, and spousal notification requirements (Haffner, 1992). There is no question that aspects of this debate continue as you read this.

For example, in 1995 bills were introduced in some states and nationally to ban a specific method of late abortion, called intact dilatation and extraction. Opponents dubbed this procedure "partial-birth" abortion. Some states have adopted bans on partial-birth abortions, and debates about it continue within the federal government. In addition, some abortion opponents have an agenda to make the fetus a child. They label later abortion as infanticide in an attempt to have abortions banned (Sonfield, Dalal & Nash, 2000).

People who oppose legalized abortion have unsuccessfully tried to completely outlaw abortion services. However, they have been successful at limiting the availability of abortion under many circumstances.

For example, in 1998 the U.S. Congress passed a $500 billion appropriations bill. It contained many restrictions on abortion. The bill prohibited the following:

- Abortion coverage for workers insured by the federal government

- Abortions for women in federal prisons

- Abortions in overseas military hospitals

- Federal or local funding of abortions in the District of Columbia

- Medicaid funding of abortions, which primarily affects women with disabilities or low income

The one area in which there has been the most similarity among states is in the treatment of minors for sexually transmitted infection. In all states it is possible for minors to consent to their own treatment for sexually transmitted infection, and in most instances confidentiality is maintained. This raises an important point for sexuality educators, though. It is one thing to tell students what the law is in a given geographical area and another to tell them what is likely to happen in practice. The law may provide for confidential treatment, but if the people at the local clinic choose to call the parents after you have told the young person that this will not happen, you will have lost credibility and the child or adolescent may feel betrayed. It is therefore wise to check out the procedures at local clinics regarding the treatment of minors before telling young people what is legal and what is not.

A final consideration for access to treatment and services has only come up in recent years—reproductive health care information and services at schools. Because of the AIDS epidemic, some school districts allow condom distribution at schools. For example, in 1991 the New York City Board of Education voted to require condom distribution on request, and without parental consent, at the city's high schools. Students could get a free condom from any specially trained teacher or the school nurse. The only students who could not receive them were those whose parents objected in writing.

A related development is the increase in the number of school-based clinics. Services in such clinics vary widely, but often include health screening tests, care for minor ailments, and sometimes reproductive information and services. Interestingly, studies indicate that when contraceptives are provided by school-based clinics there is no increase in sexual activity and a small decrease in the number of pregnancies (Flax, 1991).

The Law and Sexual Discrimination

Discrimination against people on the basis of certain sexual behavior or preferences is increasingly becoming an issue of law. One example is the ban against schools' discriminating against pregnant students or teachers (Schools can't discriminate against pregnant students, teachers under Title IX rules, 1975). Early regulations applied only to public schools, but in more recent years have related to private schools and business settings as well.

Some of the readers of this book may recall the days when school districts prevented pregnant girls from continuing their studies. Now, a school may not exclude a pregnant student from any class or activity unless she chooses not to participate. Although it may offer separate classes for pregnant students, attendance must be voluntary and the classes must be comparable to those offered to nonpregnant students.

For students, teachers, or other employees, a school must grant leaves of absence for pregnancy, childbirth, and abortion and reinstate a student or employee to the same status when she returns. In other words, a pregnancy is now treated much the same as any other medical condition; it is the individual and the physician who determine when the person may work or participate—not the school or the employer.

Of course the previously discussed laws relating to sexual orientation, various sexual behaviors, minors, and abortions can also be viewed as forms of sexual discrimination—depending upon your viewpoint. It does appear that state governments and the federal government will play an increasingly important role in affirming or restricting rights related to sexuality.

Legality, the Internet, and Information about Sexuality

Should sexually explicit materials be censored and controlled? There are varying opinions on this. In an attempt to keep sexually explicit materials on the Internet away from the millions of users under age 17 in the United States, Congress passed the Online Protection Act. It forced Web sites that contain sexually explicit material to collect a credit card number or some other form of adult identification from viewers. The law made it a crime to knowingly communicate to a minor "for commercial purposes" any online material that is "harmful to minors." It did not touch areas not

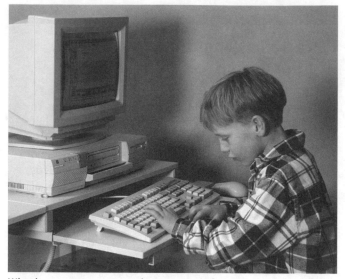

Whether or not to control access to information about sexuality on the Internet remains a controversial issue.

on the Web, such as e-mail or Usenet newsgroups. It also did not touch noncommercial sites or operations based outside the United States. In February of 1999, a U.S. district judge extended indefinitely a preliminary injunction against the act, ruling it violated free speech. In 2000, a federal appeals court struck down as unconstitutional Congress's second attempt to criminalize speech on the Internet (ACLU v. Reno II victory! Appeals court rejects Congress's second attempt at cyber-censorship, 2000). This law is controversial. Some people feel it is in society's best interest to protect children from sexually explicit materials. Free speech advocates, on the other hand, challenge the law on constitutional grounds, saying it would affect everyone on the Web.

A major related event occurred in 2003 when the U.S. Supreme Court upheld a federal law requiring public library personnel to install pornography filters on all computers providing Internet access, as a condition of continuing to receive federal subsidies and grants (Greenhouse, 2003). The law, enacted in 2001, had been blocked by a lower court and had never taken effect. Under the law, filters are required for all library users, not just children. The law authorizes, but does not require, librarians to unlock Internet sites at the request of adult users. Many opinions exist about the wisdom of this law and how it relates to First Amendment rights to free speech.

Legality and Education about Sexuality and HIV/AIDS

In this instance we can only talk about sexuality and HIV/AIDS education in public schools, since in other settings the legal question does not arise. On a number of occasions, individuals or groups in a given community have attempted to stop school sexuality education programs on legal grounds. Their objections have included illegal use of funds for programs, the unconstitutionality of sexuality education programs, and claims that local or state school authorities have not been given the legal authority to conduct sexuality education programs.

In response, courts have upheld the legality of sexuality education programs. They have said that school authorities do have the legal authority to conduct such programs, and that sexuality education programs are a reasonable, desirable, and necessary way to deal with education and social problems. Sexuality opponents have not given up; however, the legal situation surrounding school sexuality programs seems to be strongly in support of the programs. (See Appendix B for an overview of state mandates on sexuality education and HIV/AIDS/STI education.)

An interesting (and disturbing) twist has been added to some legislation about sexuality and HIV/AIDS education. For example, in Arizona legislation required that the curriculum must promote abstinence and not include anything that "promotes a homosexual lifestyle" (Haffner, 1992). This type of legislation is disturbing to educators for many reasons. Some would argue it is not appropriate for legislators to dictate how curriculum should be handled and what it should emphasize—this is a job for boards of education and educators. Also, some opponents of comprehensive human sexuality education have interpreted this type of legislation to mean that homosexuality and other sexual behaviors could not even be discussed. Still others have indicated that educators could not even imply that students need to make decisions about their sexual behavior—after all, the only decision was abstinence.

In 1996, the federal government attached a provision to popular welfare reform law establishing a federal entitlement program for abstinence-only-until-marriage education. "Abstinence education" refers to a program that requires, as its exclusive purpose, teaching about health gains to be realized by abstaining from sexual activity. It teaches that abstinence from sexual activity outside marriage is the expected standard of human sexual activity, that sexual activity outside of marriage is likely to have harmful psychological and physical effects, and that abstinence is the only sure way to avoid pregnancy, STI, and other associated health problems. Initially, Congress allocated $50 million in federal funds for the program each year, from 1998 through 2002.

With no real commitment to evaluating abstinence-only-until-marriage programs, Congress will still likely allocate more funds for such programs. This is happening in spite of many research studies showing no positive behavioral impact from abstinence education programs. It is clear that politics and ideology—and not science—are guiding the policy agenda in sexuality education (Further funding for abstinence-only-until-marriage programs, 2000). This debate continues, and it will be interesting to watch the results.

There has been a recent push for state legislators to get involved in issues in which they have never before participated. For example, Utah legislators debated what teachers could or could not say in the classroom. Their proposed bill stipulated that when teachers were asked questions about sexuality that "skirt the state approved curriculum, such as homosexuality," they must pull students aside to answer the questions or refer students to a school counselor. Although the bill passed, it was amended to clarify that it will not keep teachers from answering questions. It is not yet clear what affect this will have on classroom discussions (Notes from the field, 2002).

We have not heard the end of debates about whether it is appropriate to legislate curriculum and how it is taught. This may well be one of the hotly contested sexuality education issues for a long time.

Summary

We have only scratched the surface on the topic of the sociological side of sexuality, but we have described some of the crucial issues. We have noted that sexuality educators need to be aware of the sexuality of people of all ages, types, and conditions. Our total concept of sexuality applies to everyone. This idea has implications for the way we think about people and for the way we treat them.

Young people are sexual beings, and our recognition of this fact can facilitate healthy growth and development. They need facts about sexuality as well as understanding and support.

There has been a tendency to overlook the fact that older people are also sexual beings. Many myths of the decline or absence of sexuality in old age have existed, but for the average person in good health, sexual interest, desire, and activity continue throughout life. It is the mind and not the body that tends to get in the way of healthy sexuality for older people.

For many people, there are still strong emotional feelings and myths related to the topic of sexuality and racism. There are no inherent racial differences that have significance for human sexuality, but those working in sexuality education programs need to be aware of the emotional potential of this topic.

The physically and mentally challenged are sexual beings too, but in the past society has not looked at them this way. In our haste to see to their basic physical and security needs, we have tended to forget about their sexuality. Concerns related to sexuality are often very basic for physically or mentally challenged people and need attention.

Ill people do not lose their sexuality just because they are ill. The need for considering ill people as sexual beings should also be addressed in sexuality education programs.

A wide variety of lifestyle possibilities exists today. Couples may choose nonparenthood, living together without being legally married, and living in clusters, groups, and communes, among other possibilities. Marriage contracts can specify agreements about a variety of things; they force consideration of many issues we are often hesitant to look at because of our immediate emotional involvement.

Legality and sexuality relate to each other in several ways. Examples include the legal regulation of sexual behavior, laws regarding access to treatment and services related to sexuality, laws regarding sexual discrimination, and the legality of education about sexuality and HIV/AIDS. For the most part, the legal system is supportive of sexuality education programs.

References

ACLU v. Reno II victory! Appeals court rejects Congress' second attempt at cyber-censorship. American Civil Liberties Union Freedom Network (June 22, 2000). Available: http://archive.aclu.org/features/f101698a.html.

Bernstein, N. R. Sexuality in adolescent retardates, in *Atypical adolescence and sexuality*, Sugar, M., ed., 44–56. New York: W. W. Norton, 1990.

Bullis, R. K. Gag rules and chastity clauses: Legal and ethical consequences of Title X and the AFLA for professionals in human sexuality, *Journal of Sex Education and Therapy*, 17, no. 2 (Summer 1991), 91–102.

Cross, R. J. What doctors and others need to know: Six rules on human sexuality and aging, *SIECUS Report*, 17, no. 3 (January/February 1989), 14–16.

Drummond, T. The marrying kind, *Time*, 157, no. 19 (May 14, 2001), 52.

Flax, E. Comprehensive reproductive health care at clinics advocated, *Education Week*, 10, no. 27 (March 27, 1991), 6–7.

Further funding for abstinence-only-until-marriage programs. Sexuality Information and Education Council of the United States (May 22, 2000). Available: http://www.siecus.org/policy/PUpdates/pdate0011.html.

Greenberg, J. S. *Health education: Learner-centered instructional strategies*. 2nd ed. Dubuque, IA: William C. Brown Communications, 1992.

Greenhouse, L. Justices back law to make libraries use Internet filters. *The New York Times* (June 24, 2003). Available: http://www.nytimes.com.

Haffner, D. W. Overturn the Gag Rule now, *SIECUS Report*, 19, no. 5 (June/July 1991), 7.

———. 1992 report card on the states: Sexual rights in America, *SIECUS Report*, 20, no. 3 (February/March 1992), 1–7.

Kenney, A., Forrest, J. D. & Torres, A. Storm over Washington: The parental notification proposal, *Family Planning Perspectives*, 14, no. 2 (1982).

Knocking on the bedroom door, *Time* (July 14, 1986), 23–24.

Kreinin, T. A priority: Quality sexual health for older Americans, *SIECUS Report*, 30, no. 2 (December 2001/January 2002), 4–9.

Law ban of homosexuals upheld, *Birmingham News* (August 27, 1985).

Minors and the right to consent to health care. The Alan Guttmacher Institute Issues in Brief (2000). Available: http://www.agi-usa.org.

Murphy, D. E. Gays celebrate, and plan campaign for broader rights. *The New York Times* (June 27, 2003). Available: http://www.nytimes.com.

Notes from the field, *SIECUS Developments* (Winter/Spring 2002), 2.

Papadopoulos, C. Sex and the cardiac patient, *Medical Aspects of Human Sexuality*, 25, no. 8 (August 1991), 18–21.

Poponoe, D. & Whitehead, B. D. Should we live together? The National Marriage Project (2000). Available: http://marriage.rutgers.edu/SWLT.htm.

Rothenberg, D. L. Intimacy in the wake of surgery, *Lear's* (April 1991), 41–43.

Schiavi, R. C. Sexuality and aging in men, *Annual Review of Sex Research*, 1 (1990), 227–49.

Schools can't discriminate against pregnant students, teachers under Title IX rules, *Family Planning/Population Reporter*, 4 (August 1975), 82.

Sherwin, B. B. The psychoendocrinology of aging and female sexuality, *Annual Review of Sex Research*, 2 (1991), 181–98.

Sonfield, A., Dalal, A. & Nash, E. The states in 1999: Actions on major reproductive health-related issues, *The Guttmacher Report on Public Policy*, 3, no. 1 (February 2000), 5–7, 14.

Vermont backs gay civil union bill. Sexuality Information and Education Council of the United States (2000). Available: http://www.siecus.org/policy/PUpdates/pdate0009.html.

Suggested Readings

Late-term abortions: Legal considerations. The Alan Guttmacher Institute (2000). Available: http://www.agi-usa.org/pubs.

Nash, E. The states in 2000: Major actions on reproductive health-related issues, *The Guttmacher Report*, 3, no. 5 (October 2000), 9–11.

Recent abortion legislation. Sexuality Information and Education Council of the United States (2000). Available: http://www.siecus.org/policy/PUpdates.

Sexuality in middle and later life, *SIECUS Report Supplement* (December 2002/January 2002), 1–6.

Should sexual health education teach *only* about abstinence? Sex Information and Education Council of Canada (2000). Available: http://www.sieccan.org/.

Smith, W. Welfare reform's provision for abstinence only until marriage programs, *SIECUS Report*, 30, no. 4 (April/May 2002), 30–32.

States act to require accurate information in sexuality education, *The Guttmacher Report on Public Policy*, 2, no. 5 (October 1999), 11.

Teenagers' right to consent to reproductive health care. The Alan Guttmacher Institute (2000). Available: http://www.agi-usa.org/pubs/.

Cases for Part 2

The cases in this section are designed to use the information included in Chapters 5, 6, 7, and 8. Case 1 requires you to use knowledge about contraception: the various options available, the advantages and disadvantages of each option, and their effectiveness. This information appears in Chapter 5, but you must use this knowledge in conjunction with other concerns in order to answer the questions at the conclusion of Case 1. For example, your feelings about touching your genitalia, your religious convictions, and your feelings about interrupting sexual activity once it has begun will all influence your answers.

Case 2 is concerned with justifying family-life education as a part of a total sexuality education program. Chapter 7 discusses this point in some detail, and references to family life are made in Chapters 6 and 8.

Case 3 focuses on parenthood. As described in Chapters 6, 7, and 8, parenthood has its joys and sorrows. This case asks you to use this information about parenthood to determine its effect on a person's lifestyle.

Case 1

Staying Safe: Choosing a Contraceptive

Frankie and Johnny were sweethearts. They were also lovers who shared a sexual relationship and decided they had better do something to prevent Johnny from becoming pregnant. Approaching their problem intelligently, they consulted with Johnny's gynecologist, Dr. Hy I. Cue. During this consult they learned all about the various birth control options. In fact, they learned everything that you just learned in Chapter 5. However, Dr. Cue would not tell them which method of contraception to use. "This decision depends on many factors. I can't decide these factors for you. That is something both of you need to do," advised Dr. Cue. Frankie and Johnny went home to discuss their choice of birth control.

1. What were the other "factors" to which Dr. Cue was referring?

2. Which of these other factors would be of major concern to *you* if you were making this decision? Why?

3. Which of these factors would be of only minor concern to you? Why?

4. If Frankie and Johnny agreed with your ranking of major and minor concerns, which method of contraception do you think they would choose? Why?

Case 2

Taking the Sex from the Family: Justifying Family-Life Education as a Part of Sexuality Education

County Health Commissioner R. U. Smart has decided that the alarming increase in sexually transmitted infection, out-of-wedlock pregnancy, and abortion in the county indicates a need for a sexuality education program. He has asked Dee Crease, the county health education department head, to develop such a program. Ms. Crease was to describe the program she developed to the other health department heads and convince them to recommend its funding. At the meeting of the department heads, Dee Crease presented a program that related specifically to three topic areas:

1. Causes, signs and symptoms, treatment, and prevention of sexually transmitted infection

2. Contraception, birth, and pregnancy

3. Types of abortion, and county abortion facilities and services available

However, in addition to these topics, she included three more:

1. Parenthood education

2. Family-life education

3. Communication skills

One of the department heads, Izzy Silly, objected to including the second list of topics in a program designed to respond to increases in sexually transmitted infection, out-of-wedlock pregnancy, and abortion.

What could, and should, Dee Crease say to provide the rationale for including parenthood education, family-life education, and communication skills in her program?

Case 3

Parenting S.O.S.: Lifestyle Changes Resulting from Parenthood

Justin B. Cause (called Just by his friends) was ecstatic. He had just learned that his wife was pregnant. This was to be their first child, and they were both extremely excited. But

Just started to get scared as he adjusted to the new situation. When he realized the immense responsibility associated with parenthood and the changes that would be required in his life, he became awestruck. Could he do justice to this prospective addition to his family? Could he still function well as a husband? Would the fun he had during his leisure time be eliminated? Was his salary sufficient to provide for the newborn?

May B. Cause, Justin's wife, was similarly concerned: Could she be both a good mother and good wife? Would her career suffer? Would her leisure time enjoyment be diminished? Should she work or be a homemaker?

The Causes decided to talk with their friends, relatives, clergy, and others to either verify their concerns or alleviate them. What do you think they found out?

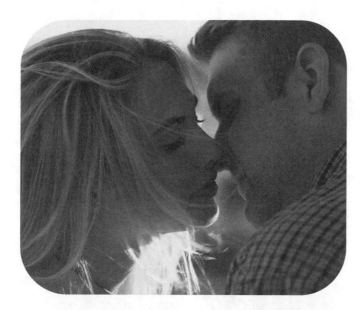

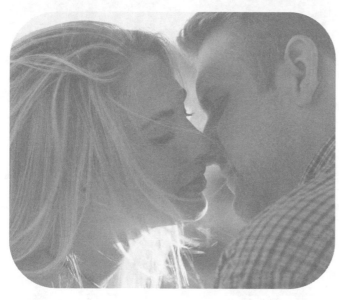

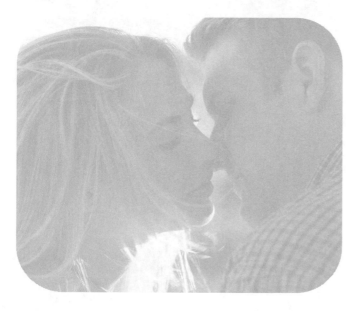

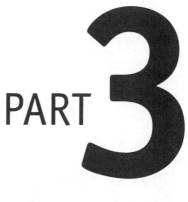

PART 3

Sexual Decision Making

Chapter 9
Sexual Morality and Decision Making

Chapter 10
Alternative Sexual Behaviors

Sexual Morality and Decision Making

Key Concepts

1. Morals are based on ethics, which are based on values.

2. Value systems influence the achievement of human potential.

3. Few sexual topics are free from considerations of morals, ethics, and values.

4. Sexual decisions often need to be made.

5. Decision making is a process that can be learned.

6. The decision-making process can be applied to sexuality.

Morals, Ethics, and Values

At the beginning of this chapter it is imperative that we establish a framework from which to discuss such controversial topics as morality and ethics. Without definitions of these terms, we (your authors) might be writing about one thing, but you may be relating our words to a completely different concept. Obviously, this is not an effective way to communicate.

Betty and Ted can serve as an example. Betty and Ted are going to celebrate their tenth wedding anniversary this year. For all but the last 6 months, their sexual relationship has been as satisfying as the rest of their marriage. However, since Ted took that new job—working with formaldehyde in the local factory—their sexual relationship has changed. Betty is no longer sexually aroused; she is not interested in having sex with Ted. Realizing something is "wrong with her," Betty became unsure of herself and embarrassed. Fortunately, Betty and Ted became so concerned about Betty's "sexual problem" that they sought the help of a trained sexual therapist. It was not long before the therapist realized that Betty did not have a sexual dysfunction, she just could not stand the smell of

formaldehyde on Ted and was so turned off she had no interest in sex. In fact, the therapist told them, if Betty could become aroused while smelling formaldehyde, that would really be unusual. Perhaps *then* she would have a sexual dysfunction! Now that Ted recognizes *he* is the problem—not Betty—he washes carefully to remove the smell that was so offensive. Sometimes it is easy to correct erroneous conclusions.

To prevent erroneous conclusions from this chapter's consideration of morality and sexuality education, we therefore offer the following definitions:

1. *Morality.* Concerns concrete decisions for specific situations. The question is asked, "What should be done?" or "What's a good thing here?"

2. *Ethics.* Refers to the rationale behind each decision, the underpinnings of moral decisions. Ethical issues are general. Theoretical questions are asked rather than questions relating to specific situations.

To illustrate the distinction between morality and ethics, imagine a situation in which you are attempting to talk your date or spouse into participating with you in a sexual act in which that person does not want to participate. Are you acting morally? That is, is your behavior in this specific situation correct? To answer this question, we must have some guiding principles to apply to this situation by which we can evaluate your behavior. These guiding principles—ethics—might include the following:

1. Sexual behavior should not be forced on anyone.

2. Sexual behavior between consenting adults is acceptable.

3. Fidelity (faithfulness) in marriage is a must.

4. Marriage partners and loved ones need to be responsive to each other's needs.

---

morality   Answers the questions of what is the right or good thing to do.

ethics   The rationale behind decisions regarding morality; the use of guiding principles.

You can see that applying these principles first necessitates the gathering of more information. Are the people in this situation married? Do they love each other? When did they last participate in this sexual behavior? And so on.

Even when we have such guiding principles and apply them to a given situation (such as using ethics to make moral decisions or behave morally), the decision made is difficult to classify as right or wrong. For example, it appears in the situation described above that principles 1 and 4 may be in conflict. Don't loved ones have a responsibility to meet each other's needs? On the other hand, should people be expected to participate in sexual behavior even when not in the mood or when it contradicts their needs? This leads us to another distinction, between rule ethics and situation ethics:

1. *Rule ethics.* Guiding principles that are to be used in all situations to arrive at moral decisions. The set of rules, ethical principles, is exhaustive enough to be able to be applied regardless of the situation. These principles are explicit, specific, and all-encompassing.

2. *Situation ethics.* Recognizes that no one situation is exactly the same as any other. Therefore, no one set of rules can apply to all situations. Consequently, the situation ethicist will carefully review, analyze, and evaluate each situation that requires a moral decision to determine which ethics are applicable.

For example, if the rule ethicist believes that killing is wrong, he or she will apply this ethical principle in all situations and might be expected to conclude that war is never justified. On the other hand, the situation ethicist would look carefully at each war to determine whether it is justified. If it is a "just war," the situation ethicist would describe that war as moral. If it is not a "just war," the situation ethicist would judge it to be immoral. So, for example, since killing is immoral and Hitler was killing Jews, war with Germany (even though it required killing Germans) was moral.

Although **values** are neither morals nor ethics, what we value is very important in deciding moral and ethical issues. In our example of the partner who wished to engage in a particular sexual activity when the other did not, our decision about morality would depend on which we value most: freedom or responsibility. If we value freedom most, we might

---

Ethical Principles and Values

List five ethical principles that you are willing to use to guide you in your sexual behavior.

1. _____
2. _____
3. _____
4. _____
5. _____

Each of the ethical principles you decided on was chosen by employing your values. Write down the value that led you to choose each principle you listed.

1. _____
2. _____
3. _____
4. _____
5. _____

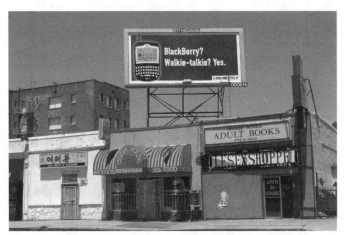

Should adult book stores, located in residential areas or within a few streets of schools, be allowed? Is their existence moral? With some restrictions on location, what can be sold (for example, no child pornography), and what can be openly displayed (for example, in a store window), the courts have ruled these stores legal. What do you think?

---

rule ethics   Guiding principles that are applicable to all situations.

situation ethics   Guiding principles that are applicable to individual situations and circumstances; no one set of rules applies to all situations.

values   An estimation of the worth ascribed to something.

decide that any coercion of one partner by the other is immoral. If we value responsibility most, we might conclude that loved ones need to be responsive to each other's needs and, therefore, that coercion (or persuasion) may be moral. Further, if we are situation ethicists, we will scrutinize the situation and use our values to determine which ethics (guiding principles) to apply and which to disregard.

As you probably recognize by now, the area of sexual morality is fraught with difficulty. It would be inappropriate—and impossible—for us to prescribe a set of values, ethics, or moral behaviors for you. Our intention in this chapter is to help you explore your own values and ethical principles so that you may apply them in specific situations, thereby acting morally.

Value Systems and Human Potential

The use of values clarification techniques in educational settings has become common in recent years, even though their use has not been without controversy. In perhaps an overly simplified way, the basic purpose of values clarification techniques is to help people understand themselves and others better by understanding the derivation and use of value systems. Advocates of a **values clarification** approach to education ask qualifying questions: How do you know that you really value something? What is involved in the process of valuing?

Answers to these questions were provided by Raths, Harmin, and Simon (1966), who developed a model of valuing consisting of seven subprocesses that has been utilized by many sexuality educators:

Prizing *one's beliefs and behaviors:*
1. *Prizing and cherishing*
2. *Publicly affirming, when appropriate*

Choosing *one's beliefs and behaviors:*
3. *Choosing freely*
4. *Choosing from alternatives*
5. *Choosing after consideration of consequences*

Acting *on one's beliefs:*
6. *Acting*
7. *Acting with a pattern, consistency, and repetition*

It might be said that in order for something to be a value, the person who claims it as a value must have gone through these seven steps or processes and must be willing to continue to do so.

The role of sexuality educators is not to tell others what they ought to do, or what is right and wrong, but instead to assist people in dealing with value issues as well as with the development of value systems.

It should be noted that "values clarification" has become a buzzword in educational circles. Individuals and groups opposed to "humanistic" education or "liberal" education or sexuality education have created a great deal of difficulty for educators who have used values clarification activities in their classrooms. Even the very mention of some of the names of the developers of values clarification is enough to cause trouble in many educational settings. These opponents of values clarification argue that it is amoral teaching; that is, it accepts any values the learners come up with. These opponents have made so much trouble in this area that sexuality educators ought to think twice before employing values clarification activities. And if they are to be employed, it would probably be wise to call these activities something else (perhaps "prioritizing"). Even if the sexuality educator determines that "valuing" learning strategies are important adjuncts to an effective sexuality program, the threat that the total program could be eliminated because of the inclusion of these valuing activities may be enough to argue for their exclusion.

Many experts believe that sexuality educators need to help people develop value systems with affirmative approaches to sexuality—value systems that emphasize human relationships and responsibility. Kirkendall also pointed out the need to help people develop behavioral principles. These principles should be based on each person's values and should serve as a guide for how that person should behave in any given situation. It is certainly possible that these behavioral principles may change in time. Kirkendall (1978, 344) listed several as illustrations:

1. Individuals need the freedom to decide how far they want to go in a relationship and what they wish to make of it.

2. A relationship is composed of numerous qualities or characteristics, each making its own particular contribution, i.e., communication, mutual respect, a sense of humor, empathy, confidentiality, physical expression.

3. So far as these qualities are concerned, if one or two outpace the others too much the entire relationship is likely to be thrown out of kilter or abandoned.

4. No one wishes to feel possessed though one enjoys the feeling of being a part of a relationship.

values clarification An instructional strategy designed to assist learners in identifying their values.

Behavioral Principles

Are you able to agree with any of Kirkendall's principles? Write down the numbers of those with which you agree and disagree. Now list three additional principles that you feel would be helpful for sexuality educators regardless of where the sexuality education occurred.

1. _____

2. _____

3. _____

---

5. In establishing limits in a fulfilling relationship, individuals must be their own governors. Dependence on others to govern one's behavior will disrupt the relationship itself.

6. A reasonable degree of consistency and predictability is necessary in a continuing relationship.

7. While communication in and of itself cannot solve problems, nevertheless communication is a vital, first step in the solution of problems.

8. People have similar needs and aspirations wherever they live and work.

It should be noted that sexuality educators—in fact all educators—teach values daily. Values such as honesty, truthfulness, respect for the law, kindness, fairness, and many others are conveyed to young people as they are taught to accept full citizenship in our society. Although culture, ethnicity, race, gender, and other factors influence values, our society agrees on these common values. This argument should be presented to anyone who objects to values being a part of a sexuality education program (Greenberg, 2004).

The National Guidelines Task Force (1991), formed to develop guidelines for comprehensive sexuality education, recommended the following values as inherent in sexuality education programs:

- Sexuality is a natural and healthy part of living.

- All persons are sexual.

- Sexuality includes physical, ethical, spiritual, psychological, and emotional dimensions.

- Every person has dignity and self-worth.

- Individuals express their sexuality in varied ways.

- In a pluralistic society like the United States, people should respect and accept the diversity of values and beliefs about sexuality that exist in a community.

- Sexual relationships should never be coercive or manipulative.

- All children should be loved and cared for.

- All sexual decisions have effects or consequences.

- All persons have the right and the obligation to make responsible sexual choices.

- Individuals and society benefit when children are able to discuss sexuality with their parents and/or other trusted adults.

- Young people explore their sexuality as a natural process of achieving sexual maturity.

- Premature involvement in sexual behaviors poses risks.

- Abstaining from sexual intercourse is the most effective method of preventing pregnancy and STI/HIV.

- Young people who are involved in sexual relationships need access to information about health care services.

Sexuality education has been controversial for a long time, and it will no doubt continue to be for a long time to come. The way that sexuality educators deal with morals, ethics, and values can have a great influence on thinking about sexuality. While they should not promote specific sexual behaviors or attitudes, sexuality educators have the difficult role of helping themselves and others learn to develop value systems that will provide for sound decision making, leading to responsible sexual behavior. It is a tough job, but one that cannot be avoided by sexuality educators who realize the far-reaching ramifications of their responsibilities and opportunities.

Relation of Sexual Topics to Morals, Ethics, and Values

As you have read through this book, you have no doubt had some personal reactions to the coverage of certain topics. We would not be surprised to learn that some readers are dissatisfied with the way some topics are presented. At least part of this dissatisfaction likely stems from feelings related to morals, ethics, and values.

How many topics likely to be covered in sexuality education are free from moral considerations? It is probably safe to assume that topics related to basic biology are not too controversial, but the minute we attempt to deal with other human sexuality topics, morals, ethics, and values become involved.

In Chapter 2 we presented a historical overview of sexual thinking in earlier times. It was no doubt obvious that differences in thinking are, for the most part, based upon differences in morals, ethics, and values. Thinking about sexuality has a direct influence on personal and group

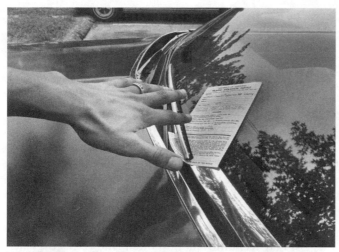

You can get a ticket for parking inappropriately. Should you also get a ticket for engaging in sexual activity inappropriately? For example, sexual intercourse without a condom. This is an ethical issue that can make for an interesting discussion.

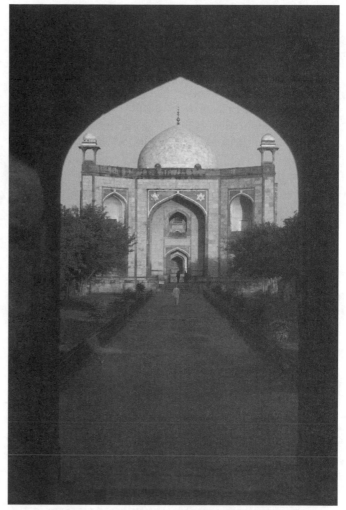

Many religious organizations support school-based sexuality education. It is not uncommon for churches, synagogues, and mosques to conduct programs for youth on topics related to sexuality.

behavior. For example, it was not just by chance that the ancient Greeks used a great deal of nudity in their artistic creations. Nor was it happenstance that according to Jewish law, women were considered unclean during menstruation and needed to take a bath after the termination of flow in order to be clean again. Such practices and beliefs of earlier times were based on morals, ethics, and values.

Let us look at some more contemporary examples. For many people, the controversy surrounding homosexuality is not based on factual observations alone but includes moral conflicts. Similarly, the reason why the controversy about the funding and legality of abortions has persisted for so long is that the moral and ethical issues surrounding the problem have prevented a resolution acceptable to all people.

Sexuality educators need constantly to be aware that almost all sexual topics are filled with moral and ethical considerations. Even when you do not think a topic is controversial, there are probably other people who disagree. An awareness of the possibility of ethical differences and a respect for these differences are always needed.

Contemporary Religions and Sexuality

In recent years most religious groups have published documents explaining their "official" stands on a variety of sexual issues. Many people have been surprised by these stands, since for so long the topic of sexuality had been either avoided in religious circles or discussed with overwhelmingly negative connotations. Countless volumes have been written on religion and sexuality in recent times, but for our purposes we simply want to point out that this type of information is

available and that it is usually far more supportive of human sexuality than religious documents have been in the past.

Religious leaders have joined the growing numbers of people who have become more willing and able to deal with human sexuality as a respectable subject. Traditional interpretations of what the Bible says about sexuality have been questioned by some people. Most of us have tended to assume that the Bible is negative and restrictive about sexuality. This is simply not the case. The Bible usually treats sexuality in a positive way. For example, the Bible deals with sexuality as an integral part of human nature, it deals with sexuality as a positive force to be enjoyed as well as controlled, and it basically says that sex is good.

In a detailed article identifying various religions' views about sexual topics, Haffner (1997) explores such controversial areas as sexual intercourse, sexual desire, gender and biological sex, physical beauty and love at first sight, fertility, sexuality in relationships, same gender sexual relations, adultery, and celibacy. Haffner concludes, "We need to understand that the Bible teaches that sexuality is a central part of being human, that bodies are good, that pleasure is good, and that men and women experience a healthy desire of each other. . . . Those of us who are people of faith must spread the gospel, literally the 'good news,' that the Bible affirms a healthy and positive view of sexuality."

Most religious denominations support sexuality education and affirm sexuality. In fact, some of the early and most effective sexuality education was offered through churches. It is clear that organized religion plays "a major role in promoting an understanding of human sexuality as one of the most affirming expressions of quality, mutual respect, caring, and love among human beings" (Haffner & de Mauro, 1991, 33). Today, religious groups recognize that sexuality is an essential aspect of humanity, that sexuality education is a shared responsibility, that there should be sexuality education in schools, that sex is God's good gift, that all persons are sexual beings, and that sexual pleasure is good. All of these points demonstrate a sharp contrast to the old restrictive and seemingly negative religious perspective. If we are to use religious information to help us and those with whom we work to make personal decisions, we owe it to ourselves and to our religions to get more of the facts straight.

Sexual Decisions

Now that we understand morals, ethics, and values a little better, it is time to turn our attention to sexual decisions and the decision-making process. As you read through our discussion of decisions, however, you should keep in mind the crucial role that morals, ethics, and values play in influencing these decisions.

As has been stated repeatedly in this book, sexuality is who and what we are, not what we do. It follows, then, that we are continually making decisions about ourselves and our sexuality. When we are young, we decide whose behavior to model, with whom to play, how to dress, and which culturally prescribed sex-role tasks to adopt. When we are somewhat older, we decide who to date, whether to pet, whether premarital sexual intercourse is appropriate, whether to obtain and use some method of contraception, and how to prepare ourselves for the future (for career, parenthood, and so on). When we are even older, we decide whether or not to marry, whether to have children (if so, how many), how to perform the marriage-partner and/or parenthood roles, how to prepare for the future (for career, security, and so on), and, often, whether to remain married or to divorce. Still later in life we must decide how to adjust to menopause (if female), how to handle a midlife crisis, how to adapt sexual desires and behaviors to a changing body, how to play the grandparent and senior citizen roles, and how to connect with past and future generations.

In making these decisions we all attempt to maximize our happiness and satisfaction. Outward appearances may belie this attempt, and the end result might be quite the opposite, but all of us make decisions that we believe will benefit us. Some decisions obviously manifest this desire, but others need some further analysis before they can be understood as an attempt at self-enhancement. For example, let us look at an unwed female adolescent who is engaging in sexual intercourse but who does not use contraception. This girl may purposely become pregnant. At first glance her decision to become pregnant appears to be anything but beneficial for her. The financial burden that either abortion or care of an infant can create, the embarrassment of out-of-wedlock pregnancy, the hassle that can be expected from parents and relatives, the physical discomfort of pregnancy, and the possible interruption of schooling are negative consequences. However, this girl may feel unloved, unwanted, and rejected by her parents. She may believe that a baby, dependent on her as it will be, will have to love her. Further, the attention she will receive when pregnant (from physicians, school personnel, family and friends, and others) may be all the love that girl believes she can obtain. Consequently, pregnancy becomes a solution for her problem: how to acquire the love and attention she needs. In the long run this solution may be dysfunctional, but, for the moment, this girl has made a decision that she believes will make her happier.

So it is with all decisions. Even if we decide to do something to consciously punish ourselves, we may believe that the punishment will relieve guilt we are feeling, or that it is in some other way necessary to make us more satisfied. If we carefully scrutinize and analyze decisions, we recognize that they are attempts at self-enhancement.

What goes wrong then? Why don't all our decisions make us happy? We shall soon explore the decision-making process in more detail, but for now let us say that many decisions are not well thought out. We often sacrifice long-term happiness for short-term pleasure. We often neglect to consider all the consequences and implications of our decisions. We too often make decisions without getting advice and guidance from others close to us or without relevant information. We often employ convergent thinking wherein we see only one solution, rather than divergent thinking wherein we consider many possible solutions.

Improving the Decision-Making Process

Of course, the sexuality educator's role regarding sexual decision making is to teach the process, not to attempt to influence particular choices. Someone once said, "Give me a fish and I eat today; teach me to fish and I eat forever." If a person learns a rational decision-making process, he or she will be able to apply that process on numerous occasions. Learners should be taught this process and provided ample opportunity to try it on nonthreatening decisions. Practice, with appropriate feedback from the sexuality educator and fellow students, will result in familiarity with the decision-making process and confidence in its usefulness.

Decision making has been described by Gelatt and colleagues (1973) as involving three steps:

1. Examination and recognition of personal values

2. Knowledge and use of adequate, relevant information

3. Knowledge and use of an effective strategy for converting this information into an action

Let us look at these steps in more detail:

1. *Values.* "Values determine what is 'satisfying' and thus help a person to set objectives. Values also dictate the actions to be taken to reach those objectives. The information that is sought, the evaluation of that information, and the weight given to various pieces of data are influenced by personal values. A person facing a decision involving a conflict of values, accompanied by strong emotion, knows [he or she] faces an important decision, one requiring skill to decide satisfactorily."

2. *Knowledge.* "Information can be divided into four parts: possible alternative actions, possible outcomes, probability of outcomes, desirability of outcomes."

3. *Strategy.* This stage "requires calculating the risks associated with each considered alternative and applying what has been learned to making the decision. . . ." (Gelatt, et al., 1973, 4). Some of the most commonly used strategies are listed as follows:

   a. *The Wish Strategy.* Individuals choose what they wish would happen. This strategy suggests that people select the course of action (make a decision) that could lead to the most desirable result, regardless of risk or cost or probability. In a horse race the choice would be the "long shot." It is easy to use this strategy. People only need to know what they desire most and to have some information about the outcomes. They do not need to know probabilities.

   b. *The Safe Strategy.* This strategy suggests that individuals select the course of action that has the highest probability of being successful. In a horse race, the choice would be the "favorite." It is a little more difficult to use this strategy. A decision maker needs to know his or her objective and to have some information about possible and probable outcomes. At the same time the person is required to be somewhat more specific about objectives and needs to investigate information about additional alternatives and their probabilities.

   c. *The Escape Strategy.* This strategy suggests that individuals select the course of action that is most likely to avoid the worst possible result. It is sometimes called the "minimax" strategy because it minimizes the maximum disaster. It escapes misfortune. It is relatively easy to use this strategy. Individuals merely need to know a little bit of information about outcomes and what they consider the worst outcome.

   d. *The Combination Strategy.* This is a combination of the wish and safe strategies. This strategy suggests that individuals select the course of action that has both high probability and high desirability (sometimes called highest expected value). Although this strategy seems the most logical and reasonable, it is the most difficult to apply.

Another effective way to make decisions involves a six-step approach (Gay, et al., 1979):

1. *Perceive the problem.* Recognizing that the problem exists is the first step in solving it.

2. *Define the problem.* Narrow the scope of the problem so that it can be solved.

3. *Get ideas about the problem.* Generate as many possible solutions as can be thought up. Do not evaluate the solutions at this point. The idea is to accumulate as many as possible.

4. *Evaluate the ideas.* Evaluate each of the ideas that were generated in order to determine the relative merits of each alternative.

5. *Act.* Choose one alternative and put it into action.

6. *React.* Evaluate the action taken and determine whether it has been effective (if so, continue it) or ineffective (in which case, choose another alternative to put into action).

One aspect of decision making that sexuality educators should emphasize is the seeking of advice from others.

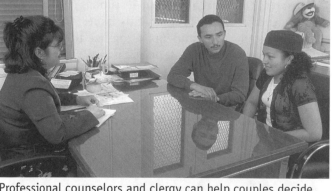

Professional counselors and clergy can help couples decide complex sexuality-related issues such as whether to marry, have children, or obtain an abortion.

Insight 9-3

Using a Decision-Making Model

Apply a model of decision making by completing the following form.

1. A problem I have that needs a solution is _____

   _____

2. More specifically, this problem entails _____

   _____

3. Possible solutions are

   a. _____

   b. _____

   c. _____

   d. _____

   e. _____

4. The best possible solution is _____

   _____

5. I will try this solution (when?) _____

6. After trying the solution, I found that _____ it worked _____ it didn't work.

7. If the solution didn't work, I will next try to _____

   _____

Notice that the word used is *advice*. Advice is to be considered and should be sought from those whose opinions are respected, but in the end only one person can make the decision. The advice obtained must be evaluated along with other bits of information. In some cases, the advice will be disregarded; in other instances, it may be the deciding factor.

The Decision-Making Process and Sexuality

Let us see how the decision-making process might be applied to a controversial area of sexuality education: abortion. First we must recognize that a personal decision is needed. Many people never even think about this issue. The sexuality educator should help students recognize the need for a citizenry aware of important societal issues.

Once the issue of abortion is raised, the problem must be defined. We actually can identify several phases of this problem. For our purposes, let us limit the problem to one of these phases, namely, should government funds be used for abortions for women who cannot afford them?

Next we must generate alternatives. Some of these might include the following:

1. No government funds should ever support abortion.

2. Only women under a specified income level should be provided government assistance.

3. All women should be provided government assistance.

4. Government assistance should be provided only to unmarried women, to women under a specified age, to women of specified intelligence, and so on. A whole range of alternatives can be generated.

We must now evaluate each alternative. To do so, we must acquire the relevant information. For example, how much government funding would be needed for each alternative? How many women would each alternative include? What are the religious, ethical, and moral implications of each alternative? What is the relevant existing legislation? What are our personal feelings? Who can we approach for advice?

Once this phase is accomplished, we must choose one alternative, observe it in action (if possible), and evaluate it some time later.

In our example, the decision-making process is applied to a societal issue, but the process can just as easily be employed for personal decision making. For example, a woman is pregnant and unwed. Should she have an abortion? We are sure that you can think of many other sexual decisions for which the decision-making process can be helpful.

Summary

Morals are based on ethics, which are based on values. Morals refer to concrete decisions for specific situations, ethics refer to the rationale behind decisions, and values are the bases for deciding moral and ethical issues.

Through values clarification techniques, people can understand themselves and others better by exploring how they know they really value something or what is involved in the process of valuing. Processes related to valuing include prizing, choosing, and acting on one's values. The role of sexuality educators is not to tell others what they ought to do, or what is right and wrong, but instead to assist people in developing morals and ethics as well as value systems.

Most sexuality education content involves considerations related to morals, ethics, and values. Sexuality educators need to constantly be aware that almost all sexual topics are controversial, even though the controversial elements might not immediately be apparent.

The official stands of most contemporary religions on sexual topics are quite supportive of human sexuality as part of total personality. Many people are surprised at this, because for so long sexuality either has been ignored in religious circles or has been discussed with negative connotations. More churches and synagogues are affirming sexuality and are recognizing that it is an essential aspect of humanity, that sexuality education is a shared responsibility, that there should be sexuality education programs, that sex is God's good gift, that all persons are sexual beings, and that sexual pleasure is good.

Sexual decisions often need to be made. At younger ages we decide whose behavior to model or how to dress, while at older ages we make decisions on dating and sexual behavior. In making these decisions we all try to maximize happiness and satisfaction. In practice, however, not all of our decisions make us happy. Many things might account for this, but one important influence is an understanding of the decision-making process.

Various decision-making models are available. Generally, the decision-making process involves perceiving the problem, defining the problem, getting ideas about the problem, evaluating the ideas, acting, and reacting.

The decision-making process can easily be applied to sexual matters. The steps indicated in this chapter are appropriate for attempting to resolve many personal and social dilemmas common today. Sexuality educators and their students will benefit by learning the decision-making process, since it has so many practical applications.

References

Gay, J., et al. *Current health problems.* Philadelphia: W. B. Saunders, 1979.

Gelatt, H. B., et al. *Decisions and outcomes: A leader's guide.* New York: College Entrance Examination Board, 1973. Excerpts reprinted with permission of the College Board.

Greenberg, J. S. *Health education and health promotion: Learner-centered instructional strategies.* 5th ed. Boston: WCB/McGraw-Hill, 2004.

Haffner, D.W. The really good news: What the Bible says about sex, *SIECUS Report*, 26 (1997), 3–8.

Haffner, D. W. & de Mauro, D. *Winning the battle: Developing support for sexuality and HIV/AIDS education.* New York: Sexuality Information and Education Council of the United States, 1991.

Kirkendall, L. A. Values and sex education, in *The new sex education*, Otto, H. A., ed. Chicago: Follett Publishing, 1978. Excerpts used by permission of Follett Publishing, a division of Follett Corporation.

National Guidelines Task Force. *Guidelines for comprehensive sexuality education.* New York: Sexuality Information and Education Council of the United States, 1991.

Raths, L., Harmin, M. & Simon, S. *Values and teaching: Working with values in the classroom.* Columbus, OH: Charles E. Merrill, 1966.

Suggested Readings

Fact sheet: Public support for sexuality education, *SIECUS Report*, 28 (2000), 29–32.

Fox, T. C. *Sexuality and Catholicism.* Scranton, PA: W. W. Norton, 2000.

Nelson, J. B. *Body theology.* Louisville, KY: Westminster/John Knox Press, 1997.

Terkel, S. N. *Finding your way: A book about sexual ethics.* Danbury, CT: Franklin Watts, 1995.

Westheimer, R. K. & Mark, J. *Heavenly sex: Sexuality in the Jewish tradition.* New York: New York University Press, 1995.

World Association for Sexology. Declaration of sexual rights, *SIECUS Report*, 28 (2000), 17.

Alternative Sexual Behaviors

CHAPTER 10

Key Concepts

1. Individual preferences in sexual behavior vary widely.

2. Heterosexual behavior has been carefully studied before, during, and after marriage.

3. Certain sexual behaviors have long had social significance.

4. Many sexual alternatives exist, although we know little about them.

5. Violent and aggressive sexual behavior appears to be increasing, but we still do not know a great deal about it.

Most people regard certain sexual behaviors as strange, abnormal, or immoral. For these people, certain sexual behaviors are emotionally charged issues. There are many ramifications of this fact for the sexuality educator: certain sexual behaviors may be difficult for some individuals to discuss; many misconceptions exist about the causes and effects of sexual behaviors; and our knowledge about certain sexual behavior is less than extensive. This poses a real educational challenge, for education is difficult when the learner has emotional blocks and misconceptions to overcome.

Before reading further, consider your feelings about sexual behaviors by completing Insight 10-1. As you thought about why you classified certain behaviors as either normal or variant abnormal in Insight 10-1, you may have noticed some emotional reactions. When handling sexuality education about a variety of sexual behaviors, it is essential for the sexuality educator to remember three things.

First, you must recognize your own feelings and consider their impact on your ability to be an effective educator. For example, if a certain topic, such as homosexuality, causes you to become emotional inside, it may be difficult for you to handle the topic with a group of people. You may need to practice talking about the topic while learning more about it in order to facilitate your objectivity. How effective would it be if the learners detected your emotional responses or saw that you have a difficult time dealing with a particular topic?

Insight 10-1

Normal and Variant Sexual Behavior

A sexuality educator must first be aware of his or her own attitudes. As a first step in your own awareness, list all of the sexual behaviors you can think of that fit into two categories: normal sexual behavior and variant sexual behavior.

Now, consider each behavior on your lists. On what grounds did you place certain behaviors in each category? How much do you really know about each behavior? Were you making rational or emotional judgments? You may recognize that you need more education about "normal" and "variant" sexual behaviors.

Second, you must remember that some learners will have emotional reactions to certain topics whether you do or not. In many cases this might be the first time that they have ever talked about some topics—particularly in groups. Your sensitivity to this is a must. In addition, you need to promote sensitivity on the part of the learners so that they will respect their own feelings as well as those of others. All feelings and statements are accepted and discussed as appropriate.

Third, learners should be helped to realize that many sexual behaviors exist on a continuum. For example, some people have tended to label behaviors as "abnormal," "sick," or "deviant" when sometimes they may exist in various degrees. If we label voyeurism as abnormal, what do people think about themselves if they sometimes enjoy looking at a person? Is this problematic? How much looking is necessary before a problem exists? We do not know and no one else does either. The point is simply that there is a need to recognize that some behaviors in themselves are not necessarily negative or a problem. What matters is how, when, and the degree to which they are used. Although this idea will probably not apply to all sexual behaviors, viewing some of them in this manner will often facilitate sexuality education.

Individual Preferences and Sexual Behavior

Masturbation

In Chapter 1 we briefly discussed masturbation and pointed out some myths and facts about this practice. People have long experienced strong emotional feelings and held many misconceptions about masturbation. In addition to its important role in healthy growth and development, masturbation also plays a role for many people as one kind of sexual outlet at various times, while some practice it throughout life. For example, some people who know the facts about masturbation and do not feel guilty about it might practice it from time to time simply because they enjoy it. Others might not usually masturbate but might find certain times in their lives, such as during separation from or illness of a spouse, when they choose to masturbate. Still others might find masturbation unsatisfactory because of personal feelings.

It is safe to say that masturbation tends to increase during preadolescence and adolescence, and that boys usually start masturbating earlier than girls. It also seems that both sexes are starting to masturbate earlier than they did a generation or two ago (Greenberg, Bruess & Haffner, 2004).

It has been suggested that, today, 99% of all males masturbate at some time in their lives and the other 1% lie. In regard to females, it is believed that 65% to 75% probably masturbate at some time. Although we do not have the evidence to support these figures with assurance, they seem reasonable, based on the fragmentary information we do have.

From an educational perspective, it may be helpful to consider five myths about masturbation along with some facts:

1. Myth: Masturbation leads to mental health problems.
   Fact: Unless someone is seriously bothered by the practice, there is no evidence that masturbation causes any mental difficulties.

2. Myth: Masturbation causes acne and other skin problems.
   Fact: Masturbation does not cause acne or skin problems.

3. Myth: Masturbation makes a male unable to have children.
   Fact: Masturbation does not affect fertility.

4. Myth: Only males masturbate.
   Fact: A majority of both sexes masturbate at some time in their lives as previously indicated.

5. Myth: Masturbation ceases after a person gets married.
   Fact: This is only true for some people.

Masturbation has been called the "solitary vice." Many people have considered it to be evil, while others have regarded it as no big deal. Some have referred to it as lonely sport at best. It is important to note that masturbation has been used effectively as part of therapy for various sexual dysfunctions. It can also be considered a healthy alternative to having a partner and is less risky than unprotected intercourse with an unfamiliar partner. Regardless of how you feel about it, it is important to keep emotions and facts separate when educating about masturbation.

Oral–Genital Contact

Fellatio is defined as oral (mouth) contact with a male's genital area. **Cunnilingus** is oral contact with a female's genital area. The familiar numerical symbol 69 is used to depict the position of two people participating in oral–genital contact at the same time. This is an excellent example of a behavior that many people think is disgusting and many other people think is wonderful. Some people learn to fear contact with such a "dirty" area of the body as the genitals; but this fear is unfounded because this area of the body can be just as clean as any other area. It has been suggested, in fact, that if oral–genital contact is unclean, it is because of the many germs in the mouth!

Homosexual Behavior

Before reading further, take a few moments to consider how strongly you feel about homosexuality by completing Insight 10-2.

Homosexuality is probably the most talked about variation in sexual behavior today. Many heterosexuals have a difficult time understanding homosexuals as people with feelings and rights. Many myths about homosexuality have developed over the years, and the facts need to be understood. One myth is that homosexuals look a lot different than other people. You have probably heard somebody claim that another person is a homosexual because "I can tell one a mile away." The fact is that only about 10% of all homosexuals are what could be termed "visible homosexuals." The other 90% look and act just like everyone else except for their sexual orientation.

Another myth is that homosexual males are effeminate and weak, while homosexual females are masculine and physically strong. In fact, sexual orientation has nothing to do with one's body type or style of movement. Male homosexuals can be found in all walks of life (yes, even football players and truck drivers), and so can lesbians.

---

fellatio   Oral contact with a male's genital area.   **cunnilingus**   Oral contact with a female's genital area.

Feelings about Homosexuality

One way to explore your feelings is to use a values grid (Greenberg, 1992). As you read over the 16 questions, place the italicized key words from each question in one square of the grid below that shows how you feel about the question. Note that in so doing you will be identifying the *degree* of your feeling and *not whether it is positive or negative*. After you complete the grid, look it over to see how strong your feelings about homosexuality are. If you can find a willing partner, share your grids with each other and discuss why you placed your responses in the respective columns. One caution: all 16 squares must be filled in, and only one key word can be placed in any one square. This process may necessitate moving key words around as you discover others about which you feel more or less strongly.

1. How would you feel if your closest *friend* told you he or she was a homosexual?
2. How do you feel about *two girls* who greet each other with a kiss after a long summer vacation?
3. How do you feel about *two boys* greeting each other with a kiss after a long summer vacation?
4. How do you feel about a person who would *beat up* a homosexual for fun?
5. How do you feel about *two girls holding hands* on the way to class?
6. How do you feel about girls wearing *boys' clothes?*
7. How do you feel about boys wearing *girls' clothes?*
8. How do you feel about *two boys holding hands* on the way to class?
9. How do you feel about *boys* who do not like *sports?*
10. How do you feel about *girls* who do like *sports?*
11. How do you feel about taking *group showers?*
12. How do you feel about a man taking over the household *chores?*
13. How do you feel about a man *hairdresser?*
14. How do you feel about a woman who becomes a *lawyer?*
15. How do you feel about going out only with a person of the *opposite sex?*
16. How do you feel about going out only with persons of the *same sex?*

How did you feel about these questions? Did any of them bother you for any reason? Why or why not? Do you have strong feelings about homosexuality?

Very Strongly	Strongly	Mildly	No Opinion

Another myth is that homosexuals lurk at every street corner waiting to pounce on innocent children and seduce them into a life of homosexuality. Although there must be some homosexuals who seduce children, there are also quite a few heterosexuals who do. Either situation is intolerable, but to blame only homosexuals for this behavior is unfair and inappropriate. A related myth is that homosexuals are not fit to be teachers. There is nothing about homosexuality that affects teaching ability. If a homosexual is preaching homosexuality in the classroom or seducing students, this is wrong; however, it would be equally wrong for a heterosexual to act similarly.

Some people regard homosexuals as mentally ill. This too is a myth. One of the problems in attempting to get a clear picture of homosexuals is that most of the literature dealing with the subject concerns homosexuals who have seen psychologists or psychiatrists. What kind of picture of heterosexuals would we get if we generalized from those who seek help with their mental adjustment? There are many perfectly happy, well-balanced homosexuals—heterosexuals often just do not hear about them. A related notion is that homosexuals obtained their sexual orientation because of problems in their early family relationships. It is obvious that a poor family relationship will influence anyone's development. But at the present time, this theory of why some people are homosexuals is far from having been proven. Many

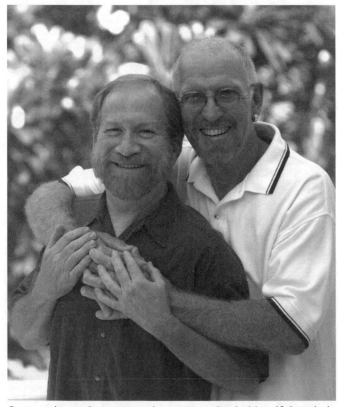

Gays are becoming more and more assertive in identifying their rights and feeling comfortable with their sexual preference.

homosexuals do not regard their sexual orientation as a "problem" that requires such explanation, since researchers are unable to explain what causes sexual orientation.

Researchers and educators are continually confronted by the biological versus environmental causation argument concerning reasons for homosexuality. However, even newer evidence of a possible biological marker for homosexuality has not cleared up the issue.

It has often been assumed that homosexuals are poor security risks. This thinking is based on the assumption that homosexuals are subject to blackmail. Although there was probably some foundation for this idea in the past, today's more tolerant and open attitudes make this possibility much less likely. Why would a publicly proclaimed homosexual be any more susceptible to blackmail than anyone else?

As can readily be seen, there is no solid foundation for any of these myths about homosexuality. Yet most heterosexuals have learned to believe that homosexuality is a second-class condition and therefore accept disparaging myths about homosexuals.

Some people argue that gays and lesbians can turn straight (heterosexual) if they wish. Such a conclusion clashes with that of major mental health groups that say nobody knows what causes a person's sexual orientation. Further, these groups indicate that there is no credible evidence that sexual orientation can be changed (Study: Some gays can go straight, 2001).

Pawlowski (1989) made suggestions about what parents might do if there were a gay child in the family. These same points apply to educators. For example, since most homosexual youths have no peer group in which they can begin to learn and understand their "different" romantic feelings, they are in need of a supportive environment in which to explore who they are. Constant negative societal messages lead most homosexual youths to grow up with a feeling that they are not worthwhile or valued human beings. To make matters worse, when parents (and perhaps even friends) learn that a young person is gay or lesbian, they frequently view this as a tragedy. The real tragedy, however, is that family messages about homosexuality are so frequently negative and condemnatory that homosexual children often turn away from their parents for love and understanding.

Educators (and hopefully parents too) can help by emphasizing that no one should ever exploit, take advantage of, or force sexual feelings or desires on someone else. We must encourage and respect whatever sexual feelings young people develop. We need to help them feel good about who they are and what they feel. We must help young people realize that when there are strong sexual feelings, some of them may be for members of the other sex and some may be for members of the same sex. Varying degrees of these feelings are normal, and they may also fade or increase at different times in life. It is entirely possible that an educator who handles the topic of homosexuality in this way may help prevent a number of adjustment problems for homosexual and heterosexual young people.

It is hard to know exactly how many homosexuals there are in our society, but contemporary estimates place the population between 2% and 10%. This means that (statistically speaking) some of your friends or classmates are homosexuals, and probably some of your teachers are too—even some of your professional colleagues and some of your favorite basketball team. Regardless of our own feelings about homosexuality, it is time to start treating homosexuals as individuals with the same rights, responsibilities, and feelings as others. Go back and look at your grid again. How do your feelings relate to myths and facts about homosexuality?

Heterosexual Behavior

Premarital Heterosexual Behavior

Many of our history books would lead us to believe that, in the past, Americans were sexually chaste before marriage. If we carefully read between the lines, however, we find that this is not necessarily true. Reiss (1973) informs us that, in the late 1700s in Massachusetts, one out of three women in a particular church confessed fornication to her minister (the actual number was probably higher still). The western frontier relied heavily on prostitution. The women's liberation movement of the 1870s revealed numerous sexual affairs. And the first vulcanized rubber condom for males was displayed at the Philadelphia World's Fair in 1876. These

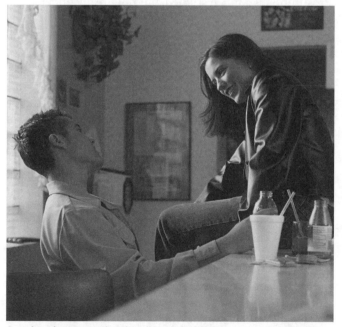

Continual communication is needed by young people to help promote positive feelings about their amount and types of sexual behavior.

are not isolated events and should make us question what we have always thought concerning the sexual purity and innocence of our forebears.

Studies done in the years between 1920 and 1945 seem to indicate that the greatest increase in rates of premarital intercourse came in the early 1900s (Bell, 1966). The so-called sexual revolution began early in the twentieth century and not in more recent years. Today's parents and grandparents, who seem so concerned about changes in sexual behavior, were in the middle of the sexual revolution in the first place. Our best research tells us that approximately 35% to 45% of females and 55% to 65% of males participated in premarital sexual intercourse during most of the first 65 years of the twentieth century.

Clearly, there are many implications here for sexuality education. Although no one seems to know for certain how to help people make responsible decisions about their premarital sexual behavior, one author prepared a list of questions for people to answer to help them determine if they are ready. Educators and parents might find these useful. Here is the list (Allgeier, 1985):

Are You Ready for Sex?

You are ready if:

1. You feel guiltless and comfortable about your present level of involvement.

2. You are confident that you will not be humiliated and that your reputation will not be hurt.

3. Neither partner is pressuring the other for sex.

4. You are not trying to:

   a. prove your love for the other person;

   b. increase your self-worth;

   c. prove that you are mature;

   d. show that you can attract a sexual partner;

   e. get attention, affection, or love;

   f. rebel against parents, society, etc.

5. It will be an expression of your current feelings rather than an attempt to improve a poor relationship or one that is "growing cold."

6. You can discuss and agree on an effective method of contraception and share the details, responsibilities, and costs of the use of the method.

7. You can discuss the potential of contracting or transmitting sexually transmitted infections.

8. You have discussed and agreed on what both of you will do if conception occurs, because no contraceptive method is 100% effective.

Communicating about Sexual Activity

Make a list of the phrases you have heard that are designed to initiate or to turn down sexual activity. Initiating phrases include such statements as, "I think I'll take a shower." Turn-down phrases are such comments as, "I have a headache tonight." When you have made your lists, note how many are straightforward and how many are euphemistic or mere hints.

Marital Heterosexual Behavior

Throughout the years the topic of marital sexual behavior has not received the attention given to premarital sexual behavior, but there are important observations and generalizations that can be made about it. For example, two general social changes have probably had a great impact on women. First, since more reliable contraceptives have been developed, the relationship between intercourse and conception is no longer beyond the control of the individual. Second, the relatively new assumption that a woman has as much right as a man to expect sexual satisfaction is widely recognized.

Other observations include the importance of communication regarding sexual matters in marriage. The old assumption that men know naturally how to perform sexually as well as know what women desire is simply not true. Communication between partners is essential. For example, for many women the need for cuddling and closeness is of greater importance than the need for intercourse itself. Some women may "exchange" intercourse for close body contact, because such contact helps meet their needs for relaxation and security.

What do we know about the frequency of marital intercourse? Today's married couples have sexual intercourse more often, experience more sexual pleasure, and engage in a greater variety of sexual activities and techniques than people surveyed in the 1950s. Precoital activity has not increased, but it tends to last longer than in earlier years. Oral stimulation of the breasts and manual stimulation of the genitals have increased as has oral–genital contact (Clements, 1994; Laumann, et al., 1994).

The frequency of sexual intercourse in marriage tends to decrease over time. For example, for newly married couples the average rate of sexual intercourse is about 3 times per week. In early middle age, the average is about 1.5 to 2 times per week. After age 50, the average rate is 1 time per week or less. This does not mean that sexual activity becomes unimportant or that marriage becomes unsatisfactory. The decrease may only be the result of biological aging, fatigue, and a decrease in sex drive (Call, Sprecher & Schwartz, 1995).

Timing of marital sexual activity contributes to possible problems. Marital sexual activity often takes place late in the evening after a long day and just before sleep. The presence of children in the family can pose additional problems to finding a time for sexual activity. Since it is often felt that a quiet and private time is needed, there may be pressure to "get sexual activity in" during the short time available after the pressures of the day's activities.

All of this is complicated by the common need to negotiate marital sexual activity. Difficulties with the language of sexuality cause communication problems. Although we have finally started to develop a public language about sexuality, most of us still do not have a private language for communicating about sexual behavior.

Need we emphasize that there are countless possibilities here for sexuality education? Almost all of the problems mentioned in connection with marital sexual behavior are related to knowledge and attitudes. Sexuality educators can have a major impact on sexual and marital happiness.

The Social Significance of Sexual Behaviors

Prostitution and pornography are perhaps the two most prominent areas of sexual behavior that have been major social issues.

Prostitution

Prostitution is a much studied, but not greatly understood, sexual variation. In a general sense, the term refers to any situation in which one person pays another for sexual gratification. Ancient history includes many examples of prostitution, so contemporary society cannot take the credit or blame (whichever is appropriate) for inventing this behavior. The debate over whether prostitution should be made legal or not and what the effects of legalization would be continues.

Is it likely that prostitution will increase or decrease in the future? Of course no one knows for sure, but various factors could influence prostitution rates one way or the other. For example, rates could increase if there are reasons for many military personnel to be overseas (servicemen have generally been good customers for prostitutes), or if the number of commercially sponsored clubs for sexual activity continues to increase. In addition, opportunities for prostitution in situations where sexual therapies are inappropriately carried out seem to be increasing.

On the other hand, rates might decrease if better programs to treat drug addicts are developed (many women have entered prostitution to get money for narcotics) or as a result of greater acceptance of various sexual behaviors within established relationships, which can result in better fulfillment

Views about Prostitution

The women's liberation movement brought a new element into the discussion of prostitution. It has been said that "prostitutes are the only honest women because they charge for their services rather than submitting to a marriage contract which forces them to work for life without pay." How do you feel about this statement? What does it say to you about prostitutes? What about the roles of females and males today? Would it matter to you who made the statement? As a matter of fact, it was made by a women's liberation leader.

of sexual needs. Prostitution will also become less popular if more people take AIDS statistics and probabilities seriously.

Adolescent prostitution has become an increasing problem in the United States. Prostitution is used as a means of economic survival. Most of these youth shun traditional work due to fear of being traced or arrested as a runaway and returned to a negative home environment. In a recent development, there have been reports of children setting up their own prostitution rings while still living at home, to earn spending money. Therapy programs for prostitutes have usually not been very successful for many reasons, particularly because many prostitutes do not feel they can receive help.

Pornography

What is pornography? No answer to this question satisfies everyone. Some people feel that pornography, like beauty, is in the eye of the beholder. Others feel that any pictures or words that have to do with anything related to sexuality are disgusting. Each of us must personally decide how we feel based on personal beliefs as well as on the facts about pornography.

The vast majority of sexually explicit material used in the United States is "adult" or "mainstream" pornography. It depicts cheerfully consenting adults and does not involve children, coercion, or violence. Studies of this kind of pornography supported the following conclusions (Harvey, 1992):

- It causes no harm and is socially and individually useful.

- It does not undermine social fabric. It is far less harmful than many other legal and acceptable things in our society (such as cigarettes, alcohol, and automobiles).

- It does not "exploit" members of our society.

- Laws against it are counterproductive. They divert resources from combating actual criminal activity and are a government attempt to legislate morality.

Donnerstein, Linz, and Penrod (1987) indicated that erotica is not the problem. The problem is violence. What research strongly supports is that the violent images, not the sexual images, are important. It is strictly the aggressive content which tends to increase aggressive behavior—not the sexual content or the sexual explicitness.

While not everyone would agree, Stein (1998) indicated that many people have accepted erotica's place in today's culture. Many people are buying materials for their own use. The many billions of dollars spent each year on sexually explicit materials show that there is a growing acceptance of pornography. However, it was interesting that in 2003 Wal-Mart decided to pull three magazines from its shelves—*Maxim, Stuff,* and *FHM.* The decision was made to make sure families felt comfortable enough to shop at Wal-Mart together (Stein, 2003).

There seems to be no debate, however, when it comes to the topic of child pornography. Unanimous opposition to this form of pornography is apparent.

How do you feel about the production, sale, and use of sexually explicit materials? Regardless of your personal feelings, education is needed about pornography and its effects, since pornography is not likely to disappear from our society in the near future.

Other Sexual Alternatives

Alternative sexual behaviors are generally classified as abnormal sexual behaviors, sexual perversions, or problematic sexual behaviors. None of these negative labels have been attached to sexual behaviors in this book, for a very good reason. The reason is that many sexual behaviors should be considered on a continuum; it is difficult to judge when a specific behavior is "abnormal" or a "perversion." Take masturbation for example. We have already established that this is a common part of growth and development as well as a generally harmless and common behavior during adulthood. On the other hand, most of us would probably think it was a little strange if someone masturbated 15 times each day. How about exhibitionism? Did you give some thought to the clothes you would wear today? You probably wore them because you wanted to look nice; yet few people would call you an exhibitionist for that reason. There are many things you can do that are exhibitionistic that would probably not be a problem or "abnormal." Somewhere along the continuum there might be problematic behavior, but who should say where that point is?

It is up to each individual to decide where various sexual behaviors fit on the continuum, but there are also important implications here for sexuality educators. We need to use care when dealing with these topics, because the descriptive words we use or even the tone of our voice can get in the way of an appropriate objective coverage of important facts. For example, if we say, "Today we are going to discuss a number of abnormal sexual behaviors," we have set the stage differently than if we say, "Today we are going to discuss some facts and feelings people might have about different types of sexual behavior." Sexuality educators need to be aware of these subtle but important differences.

Whatever labels or approaches you choose to use, you will need at least basic information about numerous sexual behaviors. In many instances, you will need more than what is provided here, but these facts should at least get you started.

Bestiality is sexual contact with animals. As you might expect, bestiality is most common among people who live on farms. It is also more common among males than females, and it is most likely to occur during adolescence. You might also hear the term *zoophilia* used to refer to this type of sexual behavior.

Bisexuals (ambisexuals) are people who enjoy sexual relationships with members of both genders. Since it has usually been thought that all of us, if left to our natural ways, are bisexual to some extent, it seems to be the process of socialization that for most people results in sexual behavior only with members of one gender. There are some people who are evenly divided between homosexual and heterosexual feelings, but most people tend to lean one way or the other.

Exhibitionism is achievement of sexual gratification by exhibiting the genitals to observers. In most cases the observers are present by accident and do not plan on the experience. Contrary to popular opinion, exhibitionists are not usually aggressive; they tend to be quiet, submissive types of people.

Fetishism is sexual fixation on some object other than another human being. Almost anything can be the object of fixation, from parts of the body to articles of clothing or certain types of material. Again, it is appropriate to mention that there is a continuum for fetishes from a mild preference to a strong preference to a necessity. You must decide for yourself at what point this might become problematic behavior.

Frottage is the act of obtaining sexual pleasure from rubbing or pressing against another person. Usually, no one notices this form of behavior since it is likely to occur in crowded places such as on an elevator or bus. Generally, no additional contact or other forms of behavior occur.

Masochism is sexual gratification from experiencing pain. Interestingly, it must be pain that is planned as part of an overall experience; accidentally hitting a finger with a hammer would not be sexually pleasurable for a masochist. **Sadism,** sexual gratification from inflicting pain on another person, is usually discussed with masochism since sadists and masochists make good partners. Masochism seems to be more common than sadism.

Nymphomania refers to an extremely high sex drive in certain women. The term has been used rather loosely; a true nymphomaniac has an uncontrollable sexual desire that must be satisfied. Most women who enjoy sexual activity a great deal are not even close to that. A similar condition in men is called **satyriasis.**

Sodomy refers specifically to anal intercourse, but throughout the years the term has been used quite broadly to refer to almost any form of sexual behavior that someone happens to think is not "normal." The term has also been used in much the same way in legal language. For example, in some places it might be legally used to refer to oral–genital contact or bestiality.

Transsexualism exists when a person believes that he or she is trapped in a body of the wrong gender. This should not be confused with homosexuality, since transsexuals want to relate sexually to members of the other gender if they can only be in a body of the "proper" gender themselves, while homosexuals want to relate sexually to members of the same gender. Although it is not a common procedure, surgery and chemical therapy can be combined to change a person's gender.

Transvestism is sometimes confused with transsexualism as well as with homosexuality. A transvestite prefers wearing clothes of the other gender and is likely to achieve sexual gratification from doing so, but has no interest in a sex-change operation or in relating sexually to members of the same gender. In most instances transvestites have quite "normal" heterosexual relationships in every way except for their tendency toward cross-dressing when alone or with an understanding partner.

---

bestiality   Sexual contact with animals.

bisexual (ambisexual)   Person who enjoys sexual relationships with members of both sexes.

exhibitionism   Achievement of sexual gratification by exhibiting the genitals to observers.

fetishism   Sexual fixation on some object other than another human being.

frottage   Act of obtaining sexual pleasure from rubbing or pressing against another person.

masochism   Sexual gratification from experiencing pain.

sadism   Sexual gratification from inflicting pain.

nymphomania   Extremely high sex drive in women.

satyriasis   Extremely high sex drive in men.

sodomy   Anal intercourse. The term is also used in legal language to refer to various sexual behaviors other than sexual intercourse.

transsexualism   Belief of person that he or she is trapped in a body of the wrong gender.

transvestism   Achievement of sexual gratification by wearing clothes of the other sex.

Troilism refers to having sexual relations with another person while a third person watches. It seems to combine elements of exhibitionism and voyeurism.

Voyeurism used in a very general sense refers to obtaining pleasure from watching people who are undressing or engaging in sexual behavior. A "Peeping Tom" is a voyeur. Generally, voyeurs are not violent and in fact are fearful of any contact with the persons they observe. You may also hear the term *scopophilia* used to refer to voyeuristic acts.

Forcible Sexual Behavior

Most of the sexual behavior variations discussed in this chapter have in common the fact that they are generally participated in by personal choice. Even though many people might consider some of the behaviors strange, there is usually no harm done to anyone involved. In contrast, such behaviors as pedophilia, necrophilia, rape, incest, and sexual abuse in general involve some degree of forcing one's will upon another. Although accurate statistics are hard to find, it appears that these forcible behaviors are increasing.

Obscene telephone callers receive sexual gratification from calling people and making obscene remarks that suggest that the person on the other end of the phone will meet them and have sexual relations. The obscene-letter writer is hoping for the same result, but in neither case is the person likely to be violent and follow up the call or letter in any other way. A more recent variation of obscene communication is done via the computer. Some people will send obscene e-mail messages for the same reasons others make obscene phone calls or send obscene letters.

Pedophilia is a form of sexual behavior that demands a child as the sexual object. Even though actual force may not be used, an adult who performs a sexual act with a child is in violation of the law.

As part of the National Health and Social Life Survey (Laumann, et al., 1994), it was found that about 12% of the men and 17% of the women surveyed had been sexually touched when they were children. The experience was reported equally by people of different ages, suggesting that there has not been an increase in rates in recent years. The females were primarily touched by men, and the males were touched more often by women but also by men. Touching

genitals was by far the most common behavior for both genders. The majority of the sample reported an experience with only one adult, but about one in three reported events that occurred with more than one person.

In the survey, family friends and relatives were the primary offenders. About 34% of respondents reported they were touched one time, 38% a few times, and 27% many times. As might be expected, only 22% told someone about this sexual contact with an older person. Those with early childhood sexual experiences were consistently more sexually active in adulthood than those without such experiences.

The most vulnerable age for sexual abuse is between 7 and 13 years. It happens to children in both rural and urban areas, in all socioeconomic and educational levels, and across all racial and cultural groups. Another study reported victimization rates of 27% of females and 16% of males (*Child sexual abuse,* 1998).

According to the National Clearinghouse on Child Abuse and Neglect Information (1998), almost 1 million children are victims of child abuse each year. Twelve percent of these (120,000) suffer sexual abuse.

Almost one-third of females and nearly 1 in 10 male high school students in Massachusetts say they have experienced sexual abuse. Those who have had such experiences are more likely to take sexual risks, including having sexual intercourse before the age of 15, having multiple partners for sexual activity, and having sexual relations resulting in a pregnancy (A history of sexual abuse elevates the Massachusetts teenagers' risk of engaging in unsafe sexual practices, 2001).

Necrophilia is a sexual variation that most people seldom hear about but that law-enforcement personnel often encounter. It is sexual relations with a dead person. There is little known about this behavior, but morticians occasionally report the disappearance of a body for this purpose.

Incest is sexual behavior between relatives who are too closely related to be legally married. The most commonly reported form is father–daughter, but in practice brother–sister probably happens more. In recent years incest has received publicity because of its role as part of an overall pattern of child abuse. It is difficult to estimate the amount of incest that occurs. The statistics given previously for pedophilia also relate to incest.

Children involved in incest are usually afraid to tell anyone about it. Educators would be wise to be aware that a child

---

troilism   Having sexual relations with another person while a third person watches.

voyeurism (scopophilia)   Achievement of sexual pleasure by watching people undressing or engaging in sexual behaviors.

obscene telephone caller   Receives sexual gratification from calling people and making obscene remarks related to meeting for sexual relations.

pedophilia   Sexual behavior that demands a child as the sexual object.

necrophilia   Sexual relations with a dead person.

incest   Sexual behavior between relatives who are too closely related to be legally married.

or adolescent may have been sexually abused if he or she exhibits one or more of the following behaviors: (1) depression; (2) low self-esteem, which may manifest itself as withdrawal or self-destructive acting out; (3) isolation from peers; (4) drug or alcohol abuse; (5) chronic runaway; (6) sophisticated or unusual sexual behavior or knowledge; (7) decline in academic performance; (8) frequent absences from school justified by the father or male guardian (Intrafamily sexual abuse—incest, 1982).

Almost every society has a taboo against incest, but incest nevertheless occurs in all social classes, in all geographic areas, and among all ethnic and racial groups. Various community organizations offer help for incest victims and their families—for example, child-protection agencies, rape crisis centers, women's centers, and organizations that offer help for parents who are under extreme stress or are frightened about their feelings toward their children. The best strategy for preventing incest seems to be to provide information to potential victims as well as to parents. This means providing sexuality education at the elementary school level and above that conveys specific information about sexual abuse. For example, children can be taught that they have control over their own bodies, and that Uncle Charlie or Aunt Mary do not automatically have the right to touch them all over. In addition, information about pedophilia and other sexual practices should be provided at the appropriate level of understanding.

Rape is a forcible act that has recently received a great deal of long-overdue attention. Rape crisis centers, workshops dealing with the topic of rape, and attention to procedures for dealing with rape survivors have become high priorities in many cities and states.

There is still a great deal that is not known about rape. Despite the substantial increase in studies of rape in the past decade, myths regarding rape are still common, with the result that it is still condoned. Let us look at a few of the myths (Greenberg, Bruess & Haffner, 2004):

Myth: Rape is an impulsive act of passion—meaning that men cannot control their sex drives.
Fact: Rapists themselves do not see rape as compulsive sexual behavior. The motive for rape is not usually sexual pleasure; it is power and violence. Sexual activity is used to carry out nonsexual needs.

Myth: Women want to be raped—meaning that women have fantasies that reflect their desire to be raped.
Fact: Rape is an act of violent aggression. No healthy individual desires to be dehumanized and violated.

Myth: Women ask to be raped—meaning they tempt the man. "She should have worn a bra." "Hitchhikers get what they deserve," and "She shouldn't have been out so late at night" are examples of this thinking.
Fact: The blame and responsibility for a criminal assault belong to the assailant, not the victim.

Myth: A woman can run faster with her skirt up than a man can with his pants down—meaning a woman can't be raped against her will.
Fact: Rape is an aggression committed under force or the threat of force upon an unconsenting person. A knife, gun, or even a verbal threat are often understandably stronger than a person's will.

Myth: You can't blame a man for trying—meaning the responsibility for stopping a man belongs to the woman; therefore, it is her fault if things get out of hand.
Fact: A criminal, not the victim, is responsible for his acts. Rape is not an impulsive act of passion. It is done for power and control.

Myth: If a woman is going to be raped, she might as well relax and enjoy it—meaning it is just sexual activity.
Fact: Rape victims experience intense psychological and physical trauma. Rape is a violent, dehumanizing, and intimate invasion of the woman's privacy and integrity as a human being. The motive for rape is power; it is not for sexual enjoyment. Rape is anything but enjoyable!

Myth: The rapist is usually of a different race than the victim—meaning rape usually reflects ethnic or racial hatred.
Fact: In most instances the rapist and the victim are of the same race (estimates indicate this is true in as many as 90%–95% of the cases).

Myth: Most rapes are committed by strangers—meaning we are safe with people we know.
Fact: It is common for the rapist and the victim to know each other, to have been acquainted, or at least to have seen each other on the street, in the grocery store, in the student union, and so on.

The Incidence of Rape

Because so many cases are not reported, statistics on rape leave a lot to be desired. Estimating rates of violence, especially sexual assault and other incidents committed by intimate offenders, continues to be a difficult task. Many factors inhibit people from reporting these crimes. The private nature of

rape   Forcible sexual intercourse with a person who does not give consent.

the event, the perceived stigma, and the belief that no purpose would be served in reporting the crime keep an unknown portion of victims from talking about the attack.

Even with the difficulties in obtaining accurate information about rapes, it is appropriate to consider the best information available. There is a wide variation in numbers, depending on the source. The U.S. Department of Justice (*Sex offenses and offenders: An analysis of data on rape and sexual assault,* 1998) indicates that each year there are about 500,000 rapes or other sexual assaults. About 32% of these are reported to a law enforcement agency. About 60% of these incidents occur in the victim's home or at the home of a friend, relative, or neighbor. In addition, an estimated 91% of the victims are female, and 99% of the offenders are male. Seventy-five percent of the assaults involve offenders with whom the victim had a prior relationship—a family member, intimate, or acquaintance. There is about one rape or sexual assault victimization of a female for every 270 females in the general population; for males, the rate is substantially lower, with about one for every 5,000 males aged 12 or older.

The *Uniform Crime Reports for the United States* of the Federal Bureau of Investigation (1996) indicate that there is one forcible rape every 6 minutes in the United States. The lowest number of rapes occurs in December, and the highest number occurs in July. Rape victims are about evenly divided among whites and African-Americans, and about 88% of the time the victim and the offender are of the same race (*Sex offenses and offenders,* 1998).

In 2001, several studies related to dating violence were reported. The U.S. Department of Justice released interesting information about the prevalence and nature of sexual assault occurring at American colleges (Fisher, et al., 2001). According to this information, about 3% of college women experience a completed or attempted rape during a typical college year. About 13% had been stalked during the previous college year.

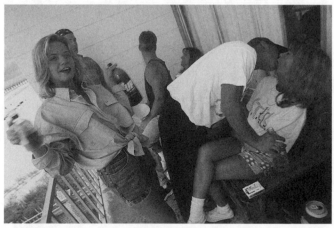

Drinking alcoholic beverages can affect judgment, leading to actions and feelings that one can regret the next day—and long after.

Of the incidents of sexual victimization, the vast majority occurred after 6 P.M. in living quarters. Nearly 60% of completed rapes that took place on campus occurred in the survivor's residence, 31% occurred in other living quarters on campus, and 10% occurred in a fraternity. Most off-campus incidents, especially rapes, also occurred in residences. Nearly 90% of the women knew the offender, who was usually a classmate, friend, ex-boyfriend, or acquaintance.

The legal definition of rape and law-enforcement procedures in rape cases differ greatly from state to state. A practical definition of rape is "forcible sexual intercourse." If a person is forced to have sexual intercourse when the person does not want to—that is rape. Sometimes only the persons involved can tell when this is happening.

In order to better understand motivations behind rape as well as to be able to more effectively assist rape victims, it is important to attempt to view rape as a forcible or violent act, not primarily a sexual one. Most rapists rape to be aggressive, to show their power, or to belittle the victim. In most instances the motivations and satisfactions are not sexual in the usual way that we think about sexual satisfactions. In fact, it is unlikely that satisfaction even occurs. Unfortunately, when we respond to the crime of rape we usually become hung up on the sexual aspects instead of the violent aspects. Rape victims and their loved ones need to be helped through difficult times in the same way that victims of other violent acts need help. Viewing rape as mainly a violent act instead of a sexual one may aid a victim's adjustment at a trying time.

Insight 10-5

Feelings about Rape

How do you feel about the following statement about rape:

Rape is certainly one of the worst things that can happen to a woman, but I believe that it isn't *the* worst. To put rape in first place, you'd have to ignore death, mutilation, disease, loss of a loved one, amputation of a limb, going blind, deafness or being mute, mental illness, paralysis, and perhaps a few other catastrophes. All of these, I think, are worse than rape, and almost every woman I've talked with agrees. Still, I'll never forget the mother who came up to me after one lecture and told me she'd rather have her daughter dead than raped. I'm afraid I wasn't very nice to her. I told her I was glad I wasn't her daughter—or son for that matter. (Storaska, 1975, 6)

Discuss your reactions with a friend of the opposite sex as well as one of the same sex. How do your feelings compare with theirs?

Fortunately, our society has shown a great deal of progress in dealing with rape. Medical and counseling services, law-enforcement procedures, and the entire legal situation has improved and will likely get even better. New laws have made it easier to convict a guilty person and have prevented unnecessary hassling of the victim. For example, since it is actually impossible to prove that a penis has penetrated a certain vagina, recent sexual offense statutes have been designed to provide for different degrees or gradations of forced sexual behavior. This allows for an easier conviction of some type of forced sexual activity without having to base an entire case on substantiation of the fact that forced intercourse occurred.

Date Rape

Date rape, or acquaintance rape, is much more common than most people realize, although by its nature it is difficult to gather reliable data on this topic. It is suspected that some incidents of date rape might be a result of poor communication, since so many people still have a difficult time talking about sexuality. At any rate, it may help those dating to realize the following: spending money on a date does not justify expecting sexual favors; just because someone participates in other forms of sexual behavior does not mean that he or she finds intercourse acceptable; and if a date uses sexual behavior as a means of proving masculinity or femininity, it might be better to date other people.

About 50% of rapes on college campuses are committed on dates. Heavy drinking of alcohol and acquaintance rape often go together (Abbey, 1991). Although women are fearful of walking alone on campus at night, the most common sexual assault is not the "stereotypical" rape attack but instead one that occurs as a part of the "normal" social environment on the campus (Ward, et al., 1991).

As many as one in four college women have had some experience with acquaintance rape. It can be even more traumatic than stranger rape because of circumstances that might make people very unlikely to believe the victim (A crime between friends—acquaintance rape, 1990).

Forced sexual behaviors are also a problem among high school students. Twenty-six percent of students in grades 8 to 12 have reported being forced into some type of sexual activity. The type of force used on dates included verbal threats, physical violence, and intimidation, with persistence topping the list (Rhynard, Krebs & Glover, 1997).

Gordon (2001) reported that 1 in 5 teen girls is physically or sexually abused by someone they are dating. The incidence of violence extended across all racial groups. Girls who experienced physical dating violence had a higher risk of substance abuse (including heavy smoking, binge drinking, and cocaine use), unhealthy weight control, and intercourse before age 15. Girls from this study also reported not using a condom during intercourse, and having three or more sexual partners within the last three months. According to a survey of over 80,000 ninth and twelfth grade boys and girls in Minnesota, nearly 1 in 10 girls and 1 in 20 boys experienced violence and/or being raped on a date (one out of ten female adolescents experience date violence and/or rape, says study of over 80,000 youths in Minnesota, 2001).

Ways to Help Prevent Acquaintance Rape

Think

Think about how you respond to social pressures and ask yourself

- What role does sexual activity play in my life?

- What role do I want it to play?

- How does alcohol affect my sexual decision making?

- How do I learn someone's desires and limits?

- How do I express my own?

Challenge the Myths and Stereotypes

- Challenge your friends who belittle rape or who accept definitions of sexuality and gender roles that allow forcing someone to have sexual activity.

- Talk with friends and give one another the opportunity to be assertive, respectful, honest, and caring.

Communicate Effectively

- Saying "no" or "yes" may be difficult, but it is important. Acting sorry or unsure sends mixed messages. The other person cannot really know how you feel without hearing it from you.

- Trust your instincts. Tell your partner what you want—or do not want—and stick with your decision.

- Listen carefully to what the other person is saying. Are you getting mixed messages? Do you understand him or her? If not—ask. Remember, yes only means yes when said clearly, not when your partner is drunk, high, asleep, or impaired in any way.

- Ask, rather than assume. You and your partner should talk about what would be most enjoyable together.

- Remember that effective and assertive communication may not always work. Sometimes people simply do not listen. However—no one ever deserves to be raped! (Acquaintance Rape: What Everyone Should Know, 2002). (Reprinted with permission of the American College Health Association.)

Date Rape Drugs

In the early 1990s the topic of date rape became even more complicated because of date rape drugs. One early date rape drug was flunitrazepam (Rohypnol). It is a prescription drug marketed legally in 60 countries around the world. It is used as a sedative hypnotic and as a preanesthetic medication in those countries. However, it is not approved for medical use in the United States (Lyman, Hughes-McLain & Thompson, 1998). Because of its sedative hypnotic action with an amnesialike effect, it is ideal for use in date rape situations. It can be administered without consent to produce disinhibition and to obtain sexual activity. It has no taste or odor when mixed with alcohol. People drugged with Rohypnol may remember nothing about what happened or have only a very sketchy memory. They are often unsure if they have been raped, except that they may wake up the next morning with genital discomfort or may be disrobed. Assailants typically claim the victims consented to sexual activity, and there is no way to know for sure. The time required for Rohypnol to reach its peak blood level is 1 hour, but it can be identified in the urine for 4 days to 30 days after ingestion (Ledray, 1996).

Another date rape drug is GHB—short for a chemical name, gamma hydroxybutyrate. It can be used by sexual predators to render their victims almost instantly helpless and to leave them with little or no memory of the attack. It is similar to the drug Rohypnol. GHB has no approved medical use, and it can cause depression, seizures, coma, and death. Kits can be purchased for making the drug at home for under $100. Many argue that GHB should be an illegal substance (Pryor warns of strong drug used by sex predators, 1998).

A third drug being used as a date rape drug is ketamine hydrochloride. It is commercially referred to as Ketaject or Ketalar. It is used medically as an anesthetic for diagnostic and surgical purposes. It produces anesthesia within 40 seconds with intravenous administration and 8 minutes with intramuscular administration. It is currently widely used by veterinarians. In the United States the popular method of use involves heating of the liquid until it turns into a white powder, which is then smoked or snorted. The full effects of ketamine occur in about 5 to 10 minutes and last up to 1 hour (Lyman, Hughes-McLain & Thompson, 1998).

In 1996, President Clinton signed a bill outlawing Rohypnol and other date rape drugs and adding 20 years to the sentence of a rapist who uses these drugs on a victim. It also included increased penalties for illegal manufacturing, distribution, dispensing, or possession of the drugs. It was the first time that using a drug as a weapon was classified as a crime in the United States.

Here are some things you can do to reduce the possibility of being a victim of a date rape drug (Lyman, Hughes-McLain & Thompson, 1998):

1. Be extra cautious on dates until you feel convinced of your companion's integrity.

2. Buy your own drinks or be present when the drinks are delivered.

3. Never leave a drink unattended.

4. Do not trust a date any more than someone else you have known for the same length of time.

5. At parties, do not drink from community punch or drink bowls.

Obviously, rape is not the only form of forcible sexual behavior even though it is probably the most highly publicized. Unfortunately, in many cases of forcible sexual behavior, fear and embarrassment often combine to prevent reporting and dealing with the situation. Various forms of forcible sexual behavior should be discussed to bring these problems out into the open. People need to realize that these things do happen, that they are not alone if they should become involved, that there are sources of help, and that abusive sexual behavior should not be allowed to continue. Raising the awareness of educators and learners can have many practical and important ramifications.

Sexual Harassment

Since the mid-1970s, the courts, popular and professional periodicals, newspapers, and books have focused on **sexual harassment.** Hundreds of articles have appeared in print, increasing national attention to the subject. It is not easy to define sexual harassment. Sometimes it is hard to draw the line between harassment and other behaviors, but it can include touching, verbal abuse, demanding certain sexual favors, or using threatening tones.

Legally speaking, there are two kinds of sexual harassment. The first is quid pro quo (Latin for "something for something") where something is to be exchanged. The second is a hostile environment, which means that speech or conduct in itself can contribute to sexual harassment (Cloud, 1998).

Defining sexual harassment in practice can be difficult. While there are legal guidelines in many instances, various people may have inconsistent perceptions. For example, Blakely, Blakely and Moorman found that more females, as compared to males, viewed ambiguous sexually oriented work behavior as harassment. In addition, those who had previously been a target of sexual harassment tended to view this behavior as a continuation of the harassment (Blakely, Blakely & Moorman, 1995).

---

sexual harassment   Unwelcome verbal, physical, or sexual conduct that has the effect of creating an intimidating, hostile, or offensive environment.

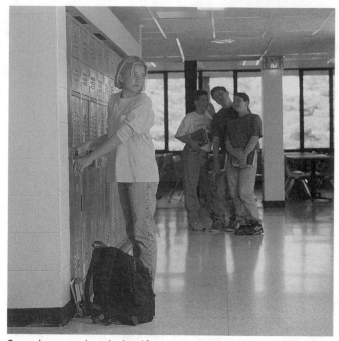

Speech or conduct in itself can create a hostile environment, which in turn is sexual harassment.

Less than 30 years ago, the topic of sexual harassment was considered by many to be a radical fringe byproduct of feminist theory. Today it is embedded in legal decisions at all levels—including the Supreme Court. About 60 new sexual harassment cases are filed every day, which result in more than 15,500 per year (Cloud, 1998).

The American Association of University Women conducted a national survey on sexual harassment in public schools in 1993 and again in 2001 (Hostile hallways: Bullying, teasing, and sexual harassment in school, 2001). They found that students in 2001 were much more likely to say that their schools had sexual harassment policies and they distribute literature on sexual harassment. As in 1993, in 2001 80% of students experienced some form of sexual harassment at some time during their school years. There was a striking increase (from 18% to 24%) in the number of boys who often experienced sexual harassment. In addition, 56% of boys said they experienced sexual harassment occasionally. Girls were more likely than boys to ever experience sexual harassment (83% versus 79%). Students who experienced sexual harassment were likely to react by avoiding the person who bothered or harassed them (40%), talking less in class (24%), not wanting to go to school (22%), changing their seat in class to get farther away from someone (21%), or finding it hard to pay attention in school (10%).

The positive effect sexuality educators can have on the frequency and severity of sexual harassment in school, at work, and in other settings is immense. The first step to being able to complain about harassment is understanding it and knowing that one is being harassed. Those who clearly understand their rights, and know about sexual harassment, will less likely become targets (Griffin, 2000).

Summary

There are many alternative sexual behaviors with which the sexuality educator ought to be familiar. Discussing these sexual behaviors sometimes requires special care on the part of the sexuality educator, because these are emotionally charged issues for many people.

Certain sexual behaviors are simply being viewed today as individual preferences. Examples are masturbation, oral–genital contact, and homosexual behavior. Certainly, not all people will agree on many aspects of these behaviors, but the many myths that have existed surrounding these topics are slowly being laid to rest. Of course, it is one thing for the sexuality educator to help people to deal with such topics on an objective level and quite another to try to deal with them subjectively.

Premarital heterosexual behavior has probably been the most studied form of sexual behavior through the years. There are many statistics and observations that shed light on this topic. Although there used to be very different male and female attitudes and behaviors related to premarital activity, in recent years the differences are becoming less prevalent.

Marital sexual behavior has been influenced by the development of reliable contraception as well as by the changing female role within the family. These situations are allowing us to learn much more about marital sexual behavior than was previously possible.

Some sexual topics, such as prostitution and pornography, have been thought to have social significance beyond that usually associated with sexual topics. Some people have thought that these two topics are real problem areas that could lead to society's ruin; others have thought they are no threat as long as they are kept in perspective.

The sexuality educator should have at least some knowledge of the wide spectrum of possible sexual behaviors. Most of us cannot be expected to be experts on all of them, so information has been provided on sexual behaviors you will most likely hear about in teaching sexuality education. When dealing with any sexual behavior, it is important to remain calm, keep an open mind, and remember that all of the behaviors collectively or individually can be placed on a continuum. People must personally choose where their behavior will be placed on the continuum, but the sexuality educator has a responsibility to help the person be in a better position to intelligently do so.

While many sexual behaviors can be viewed as a matter of personal choice, forcible behaviors such as pedophilia and rape involve forcing one's will on another person. Much needed attention has finally been given to sexual abuse, especially rape; however, we still have a long way to go in better understanding and knowing how to deal with these experiences. Many services and laws concerned with victims of sexual assault have improved.

In recent years the topic of sexual harassment has received much greater attention. While defining sexual harassment can be difficult, it is frequently experienced by many high school and college students. Sexuality educators can have positive influences on the frequency and severity of sexual harassment at school, at work, and in other settings. Those who understand more about sexual harassment are less likely to become targets.

References

A crime between friends—acquaintance rape, *Behavior Today,* 21 (1990), 1–3.

A history of sexual abuse elevates the Massachusetts teenagers' risk of engaging in unsafe sexual practices, *Family Planning Perspectives,* 33, no. 1 (January/February 2001), 44.

Abbey, A. Acquaintance rape and alcohol consumption on college campuses: How are they linked? *Journal of American College Health Association,* 39 (January 1991), 165–69.

Acquaintance Rape: What Everyone Should Know, Baltimore, MD: American College Health Association, 2002.

Allgeier, E. R. Are you ready for sex?: Informed consent for sexual intimacy, *SIECUS Report* (July 1985), 8–9.

Bell, R. R. *Premarital sex in a changing society.* Englewood Cliffs, NJ: Prentice Hall, 1966.

Blakely, G. L., Blakely, E. H. & Moorman, R. The relationship between gender, personal experience, and perceptions of sexual harassment in the workplace, *Employee Relationships and Rights Journal,* 8, no. 4 (1995), 263–74.

Call, V., Sprecher, S. & Schwartz, P. The incidence and frequency of marital sex in a national sample, *Journal of Marriage and the Family,* 57, no. 3 (August 1995), 639–52.

Child sexual abuse. Chicago: National Committee to Prevent Child Abuse, 1998.

Clements, M. Sex in America today, *Parade* (August 7, 1994), 4–6.

Cloud, J. Sex and the law, *Time,* 51, no. 11 (March 23, 1998), 48–53.

Donnerstein, E., Linz, D. & Penrod, S. *The question of pornography: Research findings and policy implications.* New York: The Free Press, 1987.

Federal Bureau of Investigation. *Uniform crime reports for the United States (1996).* Washington, DC: U.S. Government Printing Office, 1998.

Fisher, B. S., Cullen, F. T. & Turner, M. G. *The sexual victimization of college women.* Washington, DC: U.S. Department of Justice Office of Justice Programs, 2001.

Greenberg, J. S. *Health education: Learner-centered instructional strategies.* 2nd ed. Dubuque, IA: William C. Brown Communications, 1992.

Greenberg, J. S., Bruess, C. E. & Haffner, D. W. *Exploring the dimensions of human sexuality.* Sudbury, MA: Jones and Bartlett, 2004.

Griffin, M. Sexuality educators are essential to helping people understand sexual harassment, *SIECUS Report,* 28, no. 3 (February/March 2000), 5–7.

Gordon, D. Dating violence among teens widespread. InteliHealth (2001). Available: http://www.intelihealth.com.

Harvey, P. D. Federal censorship and the war on pornography, *SIECUS Report,* 28, no. 3 (February/March 1992), 8–12.

Hostile hallways: Bullying, teasing, and sexual harassment in school, *American Journal of Health Education,* 32, no. 5 (2001), 307–9.

Intrafamily Sexual Abuse—Incest, *Family Life Educator* (Winter 1982), 12–14.

Laumann, E. O., Gagnon, J. H., Michaels, R. & Michaels, S. *The social organization of sexuality: Sexual practices in the United States.* Chicago: University of Chicago Press, 1994.

Ledray, L. E. Date rape drug alert, *Journal of Emergency Nursing,* 22, no. 1 (1996), 80.

Lyman, S. A., Hughes-McLain, C. & Thompson, G. "Date-rape drugs: A growing concern, *Journal of Health Education,* 29, no. 5 (1998), 271–74.

National Clearinghouse on Child Abuse and Neglect Information. *National child abuse and neglect statistical fact sheet.* Washington, DC: U.S. Government Printing Office, 1998.

One out of ten female adolescents experience date violence and/or rape, says study of over 80,000 youths in Minnesota. Intelihealth (2001). Available: http://www.intelihealth.com.

Pawlowski, W. A gay child in the family, in *Sexuality education: A resource book,* Cassell, C. & Wilson, P. M., eds. New York: Garland Publishing, 1989.

Pryor warns of strong drug use by sex predators, *Birmingham News* (August 18, 1998), 4B.

Reiss, I. Changing trends, attitudes, and values on premarital sexual behavior in the U.S., in *Human sexuality and the mentally retarded,* de la Cruz, F. F. & La Veck, G. D., eds. New York: Brunner/Mazel, 1973.

Rhynard, J., Krebs, M. & Glover, J. Sexual assault in dating relationships, *Journal of School Health,* 67, no. 3 (1997), 89–93.

Sex offenses and offenders: An analysis of data on rape and sexual assault. Washington, DC: U.S. Department of Justice Office of Justice Programs, 1998.

Stein, J. Porn goes mainstream, *Time,* 152, no. 10 (September 7, 1998), 51–52.

———. For lad mags, the jig is up, *Time,* 161, no. 20 (May 19, 2003), 90.

Storaska, F. *How to say no to a rapist and survive.* New York: Random House, 1975.

Study: Some gays can go straight. Intelihealth Health News (May 9, 2001). Available: http://www.intelihealth.com.

Ward, S. K., Cohn, K., White, S. & Williams, K. Acquaintance rape and the college social scene, *Family Relations,* 40 (1991), 71.

Suggested Readings

Coleman, E. What sexual scientists know about . . . compulsive sexual behavior, in *What sexual scientists know about . . . brochure 2, no. 1*. Mount Vernon, IA: The Society for the Scientific Study of Sexuality, 1996.

Davis, C. M. What sexual scientists know about . . . pornography, in *What sexual scientists know about . . . brochure 3, no. 1*. Mount Vernon, IA: The Society for the Scientific Study of Sexuality, 1997.

O'Neil, R. O. What limits should campus networks place on pornography? *The Chronicle of Higher Education*, 49, no. 28 (March 21, 2003), B20.

Portellil, C. J. & Meade, C. W. Censorship and the Internet: No easy answers. Sexuality Information and Education Council of the United States. Available: http://www.siecus.org/pubs.srpt/articles'arti0001.html.

Reis, B. A guide to teaching actively about sexual orientation, *SIECUS Report*, 26, no. 4 (April/May 1998), 5–6.

———. Important points to make to students when discussing sexual orientation, *SIECUS Report*, 26, no. 4 (April/May 1998), 7–8.

Schwartz, P. Love is not all you need, *Psychology Today* (May/June 2002), 56–58, 60–62.

Cases for Part 3

The cases in this section are designed to use the information in Chapters 9 and 10. Case 1 requires you to process what you have learned about homosexuality and homosexuals as well as consider the ethical and moral discussions presented in Chapter 9, in order to answer the questions relevant to this case.

Case 2 prompts you to deal with the emotionally charged subject of violent sexual behavior. The sexuality educator needs to be prepared to handle this subject because it is so common today, is a high-interest area, and is clouded with myths. Chapter 10 provides background information that should help you satisfy Case 2.

Case 3 also relates to sexual behaviors, but this time not necessarily to violent behaviors. Explaining different sexual behaviors is something the sexuality educator frequently needs to do. Chapter 10 again relates to this case.

Case 4 gives you one of the more difficult challenges for the sexuality educator. Handling morals in sexuality education settings is always controversial. Chapter 9 ought to get you on your way, but certainly there are no hard and fast answers to the concerns raised.

Case 1

Getting Off the Middle of the Road: Developing Policy Regarding Homosexuality

Sam Mayer has just been elected mayor of his town. Mayor Mayer ran an ideal campaign, at least from his perspective. He managed to stay "in the middle of the road" on most issues. In this way he did not offend anyone and was able to get enough votes to win the election. However, now that he is in office, Mayor Mayer must resolve some thorny issues. One of these relates to the treatment of homosexuals in the town. About half of the town council advocates prohibiting avowed homosexuals from being hired for certain jobs. These jobs include those where it may be important to keep secrets, such as budget director or judge, as well as jobs that would bring homosexuals in direct contact with children, such as teacher or day care worker. The other half of the town council argues that homosexuals should not be discriminated against in any way. Mayor Mayer must provide leadership on this issue in order for it to be resolved in the best way possible.

1. What arguments do you think are offered by the advocates of prohibiting homosexuals from being hired for certain jobs?

2. What arguments do you think are offered by those opposed to restricting homosexuals?

3. What can Mayor Mayer decide that would be best in this situation? What specific policy should be proposed?

4. What is the most moral decision that can be made in this situation?

Case 2

Speaking of Violence: Separating Facts and Myths about Violent Sexual Behavior

Sam Orator has been asked to speak at a meeting of the local service club about the topic of rape. Sam has decided that he will take the liberty of broadening the topic a little and will talk about violent sexual behavior in general.

Sam needs an outline for his speech. He wants the outline divided into three areas. Please develop an outline for him, using the following headings:

1. Myths about violent sexual behavior.

2. Facts about violent sexual behavior.

3. Needed research (questions needing answers) related to violent sexual behavior.

Case 3

What to My Wondering Eyes Should Appear? Understanding a Few Sexual Preferences and Behaviors

Wanna Know and her father, Mite, were walking along a street in downtown Big City, USA, late one Saturday afternoon. Wanna noticed a man walking toward them who appeared to be around 25 years old. The man was tall and had a fairly well-developed male physique. At the same time, however, Wanna could not help noticing that he was wearing clothes she would usually expect on a female. She found herself curious, because in all her 16 years of life she had never seen a man dressed that way. Her curiosity got the best of her, and later that evening, back at home, she asked her father about the man they had seen downtown. If you were Mite, how would you explain the situation to Wanna?

Case 4

A Moral Dilemma: Morals in the Classroom

You are a ninth grade teacher who has been attempting to institute a sexuality education program in your school district.

As you expected, the road to a good school sexuality education program has not always been easy to travel. As you arrive at school one morning, Mr. Al (Always) Wright, the principal, asks you to speak with him for a few minutes.

Mr. Wright indicates that he is concerned about your efforts to promote sexuality education in the school. He is sure that the young people need some background in sexuality, but he does not feel that the school is the place to provide it, because moral issues are so closely linked with every part of the program. You attempt to explain your point of view, but he further indicates that the school is not the place for sexuality education for the following reasons:

1. It is not possible to consider sexual issues without moralizing (telling students what is right and wrong).

2. Not moralizing will not help, because if the school does not moralize, the program will be considered to be amoral.

3. Since the topic of sexuality has not been spoken of very highly, in religious circles anyway, it probably is not a proper topic for schools.

How might you respond to his points in a way that will help your school receive approval for a sound sexuality education program?

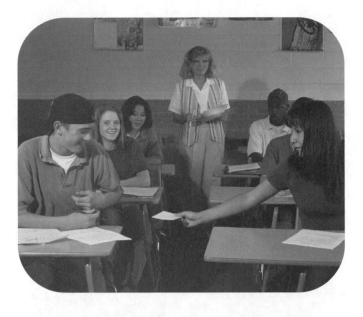
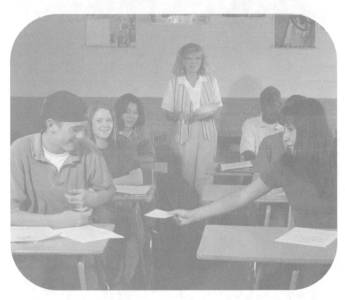
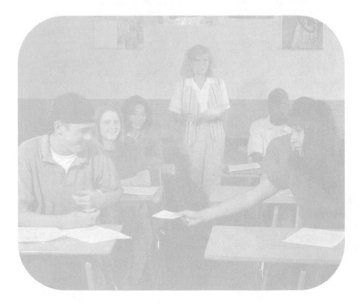

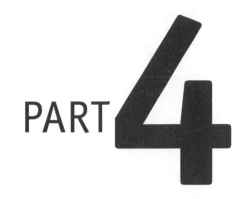
Conducting Sexuality Education

Chapter 11
Education for Sexuality: Rules of Conduct

Chapter 12
Learning Strategies for Sexuality Education

Chapter 13
Strategies for Learning and Teaching about HIV/AIDS

Chapter 14
What Should Be Taught at Different Levels and in Different Settings?

Chapter 15
The Educator and Sexual Counseling

Education for Sexuality: Rules of Conduct

Key Concepts

1. Ground rules ought to be established at the outset of a sexuality education program.
2. Certain communication skills are necessary to effectively conduct sexuality education.
3. Language usage generates complications for sexuality education.
4. Learners' needs, interests, and characteristics should be clearly identified.
5. Learners must be involved in the learning process for sexuality education to be most effective.

Sexuality education is both similar to and different from education in other content areas. Although the educational setting and the learners may be the same, the nature of the topic requires special considerations. These considerations include the establishment of specific ground rules; development of communication skills; consideration of learners' use of language; determination of learners' needs, interests, and characteristics; and the necessity of actively involving learners in the educational experience. Each of these considerations is discussed in this chapter.

Ground Rules

Both learners and sexuality educators should recognize that certain rules govern the sexuality education experience. The learners will then know what to expect from the instructor and from fellow learners. Since learners may initially approach sexuality education with some trepidation, embarrassment, or a secretive attitude, the structure provided by ground rules may be reassuring for them. They will know that aspects of their sexual lives, attitudes, and values need not be disclosed to sexuality educators. On the other hand, clear rules will keep within the bounds of propriety those learners who might otherwise take inappropriate advantage of the opportunity to discuss sex-related topics. Community leaders, administrators, taxpayers, and parents will be more comfortable knowing that the sexuality education program is being conducted within specific boundaries regarding topics, language, morality, and self-disclosure.

Since making rules requires value judgments, the rules we will recommend reflect *our* values. To help you identify *your* values, our recommended rules will be presented only after you are provided with an introduction to a situation requiring a rule and are given an opportunity to establish a rule reflective of your values. After we present the rule that makes the most sense to us, we will identify the value we hold that serves as the basis for our rule.

Rule 1: Language. In a high school sexuality education class, a student asks, "What is a blow job?" In the space provided, write a rule to govern this situation.

Now it is our turn. Our rule would state that socially acceptable terminology must be used at all times. *However,* when the correct word is not known and the learner has a question he or she wants to ask, the vernacular is acceptable. Stated differently, not knowing the socially acceptable terminology should not get in the way of learning. In this situation, the sexuality educator might answer the question and then teach the students that the socially acceptable word is fellatio. Sexual language is such an important issue in sexuality education that we devote an entire section to this topic later in this chapter.

Our value decision here is that learning is more important than propriety.

Rule 2: Disclosure. While discussing premarital sexual intercourse, the unmarried sexuality educator is asked if he or she has had such experiences. In the space provided, write a rule to govern this situation.

Our rule would state that no one may be *asked* to disclose any information about his or her private sexual behavior but that anyone may voluntarily offer such information. This rule protects those who would be threatened in a sexuality education program in which their sexual lives were expected to be open books. On the other hand, those wishing to use their sexual experiences as examples may do so *as long as the sexuality educator believes that such disclosures serve an educational purpose.* Sexuality educators are cautioned to prevent learners from showing off, bragging, or otherwise disclosing aspects of their sexual lives for the purpose of shocking the other learners. Disclosures of this nature should be prohibited.

Our value decision here is that respect for people's privacy and comfort in disclosure is more important than the benefits to be derived from analyses of specific sexual behaviors.

Rule 3: Questions. A learner asks, "How do you know if you're homosexual?" and the other learners start to laugh as one shouts out, "Don't worry Fred, we'll take you downtown after school and help you find out." Write a rule to govern this situation.

_____

_____

_____

Our rule would state that no question is silly or stupid if the person asking the question is sincere in wanting to know the answer and that, therefore, no one is allowed to ridicule anyone else for asking a question.

Although the question in our example seems elementary, many adolescents who feel close to a same-sex friend

and who are not yet much interested in the opposite sex wonder whether they are homosexuals. Further, since the onset of puberty is accompanied by sexual experimentation, it is not uncommon for adolescents to participate in sexual play with their same-sex friends. Fears of being homosexual often follow, and young people need reassurance that these sexual experiences are not unusual and do not, in themselves, indicate homosexuality. As a matter of fact, the question, how do you know if you're a homosexual? is a probing one. Researchers and theoreticians have groped with this question often. They wonder, for example, if people whose sexual outlets are restricted to same-sex partners (such as prisoners) are homosexual if they participate in sexual activity with these partners. The term *situational homosexuality* has been applied to this behavior. Further, if a person engages in sexual activity with same-sex partners sometimes and with opposite-sex partners other times, is that person a homosexual? What proportion of sexual activity with same-sex partners makes one a homosexual: any sexual activity with a same-sex partner? 50%? 70%? Some are surprised to learn that Kinsey's data indicated that over one-third of all males had participated in some homosexual behavior (Kinsey, Pomeroy & Martin, 1948). Consequently, Kinsey developed

An important rule in sexuality education is that no question is a stupid question. Program participants should feel free to acquire information about which they are curious.

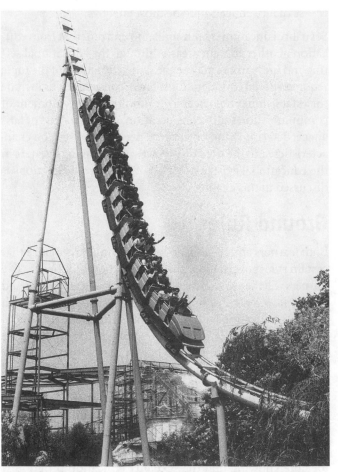

Risk-taking behavior is part of growing up. However, young people must also learn how to behave responsibly.

a heterosexual-homosexual rating scale that included the following categories:

- Exclusively heterosexual, with no homosexual
- Predominantly heterosexual, only incidentally homosexual
- Predominantly heterosexual, but more than incidentally homosexual
- Equally heterosexual and homosexual
- Predominantly homosexual, but more than incidentally heterosexual
- Predominantly homosexual, but incidentally heterosexual
- Exclusively homosexual

A good way to respond to all questions is to say, "That is an excellent question. Many young people have concerns about. . . ." No question, no matter how ludicrous it may appear to be at first glance, is silly or stupid. It may be important to the one asking the question, or its implications and ramifications may not be initially evident.

Our value decision here is that the need to learn supersedes the need to appear worldly or cool.

Rule 4: Topics. In a school setting, a student asks, "I want to improve my sexual technique. Can you show us sexual positions and ways to erotically excite our sexual partners?" Write a rule to govern this situation.

_____

_____

_____

Our rule would say that there are certain topics that are beyond the limits of the course. There are several reasons for this rule. First, some topics are so controversial that a conscious political decision may be made to exclude them from the program so as not to risk the elimination of the rest of the program. Second, some topics may best be discussed in an educator-to-learner interaction rather than in a large or small group interaction. Finally, some topics may be specifically prohibited from consideration by those responsible for administering or approving the sexuality education program. Such topics include sexual techniques, sexual intercourse positions, and even, in some school systems, abortion. It should also be recognized that whereas some topics are appropriate for some settings, others may not be. Teaching positions of sexual intercourse may make sense if one is working with a group of married adults who want to improve their sexual lives together. To teach positions of sexual intercourse to a high school sophomore group, however, would almost assure the termination of your sexuality education program.

Our value decision here is that it is more important to maintain the existence of the sexuality education program than to threaten its elimination by arguing that any topic the learners want to consider is a topic that should be studied.

Rule 5: Availability. In a community health agency setting, a learner asks the sexuality educator if a private meeting can be arranged during which the learner can discuss his or her sexual problem. The sexuality educator's schedule is very busy, and other learners have also asked for such a meeting. Write a rule to govern this situation.

_____

_____

_____

Our rule would state that the sexuality educator will make time available to meet with individuals or small groups of learners. The very nature of sexuality education, we believe, requires such a rule. Many topics studied during sexuality education are private. Other topics provide learners with new insights. And still other topics spark the intellectual curiosity of learners. In all these cases, the sexuality educator should be available for private meetings to accomplish the following:

1. Provide counsel or suggestions for referral when learners seek help with problems related to their sexuality

2. Provide reference material, or places to get such material, relative to specific sexuality topics

3. Answer questions that learners are hesitant to ask in a group situation

To assure your availability in the midst of a busy schedule, we recommend that you set aside a certain time that you publicize as your "office" hours. During this period, you should be available on either a scheduled or drop-in basis. In addition, we advise that you provide some means for learners to seek information or advice from you anonymously. Two ways to allow for this are (1) to announce a telephone number and time when you can be called when the caller need not give his or her name to get an answer, and (2) to designate a locker or mailbox in which questions can be placed for the sexuality educator to answer in the large group the next time it meets. If you provide a phone number, remember to emphasize that you will be available at that number only at specified times. It might be best to use a telephone at your place of work, although some might prefer to provide a home telephone number and be available at any time of the day or night for calls. This you must decide for yourself. An alternative to the locker or mailbox idea is to allow learners to place a telephone number or address on their questions if they want you to answer their questions privately. Further, a suggestion box can be set up in the room in which the group meets so that learners can drop in questions and suggestions for improving the sexuality education program.

Our value decision here is that answering learners' concerns and questions (whether in the large group or privately) is at the very heart of sexuality education. Therefore, sexuality educators' schedules must be adjusted to provide for this function.

Rule 6: Feelings. In a workshop for a group of elderly men and women, entitled "Becoming Comfortable Discussing Human Sexuality," some of the women said that they grew up being taught that sexuality is not a topic to discuss in public. Consequently, they felt threatened, awkward, and uncomfortable. Write a rule that will guide the sexuality educator's response to this situation.

Our rule is that all *feelings* can be expressed and will be accepted. In this example, the women should be thanked for sharing their feelings and should be told that these feelings are understandable. However, we have a corollary to this rule. The corollary is that not all *behavior* can be expressed, nor will it all be accepted. Thus, the women should be asked to accept their feelings but to continue the educational activities rather than allow these feelings to short-circuit their growth. Other illustrations of this rule come to mind. For example, a learner should be allowed to express sexual excitement, but that does not mean that he or she needs to find an immediate outlet (a sexual partner or a place to masturbate). A husband should be allowed to express a lusting for other women and his feeling should be accepted as existing. However, the actualization of that lusting (adultery) might be judged inappropriate (at least society, through its laws, judges it illegal). We are sure that you can think of other examples. The point, again, is that feelings *are;* they exist. Feelings are neither right nor wrong, good nor bad. People should feel free to express their feelings so that their feelings might be better understood. However, people should not be and are not free to behave any way that their feelings dictate. Some behavior is illegal, other behavior is immoral, and still other behavior is destructive. Since people cannot control the feelings that come to their awareness, they cannot be expected to experience only certain feelings and not others. However, people can control how they behave and what they do. The difference here is the difference between **freedom** and **license** as described by A. S. Neill (1960). One should have the freedom to do what makes sense to one, but not the license to do anything that negatively affects society, oneself, or other individuals. In a sexuality education setting, a learner might want to use slang or profane terminology but might not be allowed to use these words, because they upset the other learners or those sanctioning the program. Similarly, to feel comfortable and proud of oneself physically does not provide sufficient justification for parading around naked.

Our value decisions here are that the expression of feelings is worth the discomfort that may accompany such disclosure, and that the freedom to behave in ways one chooses is less important than the rights of others to their comfort.

Rule 7: Thoughts. In a sexuality education program conducted in a Catholic church, a learner blurts out, "I think that all methods of contraception, and I mean abortion and sterilization as well, ought to be allowed by the Pope." What rule should govern the sexuality educator's reaction in this situation?

Our rule is that, as with feelings, all thoughts ought to be allowed to be expressed. The other learners and the sexuality educator cannot deal with these thoughts unless they know of their existence. The expression of both thoughts and feelings should be encouraged. Analyzing thoughts that are brought to the group and determining their validity can contribute to learning. Even if these thoughts are contrary to the thinking of the majority of the learners, investigating them will help others identify more specifically the rationale behind their own thoughts. As with feelings, all thoughts should be accepted as existing within the learner expressing them. The task of the sexuality educator and other learners should be to ask questions to clarify the thoughts expressed and the reasoning underlying them. Once this is accomplished, others can express their thinking on the topic and their rationales. However, since all thoughts are accepted, attempts to change learners' thoughts should be discouraged. The ramifications and implications of the thoughts should be explored, but in a free society people should be allowed to think what they will.

Our value decision here is that it is more important for people to understand the reasoning process behind an opinion than to think a particular thought. Remember: give me a fish and I eat today; teach me to fish and I eat forever. Thoughts constantly change. What should be consistent is the process by which thoughts and opinions are decided.

Rule 8: Input. During a study of the abortion issue, a learner asks the sexuality educator whether abortion on demand ought to be allowed. Write a rule to govern the response of the sexuality educator in this situation.

Our rule is that decisions related to human sexuality need to be made after considering input from many sources. The sexuality educator should establish a learning environment

---

freedom   The ability to make free choices and decisions.

license   The ability to make any decisions regardless of their effects on other people or society in general.

conducive to the acquisition of such input. Certainly parents, clergy, philosophers, and others have thoughts and opinions related to abortion, for instance. Prior to deciding whether abortion on demand ought to be allowed, the advice and thoughts of these people should be sought. Topics such as premarital sexual intercourse, masturbation, homosexuality, and adultery all have social, psychological, biological, and religious implications. These implications should be identified and considered. Since learners' basic values most likely reflect those of their family, friends, and clergy, these groups of people are the keys to input for decision making once the cognitive information has been processed by the sexuality educator.

Our value decision here is that the more information obtained prior to making choices, the better the choices are likely to be. More input is better than less input.

Rule 9: Humor. During a discussion of sex-role stereotyping, a male learner, while developing the point that husbands should be sexually experienced and teach their innocent, naive wives all they know, described sexual intercourse as an art and himself as the Michaelangelo of lovers. One of the females then asked whether, as the original had done while painting the ceiling of the Sistine Chapel, the husband painted while lying on his back. The class broke out in hysterical laughter. What rule could guide the sexuality educator in responding to this situation?

_____

_____

_____

Our rule is that all facets of life, even ourselves and our behaviors, can be taken too seriously and that humor can be appropriately used to place things in proper perspective. Some would disagree and argue that sexuality is such an important aspect of living, with religious and moral significance, that it should be taken seriously. We agree. However, the use of humor to make a serious point or to help someone understand human sexual behavior and sexuality-related topics seems to us to be appropriate. Of course, excessive use of humor or humor used to belittle or demean is never advised. Our values regarding humor and sexuality education are evident throughout this book. We have used humor (at least it seems humorous to us) to make a point, to provide relief from a serious discussion, and generally to make this book more enjoyable to read. In this manner, we hope you read more of the book, pay more attention to its contents than you otherwise might, and thereby learn more.

Our value decision here is that humor is important, in particular when considering a serious issue, in ensuring that the learning process remains interesting and students remain motivated to learn.

Rule 10: Respect for diversity. You are conducting a sexuality education program for adults in a community that includes people from many different countries around the world. When you get to the topic of sexual arousal and technique, you can see disagreeable expressions on the faces of the program participants. However, the problem in deciphering the cause of these expressions is that they appear on different people's faces at different times. Write a rule to explain this situation.

_____

_____

_____

Our rule would state that the sexuality educator should recognize and respect diverse views of sexuality. Different cultures have different views of sexual issues. For example, the Thonga of South Africa believe kissing is disgusting (Masters, Johnson & Kolodny, 1992). Furthermore, whereas some societies place value on certain body parts and eroticize them (for example, the female breast), others find completely different body parts erotic. Homosexuality is an accepted lifestyle in some cultures and frowned upon in others. Considering people differ by gender, ethnicity, race, culture, experience, religion, and many other variables, it is not surprising that people have many differing views of what is sexually acceptable.

Our value decision here is that people deserve respect for their views and understanding for how these views develop. This means that people do not have to have the same views. As long as the basic values to which we have previously referred in this book (for example, respect for others, trust, and honesty) are not violated, differences related to sexuality should be accepted, and people differing from the mainstream should not be made to feel disrespected.

Communication Skills

Several important prerequisites to effective sexuality education involve communication. We will explore these prerequisite skills by identifying their significance and by describing how the sexuality educator can best use them in the instructional setting.

Listening Skills

In Chapter 7 we discussed the importance of listening skills in a group process. There are so many things that can and do interfere with listening that a conscious effort must be made to learn and use these skills. People are usually so eager to present their opinions that they do not listen carefully to the opinions of others. They are too busy organizing the words they will use to express themselves, and they cannot do that and listen at the same time. Compounding this situation is the emotion and excitement that often permeates discussions about sexuality. When people are emotionally charged, they tend to listen even less intently than otherwise.

In addition, sexual language, we will soon see, often affects the ability to listen well. Sexual terminology often inspires emotional reactions and may call up images that prevent good listening. Finally, people are often so opinionated or excited about the sexuality-related topics they are discussing that they talk for too long or present too many ideas at once. When this occurs, it is difficult for listeners to recall all but a very few of the points the speaker has made.

Other interferences in the listening process do not involve the listener at all. They involve the speaker, the message spoken, or the medium used to present the message. Let us look at one model of communication:

Sender → Message → Medium → Receiver

This model describes communication as including someone sending a message through some means to someone else. Some communication problems originate with the sender and his or her "sending skills." If the sender is not trusted, the message may not be adequately understood, because the listener may focus on hidden meanings. If the sender is known to have a particular bias, this bias might influence how the message is received. If the sender does not speak clearly or if the sender has a disturbing mannerism, these problems may detract from the effectiveness of the communication.

On the other hand, the message itself may be faulty. Perhaps the language used is confusing. For example, if two people were to discuss *sex,* what would they be discussing? The word *sex* can have very different meanings for different people. In other words, a message sent by someone may be different from the one received.

Finally, the medium by which the message is sent may be inappropriate. For example, if I wanted to express my love for you, it would be unwise for me to ask someone else (a medium in this example) to tell you that I love you. Priscilla told John Alden, and you might tell me, "Speak for yourself." Thus, those wishing to communicate need to pay attention to the way in which the message will be conveyed as well as to the other components of the communication process.

The implication for the sexuality educator is that we need good communication and listening skills in the education setting so that students and instructors can discuss thoughts and ideas effectively. Now, how do we go about obtaining these skills? A good beginning is the section on communication in Chapter 7. Another way to aid listening and communication is to require learners to start their messages with *points of agreement* or *positive statements.* The later parts of their messages can present disagreements or critical statements, but by the speaker's starting with the positive, the listener will be more apt to pay attention to what is being said. A further help in establishing good communication is to provide a glossary of terms expected to be used often during the instruction. In this way, there will be agreement on at least some of the key words being used.

Nonverbal Communication

People often communicate more by *how* they say something than by *what* they say. If, when presenting a rational, logical argument against abortion, you wave your arms, pound your fist on the desk, and contort your face, your listeners could conclude that beyond the logic of your argument lies a strong, emotional objection to abortion. If, while discussing the pros and cons of parenthood, you smile, speak softly and gently, and gesture lightly when you get to the pros, your listeners could conclude that you favor this side of the debate. If, when you are lecturing, you see one learner sitting forward in her seat staring wide-eyed at you and another learner slumped back in his chair looking around the room, you would be safe in assuming that the first learner is interested in the lecture and the second is not. These nonverbal clues provide much information for the better understanding of people's ideas and feelings.

One way to train learners to identify and interpret **nonverbal communication** is to assign each one a specific feeling to communicate nonverbally. The assigned feeling might be fear, anger, concern, bewilderment, or any other. Each learner then acts out his or her assigned feeling in front of the

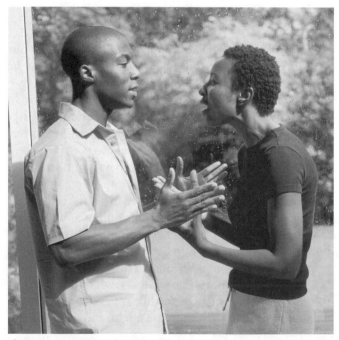

If one is attuned to it, one will see that people often express themselves without even using words.

---

nonverbal communication   Actions and body posture that send a message.

group, after which the rest of the students write down their guesses of the acted-out feeling.

Another method for teaching the identification and awareness of nonverbal communication is for learners to acquire the habit of verifying their interpretations of such communication as it actually occurs. In other words, learners should be encouraged to interrupt with a question such as, "John, your voice is low, your words are not flowing smoothly, you're perspiring, and your body is leaning away from us. I'm wondering if this means you are really unsure of these thoughts you're presenting to us. Would you tell me if I'm reading you correctly?" After establishing a routine of such interruptions, you will be amazed at how much better communication becomes.

Insight 11-1

Improving Communication

Another method for improving communication can best be explained by demonstrating it for you. Try this: Find someone for whom you will provide a pencil and paper. Stand behind this person (back to back) and describe the figure below for him or her. Be sure that you cannot be seen, that you cannot see the person's drawing, and that the other person does not communicate to you in any way (verbally or nonverbally). When you are finished with your description, note the number of mistakes that he or she has made in the drawing. Now find another person and repeat the experiment, *except* this time allow the other person to interrupt you with questions. You will probably find that the second time you describe the figure your partner will make fewer mistakes, since his or her questions help to clarify your directions. This is a demonstration of the superior effectiveness of two-way communication to one-way communication. Extrapolating these results to sexuality education, the sexuality educator should instruct learners to ask for clarification of statements before reacting to them. In other words, teach your students to ask questions so that what is said is fully understood before they express their argument or disagreement with it.

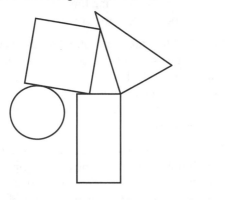

The Sexuality Educator as a Communicator

The following are some brief tips on how the sexuality educator can be a more effective communicator:

1. *Maintain eye contact with the person(s) with whom you are communicating.* Have you ever been at a party and the person speaking with you starts looking around the room at other people? Don't you get the feeling that this person is not interested in you or in what you are saying? Do not repeat such an impolite and ineffective method of communicating. Look directly at the person with whom you are communicating, both when you are speaking and when she or he is.

2. *Provide feedback.* Responding to what someone has said to you indicates you are listening and are interested in communicating effectively. Asking for feedback regarding what you have said can have the same effect.

3. *Support communication efforts of others.* Recognizing it is difficult for some people to share feelings and thoughts they have about sex and sexuality, when such communication does occur it should be reinforced. A comment as simple as, "Thanks for feeling comfortable enough to share that with me," may be all that is needed.

4. *Paraphrasing.* As we have described elsewhere in this book, summarizing what someone says to you by paraphrasing (using other words with similar meanings) demonstrates you are listening and care to communicate well.

5. *Using "I" language.* Speaking in terms of *you* rather than of other people makes for more effective communication. It is just as easy to say, "I dislike any shouting out in class," as it is to say, "I dislike it when you shout out in class." The meaning of both forms of this message is the same, but the second form places the other person in a defensive position and is accusatory. That is dysfunctional in resolving the issue being discussed.

6. *Temper constructive criticism with praise.* When it is necessary to be critical of someone, it is best to include mention of something you like or admire in that person as well. In this way, the criticism will be more easily accepted as constructive.

Building Trust

To be effective, the sexuality education experience must be based on trust. The students must trust each other as well as the sexuality educator. Since so many personal topics, opinions, beliefs, and values are involved in sexuality education, trust is a necessary condition.

There are several effective means for developing trust. The following sequence is one we have found to be effective:

Divide the class into groups of six learners each. Ask learners to think of a secret. Instruct them that they are not to tell anyone their secrets but, instead, must stand in front of each person in their groups and tell that person how they think he or she would react if told the secret. After this is done, conduct a large group discussion based on the following questions:

1. How did you feel telling others in your group how you thought they would react?

2. Did you refrain from being completely honest for fear of hurting someone's feelings? Did you refrain from saying what you really thought?

3. Did you feel good about having the opportunity to tell someone that he or she would react inappropriately? Did you want to "get even" with that person for things that person did that upset you?

4. Did you trust your group members to express their honest feelings to you? Do you think they did?

5. How can we be truthful with people while not hurting their feelings?

6. Is honesty necessary to develop trust with people?

7. Why can we be honest with some people and not with others?

Language Usage

Sexual language is often emotionally charged. As an opening activity for a workshop for the elderly conducted by one of the authors, slides were projected on a screen and the audience was asked to say the words appearing on the slides, out loud and together. The first slide was of the word *love,* and the audience loudly and clearly shouted the word. The next slide was the word *hug,* and a similar reaction greeted it. Next were *kiss, caress,* and *squeeze*—same reaction! Then appeared the words *penis, vagina,* and *sexual intercourse.* As might be expected, each of these words was repeated by noticeably fewer people than had responded to the less sexually charged words. Obviously, many in the audience were unaccustomed to saying words with sexual content out loud (at least in a group) and were embarrassed to repeat them.

When discussing sexual topics, people often find that the words themselves prevent a logical, thoughtful interaction. Since these sexual terms, or terms with sexual connotations, often evoke emotional reactions, they interfere with thoughtful discourse. Learners may be so preoccupied with their embarrassment, fear, or discomfort that they are unable to listen well or otherwise communicate effectively.

Helping learners to be more comfortable with sexual terms is a responsibility of the sexuality educator. One way of achieving this end is to teach the correct, socially acceptable terminology. This is best accomplished at an early age (before embarrassment or self-consciousness develops). Although it was some time ago, Kilander's (1968, 134–135) reasons for teaching socially acceptable terminology to children still applies:

1. If children are to learn to respect (an attitude) their bodies and body functions and organs, they will need to know respectable and dignified words to use as they speak and ask questions.

2. Normal body functions—particularly as related to urination and defecation—are less likely to acquire undesirable, shameful, and dirty connotations if words which are associated with objective, unemotional discussion are used in the instruction about them.

3. Teaching the right words and the right facts early saves a lot of unlearning later. Even while they are still young, it is good for children to know that there are correct words that can be used and that are not silly or "dirty."

4. When children enter kindergarten or first grade and come into contact with many children, their baby talk applied to bodily parts and functions may embarrass them. The ability to use correct terms should make the transition from home to school a little easier. Children get along better after they have a common vocabulary.

5. It makes it easier for young people (and adults) to bridge the language barrier in talking to adults about sex matters. The inability to use correct language is illustrated by the twelve-year-old girl who confided to her mother that she was afraid to visit the doctor because she didn't know how to tell him about personal problems—she did not know the words to use.

6. Parents and children can usually be much more objective—and therefore less emotional—about sex and its vocabulary if the correct terms are learned *before* the children have formed an emotional attitude toward sex. It is much easier to begin early with correct terminology than to wait until the children are entering puberty and adolescence.

7. When children are accustomed to calling the parts of the body by names accepted by their elders and to speaking of the body's functions from the very beginning as a matter-of-fact, decent thing, it becomes easier for them to ask—and the parents to answer—their sex questions.

The lesson for sexuality educators is clear: teach about sexual terminology and provide ample opportunity for its use so that learners will be comfortable using sexual terms. Assuming other people to be like you, how old do you think they should be when learning the terms listed in Insight 11-2?

Learning Sexual Language

Place a check in the column that indicates the educational level at which you think the word should be taught.

Word	Preschool	Elementary School	Junior High School	Senior High School	Adult
Abortion					
Abstinence					
Adultery					
Afterbirth					
AIDS					
Alimony					
Amenorrhea					
Amniotic sac					
Anal intercourse					
Anus					
Aphrodisiac					
Artificial insemination					
Autoeroticism					
Bag of waters					
Bisexual					
Birth canal					
Birth control					
Breech birth					
Caesarean section					
Cervix					
Chancre					
Circumcision					
Clitoris					
Cohabitation					
Coitus					
Coitus interruptus					
Conception					
Condom					
Contraceptive					
Cunnilingus					
Diaphragm					
Divorce					
Dyspareunia					
Ejaculate					
Embryo					
Endometrium					

Insight 11-2 (*Continued*)

Word	Preschool	Elementary School	Junior High School	Senior High School	Adult
Estrogen					
Exhibitionism					
Fallopian tube					
Family planning					
Fellatio					
Fetus					
Foreplay					
Frigidity					
Gay					
Genitalia					
Gonorrhea					
Gynecologist					
Herpes					
Heterosexual					
HIV					
Homosexual					
Hormone					
Hymen					
Hysterectomy					
Impotence					
Incest					
Infertility					
Intrauterine device					
Labia majora					
Labia minora					
Labor					
Laparoscopy					
Lesbian					
Love					
Marriage					
Mastectomy					
Masturbation					
Menarche					
Menopause					
Miscarriage					
Nocturnal emission					
Nuclear family					
Nymphomania					

Insight 11-2 (*Continued*)

Word	Preschool	Elementary School	Junior High School	Senior High School	Adult
Obscene					
Obstetrician					
Oral–genital contact					
Orgasm					
Ovary					
Ovulation					
Penis					
Petting					
Placenta					
Pornography					
Pregnant					
Progesterone					
Prostate gland					
Prostitute					
Puberty					
Rape					
Rhythm method					
Scrotum					
Semen					
Seminal vesicle					
Seminiferous tubules					
Sexual dysfunction					
Sexual intercourse					
Sexuality					
Sexually transmitted infection					
Sodomy					
Sperm					
Spermicide					
Sterility					
Syphilis					
Testicle					
Testosterone					
Transsexual					
Transvestite					
Tubal ligation					
Urethra					
Uterus					
Vagina					

Insight 11-2 (*Continued*)

Word	Preschool	Elementary School	Junior High School	Senior High School	Adult
Vaginismus					
Vas deferens					
Vasectomy					
Virginity					
Vulva					
Wedlock					
Withdrawal					
Womb					

Learners' Needs, Interests, and Characteristics

Sexual behavior lifestyles differ from person to person. There are, however, some generalities that can be made about the relationship between sexual behaviors, attitudes, and knowledge and certain demographic groupings. For example, in a landmark study of sex in America, Laumann and colleagues (1994) found that both males and females masturbate, although 85% of men as opposed to 45% of women masturbated in the year prior to the study. Education was also found to be related to sexual activity. For example, whereas 72% of men with any college education reported their last sexual encounter took between 15 minutes and 1 hour, only 61% of men with less than a high school education reported it took that long. The results were comparable with women. Seventy-four percent with any college education reported their last sexual encounter took between 15 minutes and 1 hour compared to only 60% of women with less than a high school education reporting it took that long. Oral sex was also more prevalent among the more educated respondents.

Differences were also found between racial and ethnic groups. For example, same-sex activity was more frequent for Hispanic males (8.8% reported same-sex behavior since puberty) than White males (7.6%) or African-American males (5.8%), with no Asian-American males reporting any same-sex behavior. However, rates of same-sex behavior were comparable for females regardless of race or ethnicity. Even sexual intercourse differs by demographics. For example, whereas 47.5% of females reported that the reason for their first intercourse was affection for their partner, only approximately 25% of males gave that reason. Male first sexual intercourse was most commonly motivated by curiosity about sexual behavior.

Adolescent differences regarding sexual behavior also exist. As might be expected, as teenagers get older, they become more experienced in sexual behavior. For example, whereas 38% of ninth graders report ever having experienced sexual intercourse, almost 61% of twelfth graders report having experienced sexual intercourse (Trends in sexual risk behaviors among high school students, 1998). In a study of adolescent women, 38% of 15- to 17-year-olds had ever experienced sexual intercourse, whereas 71% of 18- to 19-year-olds had; and whereas 25% of 15- to 17-year-olds reported having had sexual intercourse in the past 3 months, 48% of 18- to 19-year-olds had (Singh & Darroch, 1999). However, more experience, unfortunately, does not always translate into more caution. Surprisingly, more ninth graders used a condom during their last intercourse (almost 59%) than did twelfth graders (52%) (Trends in sexual risk behaviors, 1998).

Adolescent sexual behavior also varies by race and ethnicity, although not as much by gender as some might think. Male and female high school students report similar rates of ever experiencing sexual intercourse (49% and 48%, respectively) and being currently sexually active (33% and 37%, respectively). They do differ, however, on the use of a condom during their last sexual intercourse (63% for males, 51% for females) and on having four or more sexual partners during their lifetime (18% for males, 14% for females). In terms of race and ethnicity, African-American high schoolers are more likely to have ever experienced sexual intercourse (73%) than either Hispanic high schoolers (52%) or White high schoolers (44%). They are also more likely to have used a condom during their last sexual intercourse (64%) than Hispanics (48%) or Whites (56%). In addition, although approximately one-third of Hispanic and White high school students report they are currently sexually active, over half (54%) of African-American students state they are currently sexually active.

Recognizing that learners may differ so dramatically and that any one instructional group may be dissimilar to others, we recommend that some diagnostic evaluation be conducted prior to your commencing sexuality education. Only after determining what the learners are like can you gear a sexuality education program to their needs, interests, and characteristics. If you are teaching sexuality education in a school, perhaps the school records can also be helpful. The number of previous teenage out-of-wedlock pregnancies, data on incidence of venereal disease, and statistics on rape may be available and of help in determining the needs of your learners. Consult your town, county, city, or state records to obtain these data.

In addition to its value in helping you determine content areas to be included in a sexuality education program, knowledge of learners can provide other types of assistance. For example, if learners continue to use slang and profane terms, without knowing them well, it will be difficult for you to determine whether their intent is to shock you or whether such language is their vernacular—their standard language usage. Further, some learners may ask seemingly ridiculous questions that you must evaluate to answer. Are the questions asked to shock you? Are they asked out of ignorance or out of curiosity? At what level (depth and breadth) should the questions be answered? Knowing the learners well is necessary if you are to respond appropriately to their questions.

Involving Learners in the Learning Process

John Dewey, the famous educational philosopher, argued a long time ago for learning through experience (Dewey, 1938). Other experts and researchers concur that learning best occurs when the learner is actively involved. As someone so aptly stated, "Teaching is done by the teacher, but learning is done

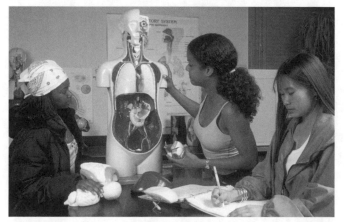

The best way for program participants to learn, and to retain that learning, is for them to be actively involved in the learning process.

by the student." The last bit of advice we offer you in this chapter is to involve your learners in the learning process. (In Chapter 12 we describe instructional strategies that can be employed for this purpose.)

For knowledge to be retained, it must be useful. The learner must internalize this knowledge and incorporate it into his or her life. The "in" word today is *relevancy.* The knowledge must be relevant to the learners. Someone once said, "Use a word three times and it's yours." Use the knowledge learned, and it will stay with you to improve your life. One way to encourage the use of knowledge is to ask learners to apply it immediately. Examples of this approach appear in books by Greenberg (2004) and Greenberg and Dintiman (1992), in which numerous scales and paper-and-pencil tests are used to provide information *to* the reader *about* the reader prior to a discussion of the topic. For example, prior to discussing the relation of self-esteem to sexual behavior, the reader might be asked to complete a self-esteem scale in order to learn more about his or her own self-esteem. Once having considered his or her own level of self-worth, the reader can be expected to be more interested in the general topic of self-esteem and sexual behavior, since he or she can now depict himself or herself in that discussion. Similarly, sexuality educators can provide learners with measures of their sexual knowledge, attitudes, and behaviors so that discussions and readings pertaining to these topics will be more interesting. With more interest, more learning will take place.

This book contains many examples of this philosophy as well. We have tried to involve you in the learning process as you read by asking you to interact with the content presented. So, for example, when a model of decision making was described in Chapter 9, you were asked to apply it to a real problem of yours by completing an Insight activity. Numerous other exercises were presented with the intent of encouraging you to use the content, so you would learn more than what you might learn from a more traditional text.

We recommend that when you conduct sexuality education, you do the same. Involve your learners with the content that is presented. Let them become immersed in it. Encourage them to use this knowledge and to determine how their lives could be improved by its use. Activate those whom you are educating.

Summary

We recommend that ground rules be established that will govern the day-to-day sexuality education group or class. Such ground rules pertain to the use of language, level of disclosure, reactions to questions, limits on topics to be studied, availability of the sexuality educator, acceptance of feelings, expression of thoughts, the need to obtain input from various people prior to sexual decision making, humor, and respect for differences.

For sexuality education to be effective, the educator must pay attention to certain communication skills. One model of communication consists of a sender, message, medium, and receiver. Each of these aspects of communication is important. Good communication involves attention to listening skills, nonverbal communication, and the need to build trust.

Sexual language is emotionally charged and often interferes with logical discourse. This is a significant problem for sexuality educators. One solution to this problem is to teach socially acceptable terminology. Learners who know the acceptable terms will be more comfortable, feel less threatened, and be less embarrassed than those unfamiliar with these terms.

The sexuality educator needs to identify learners' needs, interests, and characteristics and needs to actively involve learners in the educational process. Both of these needs pertain to providing more relevant sexuality education that relates directly to learners' lives. Without knowing the learners well, the educator will find it difficult to select content, answer questions, or evaluate learners' use of language. Without activating learners, the sexuality education experience will soon be forgotten and its content will not significantly improve the lots of those it has "educated."

References

Dewey, J. *Experience and education.* New York: Macmillan, 1938.

Greenberg, J. S. *Health education and health promotion: Learner-centered instructional strategies.* 5th ed. Boston: WCB/McGraw-Hill, 2004.

————— & Dintiman, G. B. *Exploring health: Expanding the boundaries of wellness.* Englewood Cliffs, NJ: Prentice Hall, 1992.

Kilander, H. F. *Sex education in the schools.* Toronto: Macmillan, 1968. Excerpt reprinted by permission.

Kinsey, A. C., Pomeroy, W. B. & Martin, C. E. *Sexual behavior in the human male.* Philadelphia: W. B. Saunders, 1948.

Laumann, E. O., Gagnon, J. H., Michaels, R. T. & Michaels, S. *The social organization of sexuality: Sexual practices in the United States.* Chicago: University of Chicago Press, 1994.

Masters, W. H., Johnson, V. E. & Kolodny, R. C. *Human sexuality.* 4th ed. New York: HarperCollins, 1992.

Neill, A. S. *Summerhill: A radical approach to child rearing.* New York: Hart, 1960.

Singh, S. & Darroch, J. Trends in sexual activity among adolescent American women: 1982–1995, *Family Planning Perspectives,* 31 (1999), 212–19.

Trends in sexual risk behaviors among high school students—United States, 1991–1997, *Morbidity and Mortality Weekly Report,* 47 (1998), 749–52.

Suggested Readings

Brick, P. & Taverner, B. *Positive images: Teaching abstinence, contraception, and sexual health.* Morristown, NJ: Planned Parenthood of Greater Northern New Jersey, 2001.

Brown, L. K. & Brown, M. T. *What's the big secret?: Talking about sex with girls and boys.* Boston: Little, Brown, 2000.

Hedgepeth, E. & Helmich, J. *Teaching about sexuality and HIV: Principles and methods for effective education.* New York: New York University Press, 1996.

Kirby, D. Reflections on two decades of research on teen sexual behavior and pregnancy, *Journal of School Health,* 69 (1999), 89–94.

Moore, M. J. & Rienzo, B. A. Utilizing the SIECUS guidelines to assess sexuality education in one state: Content scope and importance, *Journal of School Health,* 70 (2000), 56–60.

Okie, S. Beyond the birds and bees: Teaching children to make responsible decisions about sex, *Washington Post Health* (May 26, 1998), 12–17.

Learning Strategies for Sexuality Education

CHAPTER 12

Key Concepts

1. All decisions pertaining to instructional strategies for sexuality education must begin with clear objectives.

2. Unit plans and lesson plans, while similar, are not the same.

3. There are a variety of instructional strategies from which to choose.

In this chapter we explore instructional strategies that can be used in sexuality education. The underlying theme is *planning*. Well-planned sexuality education programs are consistent, rational, sequential, and educationally sound. Programs that are not well planned tend to be a hodgepodge of content related to sexuality without the wholeness and completeness that characterize well-planned programs. Planning involves several different people and groups and should include the use of the group-process skills and change strategies, which will be described in Chapter 16.

Learning Objectives

The cornerstone of good planning for sexuality education is well-written and explicit objectives. Decisions pertaining to content and instructional strategies cannot be made unless the purposes of the program are first specified. Once the objectives are determined, every other decision can be made with these objectives in mind. For example, the appropriate content or learning experience cannot be chosen until the objective to which it will relate is specified. An instructor who, for example, decides to use a particular film and then searches for a learning objective that the film can meet is putting the cart before the horse. Similarly, the educator who wants to use an instructional game because it is fun but does not understand the educational purpose of the game is not adhering to the basic premise of this chapter. *The objectives must be determined first.*

The focus of this section is on establishing the best way of stating objectives. However, we need to say something about the validity of the objectives first. Imagine a sexuality

---

Insight 12-1

Writing Objectives

How should objectives be stated? To begin, let us see how much information you bring to this chapter. Write three objectives for sexuality education.

1. _____

2. _____

3. _____

---

educator whose goal is to expand the sexual experiences of his or her students. This goal can be written as an objective that will meet the criteria we are about to present. However, such an objective is inappropriate in the first place. In other words, even though an objective may be stated in the right way, the objective itself may not be educationally sound. For example, an objective designed to encourage high school students to influence their parents to vote only for legislators who favor abortion on demand, even though written correctly, is not appropriate for the school setting. In Chapter 2 we discussed appropriate objectives for sexuality education programs. (Complete Insight 12-1 before reading further.)

The first criterion of good learning objectives is to focus on the learner. If your objectives are not written to express what the *learner* will be able to *do* at the end of the learning experience, you cannot determine whether the student learns anything. Are the objectives you wrote in Insight 12-1 stated in terms of what the sexuality educator will do? If so, rewrite them so that they are stated in terms of what the learner will be able to do.

If your objectives are not stated as *measurable* actions, you will not be able to determine the effectiveness of the education you conduct. Do any of the three objectives you wrote contain one or more of the following phrases?

To know	To appreciate
To understand	To realize
To enjoy	To grasp the significance of
To believe	To have the opinion that

All of these phrases indicate objectives that cannot be measured, because they are not stated in terms of observable behavior. That is, these phrases really refer to states of mind. In order to measure what a learner *understands,* for example, we would have to determine how one who understands could demonstrate that understanding by doing something. So we might ask the learner to take a test or to recite the knowledge, which will transform the understanding into a behavior that can be measured. The following phrases indicate examples of behaviors that can be measured and are therefore appropriate to include in objectives:

To describe	To answer
To list	To differentiate
To identify	To write
To interpret	To categorize
To solve	To compare
To contrast	To construct

The next consideration in setting objectives is determining how well we expect the learner to demonstrate the specified behavior. If the objective is for the learner to be able to categorize parts of the reproductive system into those of males and those of females, and we include five parts, will we be satisfied with two of five categorized correctly or will we expect all five to be categorized correctly? If we ask the learner to list three advantages and three disadvantages of the use of an intrauterine device as a method of contraception, are two correct advantages and disadvantages satisfactory,

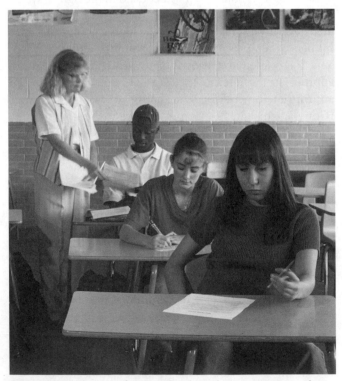

Tests are good ways of measuring knowledge. However, the learning of behaviors and skills often requires program participants to demonstrate this form of learning.

or do we expect all of them to be correct? The reason this is important is that if objectives are sequential, with the achievement of one dependent on the achievement of a previous one, the sexuality educator may want to review or reteach some content when the objective to which it relates is determined to still be unsatisfied. The following are examples of criteria that can be used to decide whether a behavior is performed well enough:

- Score 70%

- Answer four out of five

- List at least seven in 10 minutes

The final consideration in stating objectives pertains to any conditions placed on the learner. Are there any things that the learner is specifically prohibited from using or is required to use when demonstrating achievement of the objective. Here are some ways that these conditions can be phrased:

- Given a list of . . .

- Without the aid of . . .

- Using examples cited in class . . .

- Citing pertinent sex-related laws . . .

Objectives can be written about knowledge (cognition), attitudes (affect), or behavior or skills (psychomotor). As a matter of fact, many sexuality education programs include objectives in all three areas. It is hoped that knowledge will influence attitudes, which in turn will encourage learners to behave in healthier ways. Of course there are many factors that influence a person's behavior, and it is naive to assume a simple relationship between what a person knows and how that person behaves. However, appropriate knowledge is necessary for one to be well-enough informed to make sensible decisions regarding how to behave. For example, if you did not know the preejaculatory fluid contains some sperm, you would not be able to make a knowledgeable decision about whether or not to use coitus interruptus (withdrawal just prior to ejaculation) as a method of contraception.

Here are some examples of objectives that meet the criteria we have cited:

1. List three similarities and three differences between male and female sexual responses as described by Masters and Johnson.
   Behavior: list
   How well: three similarities and three differences
   Conditions: as described by Masters and Johnson

2. Given a drawing of the female reproductive system, label at least five of its parts.
   Behavior: label
   How well: at least five
   Conditions: using the drawing handed out

Insight 12-2

Writing Objectives Revisited

Now comes your opportunity to apply the information we have been discussing. Specific objectives (the kind about which we have been talking) usually stem from more general objectives. Our guess is that the objectives you wrote in Insight 12-1 could be considered general. Based on these general objectives, devise three specific ones and write them down. Bring these objectives to class; ask a classmate to evaluate your objectives, and volunteer to evaluate his or hers.

1. _____

   _____

2. _____

   _____

3. _____

   _____

A good source of further information about writing instructional objectives is Robert F. Mager's *Preparing Instructional Objectives* (1962).

---

3. In a role-playing situation, demonstrate respect for another's sexual decisions.
   Behavior: demonstrate (or act out)
   How well: that shows respect
   Conditions: in a role-playing situation

Unit Plans and Lesson Plans

Unit plans are outlines of the major components of a unit of instruction. Sexuality educators often include units of instruction on parenthood, contraception, alternate sexual lifestyles, pregnancy and birth, and many other topics. A unit plan begins with objectives for the unit. In addition, content, learning experiences, instructional material, and means of evaluation should be part of the unit plan.

A sample unit plan appears in Insight 12-3. Note that the objective is stated in such a way that it can be measured; the content is cited that is needed by the learners in order to achieve the objective; the way this content is to be presented (in learning experience) is stated clearly and succinctly; and the instructional material needed during the learning experiences is well referenced. Finally, how the learners' achievement of the objective is to be demonstrated once the learning experiences have concluded is stated in the evaluation column. Although only one objective is presented in this example, unit plans usually include many such objectives.

Lesson plans are outlines of each particular class or group session of a unit. In the unit plan given in Insight 12-3 there are two class sessions required to achieve one objective. One session involves having parents visit the learners and answer questions about parenthood. A second session entails viewing a video about parenthood and discussing it afterward. For *each* of these two sessions, a lesson plan should be written. A lesson plan consists of the following:

1. *A student objective.* What the learners should be able to do at the end of the lesson.

2. *Teacher objectives.* What the teacher is attempting to accomplish.

3. *Learning activities.* In more detail than on the unit plan. For example, include the time to be spent on each activity.

4. *Instructional materials.* All materials needed to complete the lesson.

5. *Means of evaluation.* To determine if the *student* objective has been met.

Table 12-1 presents a lesson plan for the parents' class visitation referred to in Insight 12-3.

---

unit plan   Outline of a major portion of study, or unit, from which lesson plans can be derived.

lesson plan   Outline of a particular class session.

Insight 12-3

Unit Plans

To test your understanding of how to write a unit plan, write two more objectives below and the content, learning experiences, instructional materials, and means of evaluation pertaining to each objective. Remember, first you need the objective; then you can decide on other components of the unit.

Objective	Content	Learning Experiences	Instructional Materials	Evaluation
1. To list three advantages and three disadvantages of parenthood.	Advantages of parenthood: 1. Able to give love 2. Leave something when you die 3. Can have someone to play with 4. Enjoy molding another person Disadvantages: 1. Costly 2. Time consuming 3. Decreases freedom 4. Great responsibility	1. Invite parents of three of the students to class to serve as a panel to answer questions regarding the advantages and disadvantages of parenthood. 2. Show video and discuss.	Video: *Preparation For Parenthood,* from Human Relations Media, 175 Tompkins Avenue, Pleasantville, New York. Purchase Price: $85.00.	Assuming you are counseling a friend who is contemplating becoming a parent, write three advantages and disadvantages of parenthood that you would want him or her to consider.
2.				
3.				

As you can see in Table 12-1, in a lesson plan, the time devoted to each activity is stated in the actual time rather than in the number of minutes. This helps the sexuality educator during the lesson to glance at the lesson plan and determine whether it is proceeding as planned. In addition, since the lesson plan contains all the instructional material needed for that lesson, the educator can readily gather this material prior to that lesson and remember to bring it to class.

Some final words are needed regarding unit plans and lesson plans: Remember, these are only plans. You need not adhere to them during the lesson if something good is happening. For example, if you planned one learning activity to run 10 minutes, but after this time it is still going well and is not completed, do not hesitate to let it go longer. It has been said that teaching is an art rather than a science. This means that you can—and in fact are expected to—make adaptations during class. A good example of this occurred in a class one of your authors observed. The teacher carried into the classroom a stack of instructional materials at least 4 feet high; one could only wonder what in the world this teacher would do with all this material. What she did was to place it aside as the students (seventh graders) began discussing drugs. During the class session prior to this one, a student had asked to take home a pamphlet about drugs and had read that a baby can be born addicted. When the student asked about this in class, the instructor demonstrated her teaching art. She abandoned her planned lesson, reached for materials regarding the placenta and fetal development, and proceeded to a sexuality education lesson. She took advantage of what has been called the **teachable moment.**

teachable moment   A time when learners are interested in a topic and motivated to learn about that topic.

Table 12-1 Sample Lesson Plan

Teacher Objective	Time (actual)	Learning Activity	Instructional Materials
To motivate the students to be interested in the topic	10:05–10:08	Give each learner a doll and explain that this is his or her baby. Each learner is going to have to care for it for 48 hours.	30 dolls
To introduce visitors	10:08–10:10	Tell learners the name and number of children of each parent.	Notes about parents on an index card
To have parents describe their parental experiences	10:10–10:19	Each parent takes 3 minutes to describe his or her thoughts and feelings regarding parenthood.	None
To allow students to have their questions answered	10:19–10:35	Students will ask questions of any one or all of the parents. Parent answers will be limited to 90 seconds, to allow for many questions.	None
To evaluate achievement of the student objective	10:35–10:50	Role-play: *One student is the husband; another the wife who is pregnant. They are deciding whether to raise the child or to give it up for adoption. To make a decision, they are considering the pros and cons of parenthood.*	None

---

Insight 12-4

Lesson Plans

Choose one lesson that relates to an objective you wrote for the unit plan in Insight 12-3. Write a lesson plan for that objective on the form below. Use the lesson plan presented in Table 12-1 as a guide.

Student Objective

_____

_____

_____

Teacher Objective	Time (actual)	Learning Activity	Instructional Materials

However, if you find that you need to change your lessons often, you probably are not planning well. Your lesson plans should be used to improve the planning process. To use them in this manner, you should make notes on the lesson plan right after the lesson is taught. Note whether the learning activities were effective, whether the time spent on each activity was sufficient, whether the evaluation procedure served its purpose, and so on. The next time this lesson is taught, a new lesson plan should be developed that uses the information obtained from the previous lesson. In this way, each lesson should be better than it was the last time it was taught. This is probably the major benefit to writing unit and lesson plans—to continually improve the sexuality education you conduct.

Instructional Strategies

There are many different ways in which a sexuality educator can conduct learning experiences; here, we describe a number of instructional strategies. For each strategy defined and described, an example is given to show how this strategy can be employed in one or more sexuality content areas. The use of these instructional strategies is limited only by your own creativity and initiative. It is our expectation that as these strategies are described you will already be relating them to specific lessons. However, this is not a cookbook approach to sexuality education. There are just too many variables in any one situation for us to be able to tell you specifically "how to do it." Different teachers have different philosophies, different strengths and weaknesses, and different administrative edicts limiting them in what they can do. Different learners have different needs and interests, different past experiences, different intelligence levels, and so on. Teaching is an art requiring a great deal of preparation but requiring creativity as well. The information about instructional strategies that follows will provide you with seed for the field, but you must decide where and when to plant it.

Case Studies

One way to present content is to place it within a story. A **case study** is a story that can be analyzed and from which learning can occur. The important thing to remember about case studies is that they must be complete, having a beginning, middle, and end. The case study can be presented in many forms. Handouts on which the story is presented can be given to the class. Films, videotapes, or other media can be used to present the case. The case can even be acted out. The case study analysis should include discussion of the following considerations:

1. Whether the people in the story behaved as the observers would behave

2. Whether the situation depicted frequently occurs or is unusual

3. Whether this situation should have occurred in the first place

4. What the implications or consequences are of the actions that were taken

Critical Incidents

A **critical incident** can be described as a case study (or story) that is interrupted at a point when an important decision needs to be made or action needs to be taken. Whereas the case study provides an ending for analysis, a critical incident requires that the reader or listener create an ending. The endings created by students can be acted out, presented verbally, or written down.

For example, if we began a story of Paul and Donna, but stopped the story at the point when Paul told Donna that if she did not have sexual intercourse with him he would not date her any more, we would have a critical incident. We could ask the learners, what *should* Donna do? They would have to make up their own endings rather than analyze an ending that they are given.

Here is another example of a critical incident story:

Beth and Frank considered themselves to be good parents. They loved their children and tried to bring them up well. Now their parenting skills are being put to the test. Their 13-year-old daughter has just asked permission to join her friends in attending a PG-13 rated movie that contains some nudity, some violence, and some profanity.

What do you think they'll say?

What would you say?

Brainstorming

When a range of ideas or solutions needs to be generated, **brainstorming** is an effective method to employ. This instructional strategy asks learners to supply any and all ideas that come to mind relative to the issue being discussed. The ideas are recorded (on paper or chalkboard) but are not evaluated until enough ideas have been generated. At that point, each

case study   A story with a beginning, middle, and end that can be analyzed to elicit learning.

critical incident   A story, similar to a case study, but one without an ending provided that can be used to elicit learning.

brainstorming   A method of generating multiple solutions or ideas.

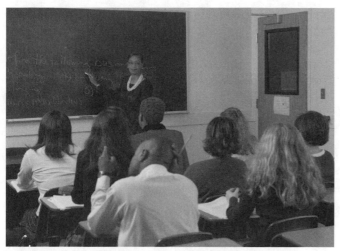
Brainstorming involves listing all responses prior to evaluating them.

idea is focused on and judged suitable or not suitable. Those not suitable are crossed out or erased, leaving a number of suitable alternatives. It is important for the learners to understand the basic rules of brainstorming.

1. Ideas or solutions are generated and listed as rapidly as possible.

2. Generated ideas or solutions must not be criticized.

3. The purpose of brainstorming is to generate many, many ideas—the more, the better.

4. After the generation phase, ideas that have common elements should be combined or modified.

5. Brainstorming should produce a number of useful ideas by having evaluated each generated idea and eliminating those not suitable.

Note that some individuals with cognitive and language deficits will have difficulty with this activity. For these learners, provide specific, concrete feedback and thoroughly review the evaluation process. Make sure that the developmental level of the participants is considered for content, vocabulary, and concepts.

This instructional strategy can be useful for controversial topics. For example, learners might be asked how society should react to homosexuals. It is conceivable that the following ideas might be generated:

1. Jail them.

2. Fine them.

3. Let them do their own thing.

4. Prohibit them from holding government security clearance.

5. Prohibit them from working with children.

6. Castrate male homosexuals.

7. Force them to have coitus with the opposite sex.

8. Force them into psychotherapy.

9. Require others to learn more about homosexuality.

After these and other ideas are listed, the sexuality educator will then teach the learners to focus on each of these ideas and decide whether to keep it on the list.

Another excellent topic to consider in this way is what an unwed teenage girl should do on learning that she is pregnant. Some of the solutions generated for this topic might include the following options:

1. Have the baby.

2. Marry the father.

3. Get an abortion.

4. Go horseback riding.

5. Give the baby up for adoption.

6. Quit school and get a job.

7. Stay in school.

8. Douche.

9. Commit suicide.

10. Enroll in a different school until the baby is born.

Role-Playing

Learning can often be facilitated by direct observation of the health-related behavior being studied. **Role-playing** involves the acting out of a situation so that the following may occur:

1. The actors may develop empathy for those who really find themselves in that situation.

2. Learners may practice behaviors in a nonthreatening, low-risk setting.

3. The implications and consequences of the behaviors can be better appreciated.

role-playing   Students acting out a scenario as a way to elicit learning.

When employing role-playing in your sexuality education classes, remember the following hints:

1. Although role-playing should be used for the spontaneous, unrehearsed acting out of a situation, the situation needs to be clearly defined so that each actor knows his or her role.

2. The audience should be assigned a specific task during their observation of the role-played situation.

3. Roles may be assigned or volunteers chosen. Assign roles when you want a particular student to develop greater empathy for people actually found in that situation. Choose volunteers to play roles when you are interested in having enthusiastic actors so that the acted-out situation is interesting for the observers.

4. Use props when available. This will aid the actors and add to the learning experience. Simple props can serve just as well as elaborate ones.

5. Keep the role-playing under 15 minutes so that sufficient time is available for discussion and evaluation. Remember, what happens *after* the role-playing is the heart of the educational experience.

Role-playing can be used in several different ways. Generally, roles are played and then discussed. The discussion usually analyzes the behavior of the role-players and specifies how observers might have behaved differently.

Role reversal is another valuable learning experience. Role reversal requires the assignment of a role to a person who in reality is the opposite of that role. For example, a sexuality educator might ask learners who believe prostitution should be a crime to raise their hands. One of these learners can then be assigned the role of a prostitute who must argue her case before a judge. Role reversal is an excellent way of helping learners to "walk in someone else's shoes."

Role-switching is still another way of adding to the sex education learning experience. Role-switching involves interrupting role-playing so that one of the observers can switch positions with one of the actors or so that two actors can switch roles. This technique allows different points of view, solutions, and so on to be presented. The discussion afterward should pertain to the implications of each actor's approach to the situation.

Regardless of which type of role-playing is employed, the processing afterward is crucial to the amount of learning that occurs. Role-playing only provides grist for the mill. What is done with this grist is most important. Thus, it is important to provide ample time for discussion, to encourage the expression of different points of view, and to allow learners to talk with each other and to argue for their points of view rather than to talk only to the sexuality educator. When the discussion has concluded, be sure to summarize the points that have been made.

Here are some excellent topics for role-playing:

- Curfews: parents versus children

- Premarital intercourse: to do or not to do, that is the question

- To marry or not to marry

- To parent or not to parent

- Discussing a sexual problem with a parent

- Discussing the impact of a disability with a partner

Buzz Groups

Small groups of learners can be organized to encourage increased opportunity for verbalization, more independent learning, and different points of view. Such small groups have been termed **buzz groups.** To achieve the goals of small-group instruction, buzz groups should consist of two to six learners. Each group should assign one of its members the role of recorder, who will keep notes about what is discussed and concluded by his or her group.

Buzz groups are most appropriately used when an open-ended topic is being studied. There should be no *one* answer but, rather, several possible solutions to the problem being discussed. When adequate discussion has occurred, the sexuality educator has two options. The learning experience can end; it may not be necessary for each buzz group to know what the other groups concluded. In fact, when the topic is a personal one that learners only feel comfortable discussing with a few people they know well, it is inadvisable to broaden the discussion beyond the buzz group. However, should you want each group to report to the others, you can have the recorder give a brief report to the total group or turn in a brief written report, which can be copied and given to each of the other groups.

Perhaps the best way to let each group in on the deliberations of the other groups is to reconstitute the buzz groups. If each original buzz group contains four learners, for example, assign each person in the group a number from one to four. After their discussion, request all the "ones" to form a group in one corner of the room, all the "twos" in another corner, and so on. This procedure will result in four groups that contain one member from each original buzz group.

---

buzz groups   Small groups of learners charged with discussing a topic.

Discussion in these new groups should pertain to reporting and discussing the original buzz group deliberations.

Here are some possible topics for buzz groups:

- When should abortions be allowed (if at all)?

- What do you think is meant by "responsible sexual behavior"?

- How are male and female sexual needs alike? How are they different?

- How do you express your sexuality?

- What would parenthood mean to you?

- How would you decide to get married or not?

- What is love?

- What would be your idea of an ideal family?

- How would you feel and behave if approached by a homosexual?

- Why do many people feel guilty about their sexual behavior?

Gaming

Gaming is an instructional experience that is fun for the learner, has rules and regulations governing it, and has a goal toward which the learners strive. Competition is often a key element in educational games, though one may compete against oneself, against other individuals, or on a team competing against another team. Since games are enjoyable to play, they often result in a level of learner involvement and interest that cannot be achieved in any other way.

Before we present an example of a learning game for sexuality education, we need to make two points. First, although there are games that can be purchased, you can also develop your own. With some time, energy, and a great deal of consideration of games with which you are familiar, you can use some principles from these games to develop your own game. For example, you can draw a football field on a chalkboard and have questions on index cards worth 5 yards, 10 yards, and 20 yards. The learners would be divided into two teams and would choose each turn whether to try a 5-, 10-, or 20-yard play (question). If they answered correctly, they would advance the yardage of the question. If they answered incorrectly, they would move back that number of yards. You could develop more detail for the game—penalties, extra points—as you wished.

Second, it is important to keep in mind that the goal is education. Fun is not the objective; learning is. Consequently, any sexuality education game chosen should have a clearly defined educational objective that the game will help the learners achieve. As an example, the following game is designed to result in students' being able to describe how the way we are perceived often determines how we behave:

Six members of the group are selected to sit in an inner circle with the remaining learners seated in a large circle around them. Each of the six inner circle learners wears a strip of masking tape on his or her forehead with one of the following roles written on the masking tape:

- *Sexy Sal*

- *Assertive Annie*

- *Chauvinist Chad*

- *Liberationist Libbie*

- *Macho Mel*

- *Ugly Eunice*

However, none of the six knows what is written on his or her masking tape and therefore does not know the role he or she is assigned. Each of the six, though, must treat the others as though they actually had the traits described on their foreheads. The role of the observers is to look for indications of each inner circle learner's actually taking on behaviors indicative of someone who possesses the trait that person was assigned. So, for example, Sexy Sal may use his sex appeal to convince one of the females to side with him.

The task of the inner circle people is to decide whether sex education should be coeducational. This game should take approximately 20 minutes. After 20 minutes, a large-group discussion should pertain to the following questions:

1. *To the inner circle learners:*
   a. *How did you feel?*
   b. *How do you think you affected the other inner circle learners?*

2. *To the observers:*
   a. *What did you notice that indicated that inner circle people acted the roles on their foreheads?*
   b. *What did you notice about how inner circle people treated each other?*

3. *To the total group:*
   a. *How can we apply generalizations from this game to everyday life?*
   b. *Have you ever been, or are you still, a victim of a self-fulfilling prophecy? Explain.*

As you can see, gaming can be both enjoyable and educational. Other sexuality education games may be found in Greenberg (2004).

Fishbowls

The game described previously employs a **fishbowl** format, that is, an inner group being observed by an outer group. Fishbowls are useful for several purposes:

1. They can be used to encourage quiet learners to become more talkative by placing these learners in the inner circle.

2. They can be used to limit the amount of verbalization on the part of talkative learners by placing them in an observer role.

3. They can be used to improve the relationship between two participants. The way to accomplish this goal is to place behind each inner circle learner an outer circle one. The outer circle learner can speak only to the person he or she is sitting behind. The outer circle person acts as a coach, advising the inner circle person what to say, ask, and so on.

4. They can be used to make large-group decisions efficiently. This requires buzz groups who send one representative into the fishbowl (inner circle) with instructions regarding what to say while the others observe the discussion of these representatives. After a short period of time, the buzz groups reconvene to give further instructions to their representatives based upon the fishbowl discussion observed. The representatives once again move into the fishbowl and come to a decision for the total group.

Here are some topics that can be discussed in fishbowls:

1. Should homosexuals be allowed to be public school teachers?

2. Is abortion murder?

3. Should mothers of preschoolers work outside the home?

4. Which sexuality education topics should we study?

5. What is obscene or pornographic?

A variation on the fishbowl technique provides for an empty chair in the inner circle. Anyone from the outer circle who wants to contribute to the inner circle's discussion can join in by sitting in this empty chair, waiting to be recognized by the members of the inner circle, saying what he or she wants to say, and then leaving the chair empty for someone else.

Sentence Completions

A good adjunct to buzz group discussions is the sentence completion technique. All this requires of learners is to write endings for incomplete sentences and be prepared to discuss these sentences in their small groups. The following are some examples of incomplete sentences:

- My body . . .

- Parents . . .

- Sex is . . .

- I think marriage . . .

- Homosexuals need . . .

- Males are . . .

- Females are . . .

- Masturbation is . . .

- Families should . . .

- Sexuality education . . .

These sentences are open-ended; there is no one correct answer. They make excellent motivators for small-group discussions.

Values Clarification

Values clarification activities are introspective activities designed to help learners identify their values. As discussed in Chapter 9, values clarification exercises are not designed to develop any particular set of values but rather to help students identify the values they already possess, so they can decide whether to keep them and how to behave more consistently with them.

One exercise requires students to rank their values. Why not try this yourself? Within each of the following groupings, identify which you would most prefer, next most prefer, and least prefer:

1. To be a married parent

2. To be a single parent

3. To not be a parent

1. To be good-looking

2. To be intelligent

3. To be wealthy

---

fishbowl   Learners organized into an inner group and an outer group as a way to elicit learning.

values clarification   A set of instructional activities designed to assist learners in identifying their values.

1. To be young

2. To be elderly

3. To be middle-aged

1. To date someone who is attractive

2. To date someone who is funny

3. To date someone who is intelligent

As with many other types of student-centered instructional strategies, the discussion following the exercise is the important aspect of the activity. *Why* a person ranks values in a certain way is more important than *what* a person's rankings are.

Another values clarification activity requires a division of students into small groups of four or five learners each. Each group has a large sheet of newsprint paper and one thick-pointed felt-tip color marker. The small group's task is to draw a house while adhering to the following rules:

1. There can be no verbal or nonverbal communication between group members.

2. The color marker must be passed from group member to group member.

3. Each group member adds one, and only one, line to the drawing.

4. The house must be completed in 20 minutes.

An example of such a drawing appears in Figure 12-1. Rather than drawings, this activity can be adapted with a felt storyboard and cutouts representative of various items around or in learners' homes.

These drawings or storyboards can then be discussed and learners asked which depictions they prefer. Such a discussion will reveal values pertaining to home life. For example, some people will prefer drawings with people in them (since drawers were not prohibited from drawing round lines, faces may have been included), indicating that home is where loved ones are. Others prefer houses that are warm and provide security (depicted by curtains on windows, the sun

beating down on the house, or smoke coming out of the chimney). Still others will prefer a large house rather than a small one, which might indicate values for material things or symbols of success.

It is important to reiterate that values clarification activities are not designed to instill any particular values in learners. Rather, they attempt to help learners clarify existing values and act more consistently with them.

Before we leave values clarification, we should reiterate what we mentioned earlier regarding this instructional strategy. There are individuals and groups of people who oppose this way of teaching. They believe that it is amoralistic to allow students to select their own values. These opponents to values clarification would prefer that a particular set of values be taught as the right ones—that is, *their* particular set of values. Regardless of your feelings about the validity of these arguments, you should know that many meaningful educational programs have been abandoned, or at least threatened with dissolution, because the instructors used values clarification activities. Therefore, we caution you to size up the community in which you find yourself teaching sexuality education and decide whether values clarification is appropriate in that setting. There is no sense in losing the entire program just because valuing activities are your preference. Sometimes common sense is the better part of valor. Additional information on values clarification may be found in Morrison and Price (1974); Raths, Harmin and Simon (1966); and Greenberg (2004).

Resource Speakers

Since the sexuality educator cannot be expected to be an expert in all sexuality-related content areas, the use of guest speakers can add a valuable dimension to a sexuality education program. Three cautions are necessary, however:

1. Make sure that the resource speaker is knowledgeable about the topic, as well as about how that knowledge relates to the learners. In short, make sure that the information presented relates to the learners' needs and interests. To alleviate your concern in this area, you should describe the learners for the resource speaker. The description should include their ages, socioeconomic levels, previous study or knowledge in the content area, and questions you obtained from them for the speaker.

2. *How* the speaker presents the topic is as important as *what* he or she says. All the speaker's expertise and knowledge is useless unless it can be conveyed to the learners in a clear and interesting way. For this reason, you will have to eliminate from your list of resource speakers people who have a great deal of experience or knowledge in a sexuality-related content area but who are boring.

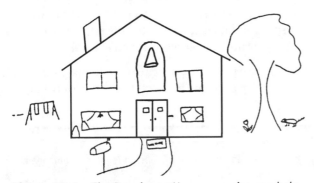

Figure 12-1   The Drawing-a-House exercise can help students identify what they value in their home lives.

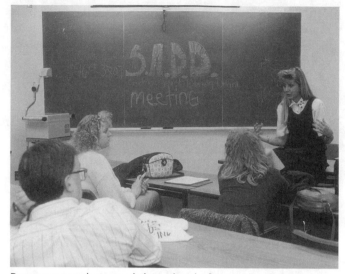

Resource speakers can bring a level of expertise or experience to the sexuality education setting that might not be available otherwise.

3. Be sure that the speaker is instructed to meet the course agenda rather than attempting to meet his or her own agenda. The speaker is there to achieve an educational objective, not to proselytize.

Here is a list of types of resource speakers and topics about which they might speak:

- Judges: Sexuality and the law
- Pediatricians: Child development
- Nurses: Abortion
- Parents: Parenthood
- Elderly persons: Sexuality and the elderly
- Vice squad police officers: Prostitution
- Planned parenthood representatives: Contraception
- Mattachine society representatives: Homosexuality
- College students: Sexual mores on the college campus
- Marriage counselors: Marital ups and downs
- School psychologists: Effects of divorce on children
- Rehabilitation counselors: Sexuality and the handicapped

- Sociologists: The family
- Historians: Sexuality and our past
- Clergy: Sexuality and religious teachings

Sexuality education is a multidisciplinary field. You can find resource speakers in many disciplines.

Refusal Skills and Assertiveness Training

One of the most important lessons students can learn is how to say, "No." This requires more than just telling them to do so. All of us, regardless of age, experience peer pressure. To be able to resist that pressure and behave in ways that we know to be in our best interest is not always easy. Refusing pressure, in a manner that maintains relationships with those pressuring us, is a skill that can be taught in sexuality education programs.

To begin, a mini-lecture on the difference between assertiveness, nonassertiveness, and aggressiveness should be conducted. Use the following definitions and distinctions:

1. *Assertiveness.* Expressing yourself, satisfying your needs, or getting what you are entitled to, but not at anyone else's expense. For example, ordering a steak cooked medium, having it delivered to your table undercooked (rare), and politely asking it to be sent back to be cooked a little longer.

2. *Nonassertiveness.* Not expressing yourself, satisfying your needs, or getting what you are entitled to in order that someone else's needs can be satisfied. For example, ordering a steak cooked medium, having it delivered to your table undercooked (rare), and eating it rare so as not to inconvenience the waiter or waitress.

3. *Aggressiveness.* Expressing yourself, satisfying your needs, or getting what you are entitled to, but at someone else's expense. For example, ordering a steak cooked medium, having it delivered to your table undercooked (rare), and loudly and obnoxiously calling the cook bad names and shouting that the steak be cooked longer. In this example, you have violated the right of the waiter or waitress to be spoken to with respect, and may have violated the rights of the restaurant patrons to a peaceful and quiet meal.

Next, have program participants role-play situations in which they have a chance to practice assertive behavior by

---

assertiveness   Expressing oneself and getting what one is entitled to without violating anyone else's rights.

nonassertiveness   Not expressing oneself and, therefore, not getting what one is entitled to because of concern regarding someone else's rights.

aggressiveness   Expressing oneself and getting what one is entitled to but at the expense of someone else's rights.

resisting pressure to do something they would rather not do. The important point here is that the student practice saying, "no"—but in such a manner as to maintain her or his relationship with the person doing the pressuring. For instance, a role-play situation can consist of a student resisting pressure to engage in sexual intercourse without using a condom. The goal in this situation would be to insist, in a friendly manner, that a condom be used. It would not be difficult for the sexuality educator to think of many other situations in which assertiveness and refusal skills would come in handy.

Instructional Media

One of the major advantages of the use of instructional media is their potential for captivating the attention and interest of the learners. Since instructional media are usually developed by experts who spend a significant amount of time and energy in planning and producing their products, these instructional aids are usually expensive. However, the expense varies a great deal; for instance, audiotapes are less expensive than films. Instructional media are abundant in the field of sexuality education, and they range, as might be expected, from the absurd to the valuable. The sexuality educator should preview material being considered prior to deciding whether to use it.

A word must be said about deciding to use instructional media: all such decisions should relate to previously identified objectives. It is never appropriate, for example, to decide to use a film, then to go about looking for a good one, and only then to search for an objective to which it might relate. First determine your objectives; then look for the best way to achieve them—a particular film might then come to mind.

There are several disadvantages in the use of instructional media. First, as previously stated, they can be quite expensive. The purchase of a film or video can cost $400 or more. The purchase of an overhead transparency series can cost the same. When budget limitations necessitate more than just ordinary caution in spending funds for instruction, media might not be the most prudent use of these funds. Second, instructional media can often be so lengthy that they take up an entire instructional session or more. Depending on the number of sessions available to you and the content you need to cover, you may not be able to spend one session observing a piece of instructional media and another session processing what has been observed. Third, instructional media tend to be used beyond their usefulness. Long after the factual content included in the media is outdated and dress, hair style, and automobiles date the media to the point of the ridiculous, companies still sell them and instructors still

use them. When one considers the cost to companies of producing media and to the instructors in purchasing them, it is not surprising that they would be squeezed to the last drop (and beyond).

One particular form of instructional media can be especially useful, however. Short films (or videos), which are relatively inexpensive, often present a situation that can be used to motivate discussion related to the situation or issue presented. These "trigger films," approximately 5 minutes in length, are excellent means of presenting critical incidents and encouraging learner participation in the resolution of these incidents.

Instructional media, then, have both advantages and disadvantages. Consequently, decisions regarding their use should be made only after consideration of the specific objectives of the program, budget constraints, time limitations, and other relevant concerns.

Learner-Centered Activities

Learning theorists tell us that learning best occurs when the learner is active in the instructional process. Other than the means of activating the learner already cited in this chapter, many other strategies can be used in sexuality education. One of these is presented here. (Others appear in Chapter 13 on HIV/AIDS.) You can devise many others yourself.

An excellent way to organize a discussion pertaining to masculinity and femininity is to instruct learners to develop two collages, each on a large sheet of oak tag or cardboard. One collage will represent the theme "A Man Is" and the other "A Woman Is." On these collages pictures, words, or actual objects may be attached; the idea is for the learners to express what they think a man and a woman are through their collages. Small-group discussions should be organized (males and females in each group) to discuss these collages.

Learner-centered activities not only result in better learning than instructor-centered activities (such as lectures) but can also be a good deal of fun.

Summary

Learning objectives must be clearly defined. Once the objectives are determined, decisions pertaining to instructional strategy, specific instructional materials, and evaluation procedures can be made. Instructional objectives should be stated so that they can be evaluated; that is, objectives should state what the learner will be able to do at the conclusion of the instruction, how well he or she will be able to do it and under what conditions.

---

learner-centered activities   Instructional strategies that actively involve students in the learning process.

A unit plan is an outline of a major component of a course of study; a lesson plan relates to one specific instructional session. Several lesson plans make up an instructional unit. Unit plans consist of objectives, content that relates to the objectives, learning experiences that present the content, instructional materials that may be used during the learning experiences, and evaluation procedures.

Lesson plans consist of teacher objectives and learning activities for a specific lesson, time allocated to each learning experience within that lesson, and any instructional material that may be needed for that lesson.

Numerous and varied instructional strategies are available to the sexuality educator. These strategies include case studies, critical incidents, brainstorming, role-playing, buzz groups, gaming, fishbowls, sentence completions, values clarification, resource speakers, assertiveness and refusal skills training, use of instructional media, and other learner-centered activities.

When implementing learning strategies for sexuality education, educators need to remember these points:

1. Good instruction requires planning.

2. Good instruction requires a sexuality educator who has knowledge of various learning strategies so that he or she can choose the most appropriate one for a given situation.

3. Good instruction requires a sexuality educator willing to be creative and to apply his or her teaching *art*.

4. Good instruction requires evaluation procedures that will result in continual improvement and adaptation.

References

Greenberg, J. S. *Health education and health promotion: Learner-centered instructional strategies.* 5th ed. Boston: WCB/McGraw-Hill, 2004.

Mager, R. F. *Preparing instructional objectives.* Belmont, CA: Fearon Publishers, 1962.

Morrison, E. S. & Price, M. U. *Values in sexuality: A new approach to sex education.* New York: Hart, 1974.

Raths, L. E., Harmin, M. & Simon, S. B. *Values and teaching: Working with values in the classroom.* Columbus, OH: Charles E. Merrill, 1966.

Suggested Readings

Barth, R. P. *Reducing the risk: Building skills to prevent pregnancy, STD and HIV/AIDS with student workbook.* Santa Cruz, CA: ETR Associates, 1996.

Harvey, S. & Goudvis, A. *Strategies that work: Teaching comprehension to enhance understanding.* Portland, ME: Stenhouse Publishers, 2000.

Hedgepeth, E. & Helmich, J. *Teaching about sexuality and HIV: Principles and methods for effective education.* New York: New York University Press, 1996.

Levine, M. *A mind at a time: America's top learning expert shows how every child can succeed.* New York: Simon and Schuster, 2003.

Pridmore, P., Stephens, D. & Stephens, J. *Children as partners for health: A critical review of the child-to-child approach.* Waltham, MA: Zed Books, 2000.

Ridini, S. P. *Health and sexuality education in schools.* Westport, CT: Bergin & Garvey, 1998.

Schenker, I. I., Sabar-Friedman, G. & Sy, F. S., eds. *AIDS education: Interventions in multi-cultural societies.* New York: Plenum Publishing, 1997.

Strategies for Learning and Teaching about HIV/AIDS

CHAPTER 13

Key Concepts

1. HIV/AIDS continues to be a health issue of concern in the United States and other countries around the world.

2. In the United States, HIV/AIDS affects minority populations disproportionately.

3. Although abstinence is the most effective way of preventing HIV/AIDS, other effective prevention methods are available to someone who chooses not to be abstinent.

4. Comprehensive sexuality education has been suggested by experts as the most effective organization of HIV/AIDS education.

Tom applied for a graduate assistantship in our department and, because of his impressive academic record and the nature of his experiences, was awarded one. He was a pleasure to have around, always smiling and willing to help in whatever way he could. It was because of his personality and conscientiousness that Tom's graduate assistantship was extended into the next year and several years thereafter.

It was during his fourth year with us that Tom began losing weight and missing some days at school. Attributing it to the flu or a similar condition, no one seemed to take much notice—that is, until Tom starting missing more days and looking emaciated. Before long, the rumor spread about Tom having **AIDS** and not having long to live. Unfortunately, the rumor was true, and before too many more months, Tom died.

With today's new medications and combinations of medications, Tom might be alive today, or at least he would have lived longer with **HIV** than he did. Of course, that troubles those of us who knew and cared for Tom. However, other issues are also troubling. Until he told us, we did not even know Tom was gay. He contracted HIV through unprotected sex. Why did he feel the need to hide his identity, and how much torment did that hiding create? More to the point, what did we (the department, the faculty, the university, and

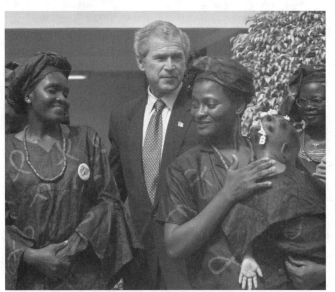

The prevalence of HIV/AIDS on the African continent was one of the agenda items during a trip to Africa by President Bush in 2003.

AIDS An incurable disease caused by the Human Immunodeficiency Virus that compromises the effectiveness of the immunological system, which can result in death.

HIV The Human Immunodeficiency Virus, which causes AIDS, thereby decreasing the effectiveness of the immunological system.

society at large) convey to Tom that led him to conclude we would reject him if we knew his secrets? And, how many others are in a similar situation to Tom's and are in torment as he was?

It is our responsibility as sexuality educators to help people like Tom by teaching the facts about HIV/AIDS; helping students explore their feelings regarding this disease and its physical, psychological, and social consequences; and teaching students how to prevent HIV/AIDS in the first place. This chapter is designed to help sexuality educators do just that.

Why a Separate Chapter on HIV/AIDS?

HIV/AIDS is a serious disease whose prevalence is of concern worldwide. It is also incurable, although the latest medication regimens significantly prolong life with the disease. For these reasons alone, HIV/AIDS deserves a separate chapter in this book.

There are an estimated 40 million people living with HIV/AIDS worldwide. Furthermore, HIV/AIDS' impact on youth is significant. More than a third of the 40 million people living with HIV/AIDS (38%) are under the age of 25 (UNAIDS, 2001). Five million people were infected with HIV in 2003. Of those newly infected, 58% will be under the age of 25 (Summers, Kates & Murphy, 2002). Alarmingly, at an AIDS conference sponsored by UNICEF, it was reported

that half of the young people in more than a dozen countries at particular risk for HIV had never heard of the virus (Edwards, 2002).

HIV/AIDS in the United States

Over the years through 2001, over 800,000 American adults and adolescents and over 9,000 children developed AIDS. Most adult and adolescent male cases were contracted through homosexual activity (55%), whereas most adult and adolescent female cases were contracted through heterosexual activity (41%), with intravenous drug use being a close second (39%). The vast majority (91%) of pediatric AIDS cases are the result of a mother passing the virus on to her child, either during childbirth or thereafter (Centers for Disease Control and Prevention, 2003).

In 2001, there were over 506,154 Americans living with HIV infection or AIDS. Of those, 5,408 were children 13 years of age or younger (Centers for Disease Control and Prevention, 2003). Table 13-1 shows the number of persons living with AIDS by region during the years 1993 through 2001.

When the HIV/AIDS data is isolated to those under age 25, it is found that whereas only 5% of males between the ages of 20 and 24 contracted HIV through heterosexual contact, 55% of females that age contracted the virus through heterosexual contact (see Table 13-2). Most male cases (61%) between ages 20 and 24 were contracted through homosexual

Table 13-1 Estimated Number of Persons Living with AIDS, by Region of Residence and Year, 1993 through 2001, United States[1]

| | Year | | | | | | | | |
Region of residence	1993	1994	1995	1996	1997	1998	1999	2000	2001
Northeast	51,559	59,225	65,382	72,142	79,904	86,008	92,054	99,450	106,601
Midwest	18,498	20,420	21,945	23,921	26,460	28,544	30,835	33,249	35,726
South	58,660	67,765	75,126	85,260	97,072	108,184	118,431	128,310	140,006
West	39,440	42,830	45,614	49,246	54,085	58,326	62,218	66,172	70,052
U.S. dependencies, possessions, and associated nations	5,615	6,212	6,644	7,166	7,943	8,646	9,266	9,836	10,443
Total	**173,772**	**196,452**	**214,711**	**237,735**	**265,464**	**289,709**	**312,804**	**337,017**	**362,827**

[1]These numbers do not represent the actual number of persons living with AIDS. Rather, these numbers are point estimates of the number of persons living with AIDS derived by subtracting the estimated cumulative number of deaths in persons with AIDS from the estimated cumulative number of persons with AIDS diagnosed. Estimated AIDS incidence and estimated deaths are adjusted for reporting delays, but not for incomplete reporting. The year 2001 is the most recent year for which reliable estimates are available.

Source: Centers for Disease Control and Prevention. *HIV/AIDS Surveillance Report, 2001,* 13, no. 2 (2003), 36.

Table 13-2 AIDS Cases in Adolescents and Adults under Age 25, by Sex and Exposure Category, Reported through December 2001, United States

| | 13–19 Years Old | | | | 20–24 Years Old | | | |
| | 2001 | | Cumulative Total | | 2001 | | Cumulative Total | |
Male exposure category	No.	(%)	No.	(%)	No.	(%)	No.	(%)
Men who have sex with men	80	(41)	889	(35)	455	(53)	12,472	(61)
Injecting drug use	7	(4)	148	(6)	65	(8)	2,414	(12)
Men who have sex with men and inject drugs	3	(2)	133	(5)	40	(5)	2,088	(10)
Hemophilia/coagulation disorder	6	(3)	763	(30)	16	(2)	675	(3)
Heterosexual contact:	8	(4)	116	(5)	73	(8)	1,059	(5)
Sex with injecting drug user	2		26		9		289	
Sex with person with hemophilia	0		2		0		4	
Sex with transfusion recipient with HIV infection	0		0		0		14	
Sex with HIV-infected person, risk not specified	6		88		64		752	
Receipt of blood transfusion, blood components, or tissue	5	(3)	98	(4)	2	(0)	111	(1)
Risk not reported or identified	86	(44)	408	(16)	214	(25)	1,518	(7)
Male subtotal	195	(100)	2,555	(100)	865	(100)	20,337	(100)
Female exposure category								
Injecting drug use	5	(3)	238	(13)	41	(7)	2,082	(25)
Hemophilia/coagulation disorder	0	(0)	13	(1)	0	(0)	16	(0)
Heterosexual contact:	57	(32)	949	(51)	289	(48)	4,569	(55)
Sex with injecting drug user	8		292		30		1,608	
Sex with bisexual male	4		50		8		313	
Sex with person with hemophilia	0		15		1		55	
Sex with transfusion recipient with HIV infection	0		2		3		27	
Sex with HIV-infected person, risk not specified	45		590		247		2,566	
Receipt of blood transfusion, blood components, or tissue	5	(3)	103	(5)	5	(1)	123	(1)
Risk not reported or identified	110	(62)	570	(30)	261	(44)	1,538	(18)
Female subtotal	177	(100)	1,873	(100)	596	(100)	8,328	(100)
Total	372		4,428		1,461		28,665	

Source: Centers for Disease Control and Prevention. *HIV/AIDS Surveillance Report, 2001,* 13, no. 2 (2003), 22.

Table 13-3 AIDS Cases and Annual Rates per 100,000 Population, by Race/Ethnicity, Age Group, and Sex, Reported in 2001, United States

| Race/Ethnicity | Adults/Adolescents | | | | | | Children <13 Years | | Total | |
| | Males | | Females | | Total | | | | | |
	No.	Rate	No.	Rate	No.	Rate	No.	Rate	No.	Rate
White, not Hispanic	11,164	13.7	2,040	2.4	13,204	7.9	33	0.1	13,237	6.6
Black, not Hispanic	13,895	109.2	7,023	47.8	20,918	76.3	113	1.4	21,031	59.6
Hispanic	6,289	43.3	1,894	12.9	8,183	28.0	26	0.2	8,209	20.7
Asian/Pacific Islander	358	8.6	69	1.5	427	4.8	3	0.1	430	3.8
American Indian/Alaska Native	152	18.8	42	4.9	194	11.7	0	0.0	194	9.0
Total[1]	**31,901**	**28.1**	**11,082**	**9.1**	**42,983**	**18.3**	**175**	**0.3**	**43,158**	**14.9**

[1]Totals include 57 persons whose race/ethnicity is unknown.

Source: Centers for Disease Control and Prevention. *HIV/AIDS Surveillance Report, 2001,* 13, no. 2 (2003), 28.

contact. These data are consistent with that found among females aged 13 to 19. However, almost as many 13- to 19-year-old males (30%) contracted HIV through treatment for **hemophilia** as did through homosexual contact (35%).

HIV/AIDS and Minority Populations

HIV/AIDS disproportionately affects minority populations. For example, whereas only an estimated 12% of Americans are African-American, African-Americans make up 38% of reported AIDS cases (Watkins, 2002). Similarly, Hispanics made up 13% of the population in 2000 but accounted for 19% of the total number of new HIV infections. Table 13-3 shows AIDS cases and annual rates per 100,000 population by race and ethnicity, age group, and sex as reported in 2001. It should be noted that the rates for African-Americans and Hispanics are significantly higher than the rates for Whites or Asian-Americans and Pacific Islanders. Rates for American Indians and Alaskan Natives are also higher than those for Whites or Asian-Americans and Pacific Islanders.

It is not being a minority that, in itself, leads to HIV infection. It is culture and society that influence transmission of HIV to minority populations. As Watkins (2002) aptly recognizes, "While race and ethnicity are not risk factors for HIV infection, they are associated with key factors in the United States that determine health status—factors such as poverty, access to quality health care, health care-seeking behaviors, illicit drug use, and high rates of sexually transmitted diseases." It then stands to reason that eliminating the risk of HIV infection among minorities involves impacting these sociological factors.

HIV and Death

Although newer medications and combinations of medications have the potential for turning HIV/AIDS into a chronic condition, the disease is presently still considered terminal. That is, myth and misconception to the contrary, although years and quality of life can be significantly extended, persons with AIDS will eventually die of complications associated with the disease. *Students need to know this.*

Through 2001, 467,910 persons with AIDS have died in the United States (see Table 13-4). Of those, 398,871 were males and 71,039 were females, although new transmissions show many more females contracting HIV than previously. In 2001, approximately 9,000 people died of AIDS.

Prevention of HIV Infection

The best method available to prevent infection with HIV is abstinence: abstaining from sexual activity with an HIV-infected partner and abstaining from intravenous drug use.

hemophilia   A blood clotting disorder that often requires regular dialysis.

Table 13-4 Deaths in Persons with AIDS, by Race/Ethnicity, Age at Death, and Sex, Occurring in 1999 and 2000; and Cumulative Totals Reported through December 2001, United States[1]

Race/Ethnicity and Age at Death[2]	Males 1999	Males 2000	Males Cumulative Total	Females 1999	Females 2000	Females Cumulative Total	Both Sexes 1999	Both Sexes 2000	Both Sexes Cumulative Total
White, not Hispanic									
Under 15	8	3	575	4	8	427	12	11	1,002
15–24	22	18	2,567	14	10	501	36	28	3,068
25–34	666	431	55,693	151	117	4,857	817	548	60,550
35–44	1,907	1,568	83,459	329	263	5,576	2,236	1,831	89,035
45–54	1,310	1,147	38,845	160	146	2,247	1,470	1,293	41,092
55 or older	542	518	16,438	56	65	1,837	598	583	18,275
All ages	4,455	3,685	197,724	714	609	15,466	5,169	4,294	213,190
Black, not Hispanic									
Under 15	41	16	1,473	28	14	1,439	69	30	2,912
15–24	55	62	2,536	79	54	1,540	134	116	4,076
25–34	920	753	34,675	581	553	12,596	1,501	1,306	47,271
35–44	2,300	1,915	53,099	1,066	945	16,322	3,366	2,860	69,421
45–54	1,718	1,629	24,925	560	550	6,127	2,278	2,179	31,052
55 or older	749	687	10,634	232	223	2,701	981	910	13,335
All ages	5,783	5,062	127,450	2,546	2,339	40,752	8,329	7,401	168,202
Hispanic									
Under 15	11	5	637	14	7	587	25	12	1,224
15–24	21	22	1,373	17	10	501	38	32	1,874
25–34	461	353	21,010	163	119	4,762	624	472	25,772
35–44	1,007	847	27,892	303	250	5,359	1,310	1,097	33,251
45–54	562	576	11,729	176	154	2,058	738	730	13,787
55 or older	290	240	4,875	50	79	960	340	319	5,835
All ages	2,352	2,043	67,557	723	619	14,236	3,075	2,662	81,793
Asian/Pacific Islander									
Under 15	0	1	19	1	1	18	1	2	37
15–24	2	1	38	1	0	8	3	1	46
25–34	13	13	743	5	3	84	18	16	827
35–44	46	28	1,181	2	8	112	48	36	1,293
45–54	23	15	578	8	2	70	31	17	648
55 or older	8	10	267	2	5	57	10	15	324
All ages	92	68	2,828	19	19	351	111	87	3,179
American Indian/Alaska Native									
Under 15	0	0	13	0	0	8	0	0	21
15–24	0	1	26	0	0	3	0	1	29
25–34	13	5	398	4	3	79	17	8	477
35–44	24	19	430	8	3	81	32	22	511
45–54	12	10	151	1	5	31	13	15	182
55 or older	2	4	50	3	1	14	5	5	64
All ages	51	39	1,070	16	12	216	67	51	1,286
All racial/ethnic groups									
Under 15	60	25	2,717	47	30	2,480	107	55	5,197
15–24	100	104	6,545	111	74	2,554	211	178	9,099
25–34	2,074	1,555	112,577	904	795	22,380	2,978	2,350	134,957
35–44	5,287	4,378	166,172	1,710	1,469	27,459	6,997	5,847	193,631
45–54	3,629	3,379	76,275	905	857	10,535	4,534	4,236	86,810
55 or older	1,592	1,460	32,284	343	373	5,572	1,935	1,833	37,856
All ages	12,742	10,901	396,871	4,020	3,598	71,039	16,762	14,499	467,910

[1]Data tabulations for 1999 and 2000 are based on date of death occurrence. Data for deaths occurring in 2001 are incomplete and not tabulated separately, but are included in the cumulative totals. Tabulations for 1999 and 2000 may increase as additional deaths are reported to CDC.

[2]Data tabulated under "all ages" include 360 persons whose age at death is unknown. Data tabulated under "all racial/ethnic groups" include 260 persons whose race/ethnicity is unknown.

Source: Centers for Disease Control and Prevention. *HIV/AIDS Surveillance Report, 2001,* 13, no. 2 (2003), 29.

This is an important message of HIV/AIDS education efforts—especially for adolescents and young adults who are in a developmental stage where sexual and drug experimentation are common. Today such experimentation carries a deadly risk of HIV and AIDS.

However, whereas abstaining from sexual activity is acceptable for some people, abstaining throughout one's life may be impractical and undesirable for others. For those who are uninfected and sexually active, maintaining a mutually faithful monogamous relationship with an uninfected partner will also prevent the sexual transmission of HIV. But each partner would also need to abstain from intravenous drug use, another high-risk behavior for HIV transmission.

There are also other ways to protect oneself from contracting an HIV infection. One of the most effective is the use of a latex condom during coital or anal intercourse and during fellatio. Unfortunately, studies show that people—youth in particular—too often engage in these activities without using a condom (Greenberg, Bruess & Haffner, 2004). In an analysis of the National Survey of Family Growth (Piccinio & Mosher, 1998), researchers investigated the contraceptive methods used by women aged 15 to 44. They found that only 23% used condoms. When broken down into various categories, younger women, African-American women, highly educated women, wealthier women, and women who never married most commonly reported the use of condoms. Yet, condom use, even among these groups, never approached 50%. In a study of adolescents' use of condoms (Ford, Sohn & Lepkowski, 2001), researchers found that condoms were used in 59% of relationships, although not necessarily during every occasion of sexual intercourse.

In addition, sex with prostitutes should be avoided, since many male and female prostitutes use injected drugs and, as a result of having multiple sexual partners, have an increased likelihood of having had sex with someone infected with HIV.

Special Considerations When Dealing with HIV/AIDS Education

The term *risk taking* is increasingly used to describe the behavior patterns of many adolescents that are responsible for many negative health outcomes. Usually included in this category are behaviors associated with violent outcomes (such as homicide), psychiatric disorders including suicide and eating disorders, vehicle use, sexual activity, and substance use. The individual behaviors are often related and the factors influencing the onset of these behaviors may be similar (Irwin, 1990).

With recognition of the interrelationships of these risky behaviors, educators are increasingly seeing the need to consider sexual behavior as part of overall health behavior. Of course, this is one of the main reasons we continually refer to the need for HIV/AIDS education and sexuality education to be part of a comprehensive health education program.

The details of changing health behavior are complicated and beyond the scope of this book; however, educators must recognize the following two principles (Turner, Miller & Moses, 1989, 265):

1. For behavior to change, individuals must recognize the problem, be motivated to act, and have the knowledge and skills necessary to perform the action.

2. To increase the likelihood of action, impediments in the social environment must be removed or weakened and inducements for change provided whenever possible.

There are some societal conflicts that have characterized America's response to the AIDS epidemic. These conflicts can interfere with effective education about HIV/AIDS. Here are some examples (Turner, Miller & Moses, 1989). Perhaps you can think of others.

Insight 13-1

Influencing Risky Health Behavior

Realizing that personal characteristics and behavior patterns of learners influence high-risk health behaviors can help educators be more effective. However, influencing negative health behaviors can be difficult. List five things you think educators can do to increase the likelihood of more positive health behaviors. Share your list with several classmates. Look for similarities and differences among the lists and discuss why items were included on the lists. Then collectively rank the three things you think represent the best ways to increase the likelihood of positive health behaviors.

1. _____

2. _____

3. _____

4. _____

5. _____

The AIDS epidemic has evoked a traditional response—it has been defined as mainly a medical problem to be solved by medical science. However, AIDS is also a social and behavioral problem. Since there is not yet a medical solution, the problem needs to be solved by social and educational means.

There is a common hesitation to discuss sexual issues. There is also a broadly accepted notion that government simply has no business dealing with sexuality. Relatedly, HIV/AIDS education efforts have been prohibited because of social barriers such as the refusal to accept condom advertising on network television, requirements that federal AIDS education materials be phrased in ways that are inoffensive to most educated adults, and attempts to use federal AIDS educational campaigns to deliver a message about desirable moral behavior.

Creative educators will need to use appropriate means to help learners deal with these social barriers to behavior change. As long as the barriers exist, it will be increasingly difficult to prevent the spread of AIDS.

HIV/AIDS Education

Preventing the contraction of HIV among youth involves various considerations. Table 13-5, "A 10-Step Strategy to Prevent HIV/AIDS Among Young People," was presented at the International AIDS Conference in 2001. Among the steps is the suggestion to increase knowledge of HIV and skills associated with HIV prevention. However, the developers recognized that having knowledge is a necessary, but not sufficient, condition to prevent HIV infection. For example, youth may know they should use a condom, but still neglect to do so. Consequently, conducting activities to end the stigma associated with HIV/AIDS is suggested, as is providing

---

Insight 13-2

The HIV/AIDS Czar

Well, we have given you a new position, the HIV/AIDS Czar. You are responsible for the government's AIDS prevention campaign. The catch is that your position is an *elected* one. That means that every four years the public scrutinizes what you did and how effective it was. They also look at how responsive to community moral standards and sensitivities you have been. After that evaluation, and after listening to criticism of your functioning by your opponent—the person running against you in the election—the public votes who should serve as Czar for the next four years.

You recognize that there are barriers to what you can do. You cannot use some sexual terms in your educational pamphlets. You cannot use some graphics in the visual materials you develop. You cannot say some things in your public service announcements that air on television and radio.

1. What compromises are you willing to make? _____

_____

2. What compromises will you never make? _____

_____

_____

3. What frustrations do you think you will encounter? _____

_____

_____

4. Would you want such a job? If so, why? If not, why not? _____

_____

_____

5. How can you help people in your community who are responsible for HIV/AIDS education overcome some of the barriers they encounter? _____

_____

_____

6. When will you offer your help to these people? _____

_____

_____

Table 13-5 A 10-Step Strategy to Prevent HIV/AIDS Among Young People

This "10-Step Strategy" was released during the International AIDS Conference in Barcelona to help countries as well as communities develop their own HIV/AIDS program guidelines based on individual situations and needs.

1. End the silence, stigma, and shame
National and community leadership must break the silence, challenge the stigma, and eliminate the shame associated with HIV/AIDS. They must have the courage to talk openly and without judgment about adolescent sexuality, about violence against girls and women, and about drug use.

Policymakers must ensure that adolescents have the information, services, and support they need. Leaders must marshal the necessary financial resources for the fight against AIDS and develop strategies based on thorough analysis of the local situation.

2. Provide knowledge and information
Young people cannot protect themselves if they do not know the facts about HIV/AIDS. Adolescents must learn the facts before they become sexually active, and the information must be regularly reinforced both in the classroom and beyond.

Increasing knowledge through schools. Good-quality education fosters analytical thinking and healthy habits. Better educated young people are more likely to acquire the knowledge, confidence, and social skills to protect themselves from HIV. Prevention education should be timely, age-appropriate, and relevant to the situations and culture of the young people and their families.

Increasing knowledge through communities. Parents as well as community and religious leaders need to recognize the importance of their own roles in providing lifesaving information and skills.

Increasing knowledge through the media. The media is a powerful weapon against HIV/AIDS. Good programming can counter popular misconceptions about adolescents, reveal the discrimination and abuse young people face, and highlight the contributions they make to their communities.

3. Provide life skills to put knowledge into practice
Young people cannot change their behavior by knowledge alone. They need skills to put what they learn into practice.

Life skills—involving negotiation, conflict resolution, critical thinking, decision making, and communication—are vital for young people. These skills will help them learn to relate to one another as equals, work in groups, build self-esteem, peacefully resolve disagreements, and resist both peer and adult pressure to take unnecessary risks. They can be taught in many creative and innovative ways, both in and out of school.

4. Provide youth-friendly health services
The services to help prevent HIV and other sexually transmitted diseases include access to condoms as well as access to voluntary HIV counseling and testing. For young women who are pregnant and HIV positive, the clinics can provide information and services to help them avoid transmitting HIV to their infants.

5. Promote voluntary and confidential HIV counseling and testing
Nine out of 10 people living with HIV/AIDS do not know they are infected. Yet studies show that young people have a strong interest in knowing their HIV status.

Voluntary and confidential HIV counseling and testing is an important tool for preventing HIV. This allows adolescents to evaluate their behavior and its consequences. For example, a negative test result offers a key opportunity for a counselor to reinforce the importance of safety and risk-reduction behaviors. Young people who test positive for HIV must receive referrals for medical care and must talk to individuals who can help them understand what their HIV-positive status means as well as the responsibilities they have to themselves and others.

Table 13-5 (*Continued*)

6. Work with young people and promote participation

Energetic, enthusiastic, and creative young people are a tremendous resource in all areas of HIV prevention and care. Their input is invaluable in developing program design and outreach, ensuring that prevention and care efforts are meaningful to their peers, and making certain that information is communicated through effective channels.

Involving young people in prevention efforts educates them about HIV and gives them a sense of responsibility and pride. With the right skills, young people are extremely effective messengers in reaching high-risk individuals and groups.

7. Engage young people living with HIV/AIDS

A major challenge in HIV prevention is to convince young people that HIV/AIDS can strike anyone. One of the most effective ways to accomplish this is to get young people living with HIV/AIDS to share their experiences.

Young people living with HIV/AIDS are in a strategic position to reinforce information about the need to adopt and maintain safe behaviors. They, more than anyone else, can convey the message that individuals must make every effort to ensure that no one contracts HIV from them.

They can also reduce the stigma associated with HIV by showing that the virus can infect anyone and can serve as effective role models for living productive lives.

8. Create safe and supportive environments

Providing young people with information and skills without ensuring that they feel safe and supported at home, at school, and in their community severely limits their ability to protect themselves from HIV.

Parents, schools, and social institutions need the knowledge and skills to create an environment in which young men and women are safe from harm, are cared for equally, and are treated with respect.

Schools and communities must condemn sexual violence, abuse, and exploitation. Governments must make sexual violence unacceptable by enacting and enforcing laws that protect young women and men from all forms of sexual violence, inside and outside of marriage, as well as imposing criminal penalties on their abusers. Media and education campaigns must encourage equality between men and women and denounce all forms of violence against women, children, and adolescents.

9. Reach out to young people most at risk

Those young people especially at high risk for contracting HIV—young men having sex with men, children living on the street, child soldiers, young refugees, children orphaned by AIDS, and others—are often on the periphery of society and face enormous difficulties obtaining help.

These individuals need access to livelihoods, education, and services to help them to build their future. Interventions must take into account the range of constraints they face and help to establish an environment marked by respect, acceptance, and stability. This is key to helping them to integrate into society.

10. Strengthen partnerships, monitor progress

Protecting young people from HIV is too big a job for any one sector of society. To make a real and lasting difference, the commitment and resources of all sectors must be mobilized, coordinated, and channeled to families and communities. There must be a commitment to bring people together at every level—community, nation, region, world—to invest in young people.

The partners must include nongovernmental and civil society organizations, including faith-based groups and the private sector; governments; young people; academic and research institutions; private foundations; bilateral donor agencies; and the United Nations and other multilateral agencies.

Defeating HIV/AIDS will also require tracking change, both in the infection rates and in the knowledge, awareness, and behavior of young people. Collecting information on their knowledge and behavior will not only help to monitor progress but will also help to identify which programs are succeeding and why.

Source: A 10-step strategy to prevent HIV/AIDS among young people, *SIECUS Report,* 31, no. 1 (2002), 8–9.

youth-friendly health services, providing confidential counseling and testing, and creating safe and supportive environments for youth.

School HIV/AIDS Education

Since students are a "captive" audience, schools are good places to educate them about HIV/AIDS. This occurs sometimes as part of a sexuality education program, and other times as part of the science and/or health curriculum. However, too often there are limitations placed on HIV/AIDS education conducted in schools. One of the more significant of these restrictions relates to **abstinence-only-until-marriage** curricula.

Abstinence-Only-Until-Marriage

At the time of this writing, President George W. Bush and Congress have funded sexuality education programs that limit instruction to preventing sexual intercourse until marriage. They argue, in spite of evidence to the contrary, that sexuality education that includes discussion of safer sex practices and contraception encourages youth to experiment with sexual intercourse. As stated by the director of public policy of the Sexuality Information and Education Council of the United States (SIECUS), William Smith, while criticizing the Bush administration's stance on HIV/AIDS prevention programs, "At the heart of the problem is the Administration's focus on abstinence-only-until-marriage programs that prohibit educators from giving information to young people that they can use when they become sexually active—and at risk for HIV/AIDS" (Edwards, 2002). The support for limiting HIV/AIDS education programs to an abstinence-only-until-marriage approach is a political one. Politicians have voted to provide the majority of money to these programs. Smith presents his view of the reason for this political decision (Smith, 2002):

> On the whole, politicians have found it difficult to embrace prevention strategies that fall outside the realm of comfort. For example, demonstrating the proper use of condoms and making available clean needles and bleach kits run against the grain of what most politicians feel is appropriate.
>
> Yet, it is precisely these types of interventions— specifically targeted to populations with increased risk factors for HIV infection—that are culturally appropriate and seek to deal with the reality of the epidemic in America.

Comprehensive Sexuality Education

The approach to sexuality education advocated by many experts in the discipline calls for recognizing that, although abstinence is to be valued and encouraged, large numbers of youth and others will still choose to engage in sexual intercourse and other sexual activities. Therefore, education should be directed toward assisting those nonabstainers to prevent unintended pregnancies and sexually transmitted infections, including HIV. This is called **comprehensive sexuality education.** Programs of this kind include education relevant to abstinence, but also include such topics as contraception, the proper way to use a condom, and safer sex, among others. They are also comprehensive in that they include sexuality

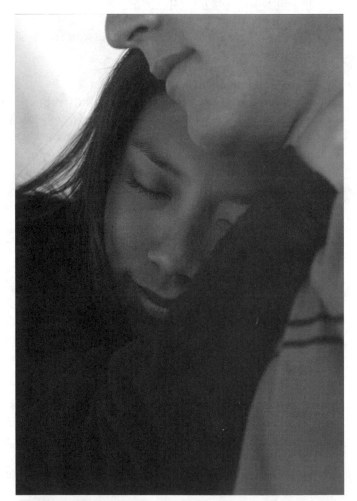

Whether we like it or not, we must recognize that many young people engage in sexual intercourse.

---

abstinence-only-until-marriage   An approach to sexuality education that restricts instruction to encouraging abstinence from sexual intercourse until one is in a marital relationship, thereby ignoring the educational needs of those who choose not to refrain from sexual intercourse.

comprehensive sexuality education   Sexuality education programs that are sequential and broad in scope. Subsequent learning builds upon previous learning.

education in the earlier grades (at the level that students can comprehend) and build upon that knowledge in subsequent grades. For example, relative to HIV/AIDS, children might learn about communicable diseases and means of preventing these diseases. High school students might consider the role of condoms in the prevention of HIV/AIDS. Even experts in the federal government recognize the value of comprehensive sexuality education programs. The Division of HIV/AIDS Prevention of the Centers for Disease Control and Prevention (2003) asserts the following:

> ***School-based programs are critical for reaching youth before behaviors are established.*** *Because risk behaviors do not exist independently, topics such as HIV, STDs, unintended pregnancy, tobacco, nutrition, and physical activity should be integrated and ongoing for all students in kindergarten through high school. The specific scope and content of these school health programs should be locally determined and consistent with parental and community values.* ***Research has clearly shown that the most effective programs are comprehensive ones that include a focus on delaying sexual behavior*** *and* ***provide information on how sexually active young people can protect themselves.*** *Evidence of prevention success can be seen in trends from the Youth Risk Behavior Survey conducted over an 8-year period, which show both a decline in sexual risk behaviors and an increase in condom use among sexually active youth. The percentage of sexually experienced high school students decreased from 54.1% in 1991 to 49.9% in 1999, while condom use among sexually active students increased from 46.2% to 58.0%. These findings represent a reversal in the trend toward increased sexual risk among teens that began in the 1970s and point to the success of comprehensive prevention efforts to both delay first intercourse among teens and increase condom use among young people who are sexually active.*

Special HIV/AIDS Educational Considerations at Different Levels and Populations

Working with Different Levels and Populations

Regardless of the educational level or the kind of population, the general goals developed by Dorman, Collins and Brey (1990) for a teacher preparation course apply to HIV/AIDS education. They are as follows:

1. To provide accurate, current information regarding HIV/AIDS

2. To engender attitudes that acknowledge personal risk for HIV infection

3. To provide skills for reducing high-risk behaviors known to contribute to HIV infection

4. To reduce unreasonable fears about the transmission of HIV

5. To foster compassionate and caring responses to people with HIV infection and AIDS

6. To confront prejudice and discrimination against people with HIV infection and AIDS, as well as against other subgroups of the population

7. To provide support for needed services for people with HIV infection and AIDS

8. To increase attention to important economic, social, ethical, legislative, legal, and psychological issues created by HIV/AIDS

In Chapter 14 we give ideas about what should be taught in sexuality education at different levels and in different settings. Much of that information is relevant here; however, now we will only mention points specific to HIV/AIDS education. Ideally, there would be integration into one comprehensive program.

HIV/AIDS Education at Different Levels

At different levels of education—with students of different intellectual, emotional, and physical development—different HIV/AIDS content should be taught. We list some of that content by grade level below.

Early Elementary School

1. Education should be designed to allay fears of the epidemic and of becoming infected.

2. AIDS is a disease that is causing some adults to get very sick, but it does not commonly affect children.

3. AIDS is very hard to get. You cannot get it by just being near or touching someone who has it.

4. Scientists are working hard to stop people from getting AIDS and cure those who have it.

Late Elementary School

1. Viruses can be transmitted from an infected person to an uninfected person through various means.

2. People who are infected with some viruses that cause disease may not have signs or symptoms of disease.

3. AIDS is caused by a virus that weakens the ability of infected individuals to fight off disease.

4. People who have AIDS often develop diseases that healthy people do not get.

5. People who are infected with AIDS live in every state in the United States and most countries of the world.

6. A small number of people have been infected when they were directly exposed to infected blood.

7. It sometimes takes several years after being infected with HIV before symptoms appear.

8. The AIDS virus cannot be caught by touching someone who is infected, by being in the same room with an infected person, or by donating blood.

Junior and Senior High School

1. The virus that causes AIDS and related health problems is called human immunodeficiency virus or HIV.

2. The risk of becoming infected with HIV can be virtually eliminated by not engaging in sexual activities and by not using illegal intravenous drugs.

3. HIV may be transmitted by sexual contact with an infected person, by using needles or other injection equipment that an infected person has used, and from an infected mother to her infant before and during birth.

4. In the past, blood transfusions have caused some people to become infected with HIV. However, since 1985 all donated blood has been tested to determine whether it has been infected with HIV.

5. Persons who continue to engage in sexual intercourse with persons who are at increased risk or whose infection status is not known should use a latex condom (not natural membrane) to reduce the likelihood of becoming infected.

6. Behavior that prevents exposure to HIV also may prevent unintended pregnancies and STI.

Table 13-6 Sources of Information and Advice about HIV/AIDS

CDC National STD & AIDS Hotlines:
1-800-342-AIDS
Spanish: 1-800-344-SIDA
Deaf: 1-800-243-7889

CDC National Prevention Information Network:
P.O. Box 6003
Rockville, Maryland 20849-6003
1-800-458-5231

Internet Resources:
NCHSTP: http://www.cdc.gov/nchstp/od/nchstp.html
DHAP: http://www.cdc.gov/hiv
NPIN: http://www.cdcnpin.org

---

7. Persons who believe they may be infected should take precautions not to infect others and to seek counseling and antibody testing.

HIV/AIDS Education in Different Settings

Religious Settings.   The topic of HIV/AIDS raises profound moral concerns. However, the opinions being expressed by religious leaders about the role of religious institutions as AIDS prevention educators is quite diverse (Lyons, 1988). Here are a few examples.

Pickerel (1988) commented on AIDS education from a Catholic perspective. She pointed out that we cannot make any decisions for our students and certainly not moral ones. It is our obligation as educators to give students as much information as possible to use when they make their decisions. We should also encourage them to use a decision-making process that helps them understand available alternatives, the consequences of the alternatives, how to discern the values underlying each alternative, and the Catholic values, ideals, and teachings regarding those alternatives. However, she also pointed out that an adolescent who disagrees with the Church's moral teachings should not be handed a death sentence because information about condoms and sterilized needles was withheld.

Pickerel further indicated that even though the official Catholic stance may be against homosexual or sexual activity outside a marital relationship, prejudice that can lead to violence or the abrogation of human rights for any segment of society cannot be condoned. She felt that education can be a wonderful way to disarm prejudice and fear. It can be helpful in producing an effective and compassionate response to the AIDS epidemic in our society and the world.

Rose (1988) commented on HIV/AIDS education from a Jewish perspective. He indicated a major Jewish guiding principle has long been saving and sustaining life, and that is the basis for HIV/AIDS education in the Jewish community. It takes precedence over other considerations, such as possible embarrassment when talking publicly about sexual behavior. Within the Jewish setting, HIV/AIDS education is about much more than prevention. Rose also indicated that efforts must encompass the human reality of AIDS, our responsibility to transcend human self-interest, and our mandate to act. These efforts also need to enable and empower us to make difficult personal decisions now and in the future.

Rose pointed out that Jews have a historic commitment to education. Ignorance is viewed as destructive. In addition, in Jewish history there are commandments about not isolating those who are sick or disabled from the community. Regarding AIDS patients, this means advocating for sufficient home and hospice resources, and giving people support and comfort rather than offering isolation or discrimination.

Rose also indicated that we need to acknowledge the level of sexual activity among teenagers and stay clear of the erroneous belief that teens will only be heterosexually active.

Table 13-7 A Sample School HIV/AIDS Policy

Preamble

State/District/School shall strive to protect the safety and health of children and youth in our care, as well as their families, our employees, and the general public. Staff members shall cooperate with public health authorities to promote these goals.

The evidence is overwhelming that the risk of transmitting human immunodeficiency virus (HIV) is extremely low in school settings when current guidelines are followed. The presence of a person living with HIV infection or diagnosed with acquired immuno-deficiency syndrome (AIDS) poses no significant risk to others in school, day care, or school athletic settings.

1. School Attendance

A student with HIV infection has the same right to attend school and receive services as any other student, and will be subject to the same rules and policies. HIV infection shall not factor into decisions concerning class assignments, privileges, or participation in any school-sponsored activity.

School authorities will determine the educational placement of a student known to be infected with HIV on a case-by-case basis by following established policies and procedures for students with chronic health problems or students with disabilities. Decision makers must consult with the student's physician and parent or guardian; respect the student's and family's privacy rights; and reassess the placement if there is a change in the student's need for accommodations or services.

School staff members will always strive to maintain a respectful school climate and not allow physical or verbal harassment of any individual or group by another individual or group. This includes taunts directed against a person living with HIV infection, a person perceived as having HIV infection or a person associated with someone with HIV infection.

2. Employment

The *State/District/School* does not discriminate on the basis of HIV infection or association with another person with HIV infection. In accordance with the Americans with Disabilities Act of 1990, an employee with HIV infection is welcome to continue working as long as he or she is able to perform the essential functions of the position, with reasonable accommodation if necessary.

3. Privacy

Pupils or staff members are not required to disclose HIV infection status to anyone in the education system. HIV antibody testing is not required for any purpose.

Every employee has a duty to treat as highly confidential any knowledge or speculation concerning the HIV status of a student or other staff member. Violation of medical privacy is cause for disciplinary action, criminal prosecution, and/or personal liability for a civil suit.

No information regarding a person's HIV status will be divulged to any individual or organization without a court order or the informed, written, signed, and dated consent of the person with HIV infection (or the parent or guardian of a legal minor). The written consent must specify the name of the recipient of the information and the purpose for disclosure.

All health records, notes, and other documents that reference a person's HIV status will be kept under lock and key. Access to these confidential records is limited to those named in written permission from the person (or parent or guardian) and to emergency medical personnel. Information regarding HIV status will not be added to a student's permanent educational or health record without written consent.

4. Infection Control

All employees are required to consistently follow infection control guidelines in all settings and at all times, including playgrounds and school buses. Schools will operate according to the standards promulgated by the U.S. Occupational Health and Safety Administration for the prevention of blood-borne infections. Equipment and supplies needed to apply the infection control guidelines will be maintained and kept reasonably accessible. *Designate* shall implement the precautions and investigate, correct, and report on instances of lapse.

A school staff member is expected to alert the person responsible for health and safety issues if a student's health condition or behavior presents a reasonable risk of transmitting an infection.

If a situation occurs at school in which a person might have been exposed to an infectious agent, such as an instance of blood-to-blood contact, school authorities shall counsel that person (or, if a minor, alert a parent or guardian) to seek appropriate medical evaluation.

5. HIV and Athletics

The privilege of participating in physical education classes, athletic programs, competitive sports, and recess is not conditional on a person's HIV status. School authorities will make reasonable accommodations to allow students living with HIV infection to participate in school-sponsored physical activities.

Table 13-7 (*Continued*)

All employees must consistently adhere to infection control guidelines in locker rooms and all play and athletic settings. Rulebooks will reflect these guidelines. First aid kits must be on hand at every athletic event.

All physical education teachers and athletic program staff will complete an approved first aid and injury prevention course that includes implementation of infection control guidelines. Student orientation about safety on the playing field will include guidelines for avoiding HIV infection.

6. HIV Prevention Education

The goals of HIV prevention education are to promote healthful living and discourage the behaviors that put people at risk of acquiring HIV. The educational program will:

- be taught at every level, Kindergarten through grade twelve;
- use methods demonstrated by sound research to be effective;
- be consistent with community standards;
- follow content guidelines prepared by the Centers for Disease Control and Prevention (CDC);
- be appropriate to students' developmental levels, behaviors, and cultural backgrounds;
- build knowledge and skills from year to year;
- stress the benefits of abstinence from sexual activity, alcohol, and other drug use;
- include accurate information on reducing risk of HIV infection;
- address students' own concerns;
- include means for evaluation;
- be an integral part of a coordinated school health program;
- be taught by well-prepared instructors with adequate support; and
- involve parents and families as partners in education.

Parents and guardians will have convenient opportunities to preview all HIV prevention curricula and materials. School staff members shall assist parents or guardians who ask for help in discussing HIV infection with their children. If a parent or guardian submits a written request to a principal that a child not receive instruction in specific HIV prevention topics at school, and assures that the topics will be discussed at home or elsewhere, the child shall be excused without penalty.

The education system will endeavor to cooperate with HIV prevention efforts in the community that address out-of-school youth and youth in situations that put them at high risk of acquiring HIV.

7. Related Services

Students will have access to voluntary, confidential, age and developmentally appropriate counseling about matters related to HIV infection. School administrators will maintain confidential linkage and referral mechanisms to facilitate voluntary student access to appropriate HIV counseling and testing programs, and to other HIV-related services as needed. Public information about resources in the community will be kept available for voluntary student use.

8. Staff Development

All school staff members will participate in a planned HIV education program that conveys factual and current information; provides guidance on infection control procedures; informs about current law and state, district, and school policies concerning HIV; assists staff to maintain productive parent and community relations; and includes annual review sessions. Certain employees will also receive additional specialized training as appropriate to their positions and responsibilities.

9. General Provisions

On an annual basis, school administrators will notify students, their family members, and school personnel about current policies concerning HIV infection, and provide convenient opportunities to discuss them. Information will be provided in major primary languages of students' families.

This policy is effective immediately upon adoption. In accordance with the established policy review process, or at least every three years, *designate* shall report on the accuracy, relevance, and effectiveness of this policy and, when appropriate, provide recommendations for improving and/or updating the policy.

Source: Someone at school has AIDS: A complete guide to education policies concerning HIV infection. Arlington, VA: National Association of State Boards of Education, 2001.

It is an especially frightening time to come of age sexually. It is more important than ever to affirm sexuality as a positive part of human experience, and to link it with respect for oneself and genuine caring for others.

Webster (1988) commented on HIV/AIDS education from a Protestant perspective. He indicated Protestants have been known for their programs of social concern, and that AIDS requires churches to put into practice all the social love and concern they can. People should be kept within the life of the church community, whatever their illness. It is in trying times that patients and their families most need the support and counseling of spiritual leaders.

Webster further indicated that education of the various segments of the church community is necessary. As much as possible, parents and children should be educated together. There is a need for human sexuality education before effective and responsible AIDS education can be presented. Basic information as well as addressing highly sensitive issues are needed. The need is so great that it makes sense for churches and schools to join together to provide adequate services and education.

Webster also pointed out that sermons can be an important vehicle for HIV/AIDS education. Emphasis could be directed to the Biblical basis for a church's response to an epidemic. The story of the Good Samaritan would also remind us to help others. Jesus wept with lepers and prostitutes. Today he would certainly go with persons with AIDS and their families.

Obviously, the above three examples from religious settings should not be interpreted as reflecting a consensus within any religious denomination. They do, however, give us some interesting food for thought.

Settings for Individuals with Developmental, Learning, or Mental Disabilities.   The fear of AIDS has created an environment in which sexuality education is "in." Stiggall (1988) pointed out that students with learning or developmental disabilities should not be left out—especially since so many of them have poor self-esteem and are at greater risk than their nondisabled counterparts of being sexually exploited. Reading skills are often limited, so getting information from the usual printed materials is difficult. Many lead protected lives and use poor judgment in relationship development.

Stiggall indicated that people in this special population need the same information as everyone else—that AIDS is dangerous, that it can happen to you, that a person can have AIDS and not know it, and that you can prevent AIDS. Since persons with developmental and learning disabilities are especially influenced by authority opinions, educators must strive for a balance: present factual information, be explicit and honest. They should not teach in a manner that frightens, engenders paranoia, or promotes homophobia.

When working with persons with learning disabilities, educators can do a number of things to make learning more effective. For example, information should be as concrete and explicit as possible. Teaching approaches must not rely on reading skills—audiovisuals, models, and pictures are essential and effective. Learning should take place over a longer period of time with short sessions. Repetition and simple language also help. Using role-plays to practice saying no, talking about lower risk practices, and demonstrating effective communication skills can be very successful.

Settings for Individuals with Sensory or Physical Disabilities.   Disabled people have the same needs as anyone else for education about HIV/AIDS, but they do have some special concerns. Simpson (1988) indicated that the assumption that people with disabilities are not or should not be sexual is a source of many problems. They may get negative messages or an absence of messages—when no mention is made of sexual matters. Therefore, a young person may be discouraged from dressing to attract and rarely sees disabled adults as sexy role models.

Self-esteem is a primary issue to be incorporated in any HIV/AIDS training for these populations. Young people with visual impairment need help learning to dress attractively, along with assistance in finding alternatives to the visual flirting cues we often depend on. Hearing impaired youth may not be comfortable in a typical romantic setting—with low music (which they probably cannot hear). Educators need to help disabled youth find appropriate ways to express their attractiveness and interest in romantic relationships. Obviously, this can contribute to a positive self-image.

Simpson also reminded us that disabled youth typically receive little or no formal sexuality education. This increases the chances for sexual misinformation to be shared with others. In combination, negative messages about their own sexuality, social difficulties, and a lack of education can make disabled people more likely to engage in risk-taking behavior.

Language should be simple and clear, and graphics should be well done. Modified materials, such as using large print or braille, may be needed. Dealing with myths, particularly the one that people with disabilities are not at risk for HIV infection, is a good way to get the interest of learners.

Materials should be in as many sensory modes as possible. For example, this includes the use of tactile as well as visual materials, role-plays, small and large group discussions, and other innovative techniques. Lifelike, lifesize models can be particularly helpful. For many disabled youth, explanations and demonstrations will need to be more explicit and lengthy than might be true for the nondisabled. Disabilities can affect the ability to use contraception. In private, disabled individuals might need help putting on a condom or inserting foam.

While it is a good practice with any learners, with disabled learners it is especially wise to ask for constant feedback to be sure they understand you and the materials you use. Since time is usually limited, be sure to cover the top priorities. For example, it is more important for learners to understand AIDS transmission than all the details of reproduction.

Teaching Suggestions

Experts state that school-based HIV/AIDS education is most effective when conducted as part of a comprehensive health education program that also includes sexuality. Teaching suggestions offered include the following (Laing & Yarber, 1994):

1. Consider the needs of all students by recognizing that some students may be practicing risky sexual and injecting-drug use behaviors. Hence, not only should abstinence be emphasized, but discussions about other prevention methods such as condom use are necessary.

2. Present the material in a nonjudgmental, objective manner. A responsible health lifestyle should be emphasized. Classroom learning is enhanced if students believe that the environment is safe for discussion.

3. Employ teaching strategies that decrease student denial. Many people choose not to protect themselves from STDs because they feel that such planning indicates an intention to be coitally active. Attempts to counter this include an emphasis on the benefits of planning, and that such planning is actually an indicator of responsibility. Also, some students deny that their friends or persons in their community have actually acquired STD/HIV. If possible, utilize a young adult with an HIV infection as a guest speaker or show videos with young adults describing their experience with STD/HIV. Local statistics indicating the prevalence of STD/HIV in adolescents would be valuable.

Instruction should begin at the early grades (in elementary school) and become more extensive in the later grades—each grade building on the instruction that occurred in earlier grades. HIV/AIDS education should include instruction in the three learning domains (Laing & Yarber, 1994):

1. KNOWLEDGE.
   . . . students need accurate knowledge about the health behaviors related to STD/HIV. Content emphasis should be limited with minimal information about biomedical aspects. Specifically, STD/HIV education should inform students about:

   • The health problems caused by STD/HIV.
   • How STD/HIV are transmitted and ways they are not passed.
   • Ways to avoid STD/HIV.
   • The major symptoms of STD/HIV infection.
   • What to do if an STD/HIV infection is suspected.
   • Where one can get STD/HIV information, counseling, and testing.
   • Ways to get a sex or drug-using partner to a doctor.
   • What can be done to help stop the spread of STD/HIV.

   • Who can provide support and information in helping one avoid STD/HIV. (Yarber 1993)

2. ATTITUDE.
   . . . an open, safe atmosphere in the classroom encourages discussion and acceptance of issues related to prevention of STD/HIV. Students need to know that STDs can affect anyone who practices risky behavior, regardless of age, sexual orientation, socioeconomic status, ethnicity, or living location (large city or small town). Hopefully, such discussion will result in less guilt, shame, and fear that may be associated with STDs, and students would therefore be more likely to seek prompt medical care. Educational efforts should also be directed toward student *acceptance* of (1) the personal possibility of contracting STD/HIV if one practices risky behavior, (2) using prevention measures, (3) responsibility toward sexual partners, and (4) greater support and compassion toward persons with STD/HIV.

3. BEHAVIOR.
   Many students lack adequate skills to prevent STD/HIV. For example, they may not be able to communicate with a dating partner about STD/HIV prevention, they may not be assertive enough to refuse sexual activity, or they may not be able to acquire condoms. Hence, major efforts should be directed toward increasing student skills through, for example, role-playing and decision-making and problem-solving scenarios.

An example of an innovative and effective HIV/AIDS education program is the one conducted by the California schools. Health, English, and language arts teachers collaborated to write lesson plans that integrated HIV/AIDS education—education that was mandated by the state—with the core literature used in California schools. This resource is called *Health Connections: AIDS Education Lessons*. The lesson plans focus on AIDS-prevention skills such as problem solving, decision making, conflict resolution, dealing with peer pressure, and assertiveness. This resource can be obtained for a minimal cost by writing to the Healthy Kids Resource Center, 313 West Winton Avenue, Haywood, CA 94544-1188, or by calling (510) 670-4581.

Program Assessment

Once an HIV/AIDS education program is conducted, it should be evaluated. As we will discuss in Chapter 17, evaluation provides the information needed to improve the program's effectiveness. Table 13-8 presents a detailed means of evaluating an HIV/AIDS program's content, the presentation of student material, and background for teachers.

Table 13-8 Checklist to Evaluate Curricula

This checklist to evaluate curricula includes 63 specific criteria/performance standards. It presents essential topics and components to include in the curriculum (regular typeface) as well as health-enhancing behaviors that curricula should promote and encourage (italic typeface).

STUDENT CONTENT

The STD/HIV Problem

1. The "Hidden" STD Epidemics
____STDs are the most commonly reported infectious diseases in the United States
____STDs are hidden for many reasons
____There are negative outcomes as a result of the hidden nature of STDs
____The STD/HIV risk for sexually active teenagers is underestimated
____The STD prevalence among teenagers is underestimated
____Sexually transmitted infections (STIs) is a new term used to describe STDs

2. STDs
____Over 25 STDs, including HIV/AIDS, currently exist
____Certain STDs have a particular impact on teenagers
____Teenagers have a greater chance of contracting STDs, other than HIV
____Teenagers are concerned about STDs and HIV

3. Size of Problem
____The prevalence of STDs
____The estimated number of new STD/HIV cases annually
____The number of people in the United States infected with STD/HIV
____The increase or decrease of STD prevalence
____The status of HIV/AIDS in the United States and around the world

4. People with STD/HIV
____Behavior, not sexual orientation, is a risk factor for STDs
____Infections occur in all communities and population groups
____Teens and young adults account for two-thirds of STD cases
____Teenagers and young adults are at great risk for specific reasons
____STDs have a greater impact on heterosexual men and women, as well as men who have sex with men, than on women who have sex with women
____Individuals in underserved communities and communities of color are disproportionately affected by STD/HIV

5. Problems Caused by STD/HIV
____Untreated and incurable STDs have health consequences
____Health damage is more serious for women and infants
____STD/HIV impact lives and relationships, finances, research and health care priorities, and prevention efforts

6. Reasons for the STD/HIV Problem
____Risky behaviors
____STDs are often incurable and difficult to treat
____Emotional factors, such as guilt and shame, prevent people from getting treatment
____Social and economic barriers prevent people from getting treatment
____Public silence
____Inadequate education, health care, and support

STD/HIV Transmission

7. STD Organisms
____STD/HIV are usually found in body fluids
____An individual can have more than one STD infection at a time

Table 13-8 (*Continued*)

8. Sexual Transmission of STD/HIV

____STDs are most often transmitted through sexual intercourse

____STD/HIV are contracted during contact with an infected person

____Sex is defined in a variety of ways

____STD/HIV are more easily transmitted from men to women than from women to men

____Vaginal intercourse involves risk

____Anal intercourse involves risk

____Oral sex involves risk

9. Sexual Relationships

____People with one partner can be at risk

____People who do not know if their partner is sexually exclusive are at increased risk

____People who have multiple partners are at increased risk

____People with certain types of partners are at increased risk

____Teenagers with much older partners are at increased risk

____People who have an early sexual initiation are at increased risk

10. Blood Transmission of STD/HIV

____Blood-to-blood transmission is the second most common way STD/HIV are contracted

____People who share injection drug needles and equipment are at increased risk

____Health care workers handling HIV-infected blood are at increased risk

____People who have their bodies tattooed and pierced are at increased risk

11. Mother-to-Child Transmission

____STD/HIV are sometimes passed from mother to child

____The child of a pregnant HIV-infected mother is at increased risk

____A child who is breast fed by an HIV-infected mother is at increased risk

____Medical treatment is available to reduce such a child's risk for contracting HIV

12. Increased HIV Risk with STD Infection

____People with an STD are at increased risk of contracting HIV

____People with HIV and an STD are at increased risk of transmitting HIV

13. STD Transmission without Sex or Injecting Drug Use

____STD/HIV are not transmitted in certain ways

____HIV-infected individuals should not donate blood, bone marrow, organs, semen, or tissues

____STD/HIV are not transmitted through casual, non-sexual contact

____Family members caring for a person with HIV/AIDS are not at risk

____Unreasonable fear exists about STD/HIV transmission

STD/HIV Prevention

14. Sexual Abstinence

____Definitions of sexual abstinence

____Normalcy of sexual abstinence

____Benefits of sexual abstinence

____Risks of early sexual involvement

____Naturalness of sexual feelings

____Religious and societal support for sexual abstinence

____Factors to consider prior to sexual intercourse

____The value of delaying sexual intercourse

____There are intimate behaviors other than vaginal intercourse, anal intercourse, or oral sex

____*People desiring to abstain from sexual contact are encouraged to adhere to their decision*

____*People are encouraged to support peers who choose to abstain from sexual contact*

____*People are encouraged to consider all factors when deciding to have sexual contact with someone*

Table 13-8 (Continued)

15. Mutual Sexual Exclusivity

____Definitions of mutual sexual exclusivity

____Benefits of mutual sexual exclusivity

____Risks involved in having multiple partners

____Exclusive relationships other than marriage do exist

____A partner who is not sexually exclusive or uses injection drugs puts the other partner at risk

____*People are encouraged to avoid multiple sex partners*

____*People are encouraged to delay sexual contact until they are able to form a long-term, mutually exclusive relationship*

____*People who are sexually involved and want to remain so are encouraged to establish and/or maintain a mutually exclusive relationship*

____*People are encouraged not to have sexual contact with partners who do not agree to remain sexually exclusive*

16. Condom Use

____When an individual should use a condom

____Types of condoms people should use

____How to use a condom

____Effectiveness of condoms in preventing the spread of STDs

____Condoms are FDA approved

____How to discuss condom use with a partner

____How and where to acquire condoms

____The dangers of nonoxynol-9

____Research is needed on the female condom for STD/HIV prevention

____*People are encouraged to use latex or polyurethane condoms consistently and correctly*

____*People are encouraged not to use nonoxynol-9 with condoms*

____*When couples cannot use a male condom, they should consider using a female condom*

17. Careful Partner Selection

____Value exists in the careful selection of a partner

____Value exists in knowing if a partner is at risk for STD/HIV

____A partner's STD/HIV status is not certain as a result of appearance, familiarity, or reputation

____Certain people are at increased risk for STD/HIV

____Some STD/HIV-infected people are dishonest about their infection status and sexual history

____*People are encouraged to carefully select partners and to avoid sexual contact with people who might be at high risk for STD/HIV*

____*People are encouraged to seek STD/HIV testing of their partners and themselves*

____*People are encouraged to look for STD/HIV symptoms on their partners as one, but not a completely accurate, way of judging possible infection*

____*People are encouraged to get contact information from partners they do not know well*

18. Avoid Injecting and Other Drugs

____Injection drug use involves risk for STD/HIV

____Mixing alcohol, drugs, and sex involves risk for STD/HIV

____"Date-rape" drugs involve risk for STD/HIV

____*People are encouraged to identify and resist the pressure to use drugs*

____*People are encouraged not to use injection drugs*

____*People using injection drugs should not share needles, syringes, and other equipment*

____*People addicted to drugs are encouraged to seek professional help*

19. Vaccines

____Hepatitis B is the only STD with a vaccine

____Efforts are underway to create an HIV vaccine

Table 13-8 (Continued)

20. Other Prevention Methods

____Alternatives to intercourse, such as masturbation and massage, significantly minimize the chance of contracting STD/HIV

____Laws require the disclosure of STD/HIV infection to sex and injection drug partners

____Laws require the screening of donated blood, semen, tissues, and organs

____Donation of a person's own blood for his/her own surgery will prevent the risk of contracting an STD or HIV

____*People infected with STD/HIV are encouraged to avoid exposing others*

____*People are encouraged to limit partner affection to such activities as hugging, massaging, and/or masturbating until criteria are met for more intimate sexual behavior*

____*People are encouraged not to allow blood, semen, or vaginal fluids to touch their genitals, mouth, or anus*

____*People are encouraged not to engage in open-mouth kissing of an HIV-infected person*

____*People who are infected with STD/HIV are encouraged not to use injection drugs and not to share injection equipment*

____*People at high risk for HIV are encouraged not to donate blood, bone marrow, organs, semen, and tissues*

____*Pregnant women are encouraged to get tested for HIV*

____*HIV-infected women are encouraged to seek medical care before and during pregnancy; they should not breast feed*

____*Women thinking about becoming pregnant should know if their partner has an STD or HIV*

____*Women planning to become pregnant should avoid sexual contact with anyone who has practiced risky sexual behavior or used injection drugs*

____*Pregnant women are encouraged to insist that male partners use a condom if they have practiced high-risk behavior or have an uncertain STD/HIV-infection status*

____*People seeking body tattoos and piercing are encouraged to ask the parlor staff people about their license and if they follow regulations, such as sterilizing their equipment*

____*People who bleed during sports are encouraged to stop participating until the wound stops bleeding and until it is properly cleaned and securely bandaged*

21. Communicating Prevention to Others

____There is a need for and a value to communication

____There is a need to communicate values

____There is a need to be certain of beliefs and values

____People should suggest ways to improve communication about sexuality-related issues

____People should avoid negative peer pressure

____People should suggest ways for others to resist negative peer pressure

____*People are encouraged to clarify their values and stand by the health-enhancing ones*

____*People are encouraged to learn how to resist negative peer pressure*

____*People are encouraged to avoid and/or leave situations involving negative peer pressure*

____*People are encouraged to rehearse good communication skills*

____*People are encouraged to talk about STD/HIV prevention with possible partners*

____*People are encouraged to seek the sexual and injecting drug history as well as the STD/HIV infection testing and status of a possible partner*

____*People are encouraged to be honest with possible sex and drug injecting partners about their past sexual behavior, injecting drug use, and STD/HIV testing and status*

____*People are encouraged not to have sex with a person who will not talk about STD/HIV prevention*

____*People are encouraged to talk with their parents or other adults about good communication skills relating to HIV/AIDS prevention*

22. Choosing Friends Wisely

____Influence of peer norms and friends is important

____Friends who support preventive and risk-reduction behaviors are important

____*People are encouraged to choose friends who are supportive of avoiding STD/HIV risk behavior*

Table 13-8 (Continued)

23. Help to Avoid STD/HIV

_____Value exists in the encouragement and support of others

_____People need to know who might help them avoid STD/HIV

_____*Teens are encouraged to talk with their parents or other supportive adults about sexuality, growing up, and STD/HIV prevention*

24. Taking Responsibility for Health and the Health of Others

_____There is a value in individual efforts to control STD/HIV

_____People should serve as responsible role models

_____People should serve as accurate information sources

_____People should support STD/HIV control efforts

_____People should support friends with STD/HIV

_____People should keep informed about STD/HIV

_____*People are encouraged, in taking responsibility for their own health, to avoid STD/HIV, pay close attention to their own bodies, seek medical care if STD/HIV are suspected, avoid spreading STD/HIV if they are infected, and get partners to treatment*

_____*People are encouraged to practice STD/HIV prevention to be a healthy role model as well as for personal safety*

_____*People are encouraged to create an HIV/AIDS resource center in their school or town*

_____*People are encouraged to continue being friends with those having STD/HIV*

_____*People are encouraged to organize fund-raising drives or to contact a local STD/AIDS agency to see what they can do*

_____*People are encouraged to serve as STD/HIV volunteers*

_____*People are encouraged to stay alert to proposed legislation related to STD/HIV and to voice opinions to officials and legislators*

_____*People are encouraged to keep up-to-date about STD/HIV*

_____*People are encouraged to inform their friends that they know the latest STD/HIV facts and are willing to share them*

_____*People are encouraged to correct fallacies when talking with others*

Recognizing STD/HIV Infections

25. STD/HIV Symptoms

_____Value exists in seeing a health care provider promptly if a person suspects having STD/HIV

_____STD/HIV symptoms are often similar to other infections

_____STDs frequently have no early symptoms

_____People should know the symptoms of STD/HIV

_____People can have an STD or HIV without symptoms

_____People can transmit STD/HIV when they have no symptoms

_____Males have STD symptoms earlier than females even though they have fewer

_____*People should become aware of their bodies*

_____*People are encouraged to become alert to the symptoms of STD/HIV, especially those people having sex with more than one partner, those who share injection drug needles and equipment, and those having sex with partners at risk for STD/HIV*

26. What to Do After Suspecting STD/HIV Symptoms

_____Value exists in deciding to stop having sexual contact

_____Value exists in prompt medical treatment

_____Value exists in getting a partner to treatment

_____*People are encouraged, after suspecting STD/HIV symptoms, to stop having sexual contact, to stop using and sharing injection drugs and their equipment, to go to a doctor or clinic promptly, and to get a partner to treatment*

_____*People who have no symptoms of an STD but still suspect an infection are encouraged to see a health care provider*

Seeking STD/HIV Tests and Treatment

27. STD/HIV Tests and Counseling

_____Who should receive tests

_____Benefits and limitations of tests

_____How an STD/HIV is detected

_____There is an HIV "home test kit"

Table 13-8 (*Continued*)

_____There are confidential and anonymous tests
_____Local resources for tests and counseling
_____National hotlines and Internet resources
_____How a person can remember sources of help
_____What people can do when they have no money for tests
_____*People who have practiced high-risk behaviors are encouraged to seek counseling/tests*
_____*People who have multiple partners are encouraged to check regularly for STD/HIV*
_____*People are encouraged not to try to diagnose their own STD/HIV status*
_____*People are encouraged not to donate blood to determine their HIV infection status*
_____*People are encouraged to call their local health department to find STD/HIV medical care in their community*
_____*People are encouraged to seek STD/HIV health care even if they have no or little money*
_____*People are encouraged not to take frequent HIV tests in place of prevention and risk-reduction methods*

28. Confidential Tests and Treatment for Minors
_____For young people facing health issues, value exists in talking to parents and guardians
_____Some teens experience difficulty talking to their parents about having STD/HIV
_____There are laws that permit minors to get STD/HIV treatment without parental consent
_____*Teenagers are encouraged to talk with their parents or guardians about having STD/HIV*
_____*If teenagers cannot talk to their parents about having STD/HIV, they are encouraged to see a health care provider*

29. The Medical Visit
_____People should receive counseling about tests
_____Different types of treatment exist
_____Hotline information is available on HIV/AIDS treatment
_____*People are encouraged to refer their sex and drug-using partners to counseling and treatment*
_____*People are encouraged to tell health care providers why they suspect they have STD/HIV, what parts of their bodies they think were exposed, and when they think the contact took place*
_____*People are encouraged to ask health care providers when they can resume having sex and ways they can protect their partner if they have an incurable STD*
_____*People infected with STD/HIV are encouraged to practice sexual abstinence or low-risk behavior and never to share injecting drug needles and equipment*
_____*People diagnosed with STD/HIV are encouraged to communicate their infection status to past, current, and possible future sex or injecting drug partners*
_____*People with negative test results are encouraged to practice behaviors that prevent or reduce their chances of infection*

30. STD/HIV Treatment
_____A number of STD treatments exist
_____HIV/AIDS has no cure
_____New HIV treatments exist
_____Treatments for AIDS are available
_____The future outlook for HIV/AIDS treatment is improving
_____*People who are infected are encouraged to follow medical advice and seek support/counseling*
_____*People are encouraged not to use home remedies, mail/Internet-order products, or drugs from friends*

31. Support for People with STD/HIV
_____Value and need exists for the support of family and friends
_____Support groups and Internet chat rooms can help people infected with STD/HIV
_____Other sources exist for finding support groups

Partner HIV/STD Tests and Treatment

32. Importance of Asking Partners to See a Health Care Provider
_____It can prevent serious illness in the partner

Table 13-8 (Continued)

_____It can prevent re-infection

_____It can control the spread of STD/HIV

_____*People having sexual contact with infected partners should not resume sexual contact until all people have been cured or should practice risk-reduction if sexual contact does resume*

33. Ways of Getting Partners to Tests and Treatment

_____Take the partner to the clinic

_____Inform the partner of the infection

_____Seek the help of an STD/HIV public health specialist

_____*People who are infected are encouraged to make certain that their sex and needle-sharing partner(s) have tests/counseling*

_____*People who suspect they are infected are encouraged to take their sex or injecting drug use partner with them to the health care provider*

_____*People who suspect they are infected are encouraged to be honest with their partner, to not blame anyone, to be supportive, and to remain calm and positive*

_____*People are encouraged to cooperate with public health specialists in locating partners*

PRESENTATION OF STUDENT MATERIAL

Theoretical Approach

34. Theoretical "behavior change" models

_____Several constructs of empirically tested "behavior change" models are used in determining content and learning opportunities

Learning Domains Approach

35. Cognitive

_____The major emphasis is on health-enhancing behaviors related to avoiding STD/HIV, recognizing STD/HIV symptoms, finding STD/HIV medical help, following treatment directions, getting partners to treatment, and individual efforts to help control STD/HIV

_____The STD and HIV messages are integrated

_____There is minimal emphasis on biomedical/technical information

36. Affective

_____Health-enhancing attitudes are reinforced and supported

_____Learning opportunities related to attitudes are provided

37. Skill

_____Learning opportunities that require rehearsal of skills related to STD/HIV prevention and risk-reduction are provided

Learning Enhancement

38. Repetition

_____Major concepts are presented several times

39. Feedback/Reinforcement

_____Opportunities are provided for students to test their learning with prompt feedback and reinforcement

40. Involvement

_____Learning opportunities are provided that require a student's involvement and use of major concepts

41. Relevance

_____Information is specifically geared to teenagers based on developmental principles

42. Vocabulary

_____Definitions and pronunciations of technical and possible unknown/unfamiliar terms are provided

_____Terminology familiar to teenagers is used

Table 13-8 (*Continued*)

43. Sensitive to Diversity
____Material is congruent with cultural diversity
____Material is not condescending or prejudicial toward diverse groups

Verbal Quality

44. Readability
____Reading level is junior high school level; this includes minimal use of words with more than three syllables as well as minimal use of long and complex sentences
____Syntax is sound, with precise and simple presentation of concepts

45. Accuracy
____Information is accurate according to contemporary understanding

Visual Esthetics

46. Layout
____Pages have ample "white space"
____Print is an adequate size; layout has a logical, natural flow; and a variety of typeface fonts and colors are used

47. Graphics
____Photos, graphs, and illustrations are used to enhance student interest and understanding
____No negative, confusing, or prejudicial effects are produced

Tone of Message

48. Health-promoting
____Material emphasizes self-directed, health-enhancing behavior, including responsibility for the health of others

49. Objective
____Material does not make moral judgments, use emphatic adjectives or adverbs, contain any obtrusive style, or use offensive material
____Material includes anxiety-alleviating information

BACKGROUND FOR TEACHERS

School STD/HIV Prevention Education

50. Teenagers as a Critical Prevention Target Group
____Prevalence of teen sexual and drug-use risk behaviors is described
____Teenage STD/HIV-related attitudes and knowledge are described

51. Effectiveness of STD/HIV Prevention
____Common characteristics of most successful prevention programs are provided

52. Goal and Rationale
____The major instructional emphasis includes preparing individuals to avoid STD/HIV; to recognize STD/HIV symptoms; to access STD medical care; to follow treatment instructions, if infected; to refer all partners to medical care; and to help control the STD/HIV problem
____Desired behavioral outcomes are stated
____The value of integrating STD/HIV prevention messages is provided
____Teenagers' opinions of their need for STD/HIV information and services is given
____Parental support for school STD/HIV education and for instruction about specific topics is given

53. Curriculum Development
____Material describes rationale for conducting curriculum preparation studies, process evaluations, program effectiveness assessments, and program refinements
____Material describes local, state, and national resources that can assist in curriculum development, implementation, and evaluation

---

Table 13-8 (*Continued*)

____Material lists the traits of the most successful prevention education programs and encourages their use in curriculum development

____Suggestions are provided for working effectively with the local community, such as with an advisory committee

____Material describes the composition of an advisory committee and encourages the inclusion of student members from diverse communities

____Suggestions for gaining support and resolving conflict relative to STD/HIV prevention education content are provided

____Resources are given that can provide accurate STD/HIV information

School STD/HIV Prevention Education Implementation

54. Administration/School Board Acceptance

____Importance and value of administrative and School Board approval and support of HIV/AIDS prevention education are stated

____Importance and value of establishing a school policy for STD/HIV prevention education is given

____Suggestions for securing approval and support are provided

55. Placement within the Curriculum

____Material describes the rationale for STD/HIV prevention education as part of a comprehensive, kindergarten through twelfth grade health science education program that also includes comprehensive sexuality education

____Material provides suggestions on how to integrate STD/HIV prevention education into the curriculum

56. Lesson Plans

____A lesson plan for the curriculum that suggests daily activities is provided

____Materials needed to implement the curriculum are listed

57. Learning Environment

____Material describes and encourages the creation of a safe classroom environment in which students can discuss STD/HIV without the fear of censorship or ridicule

____Material allows students to decline participation in activities that violate their personal values

58. Presenting STD/HIV Prevention Education in Diverse Settings

____Importance of instruction addressing the entire range of needs among diverse groups is stated

____Suggestions for presenting culturally appropriate instruction are given

____Suggestions for dealing with various religious and moral views toward STD/HIV-related issues are provided

59. Instructor Qualities

____Material describes teacher competencies required to provide quality STD/HIV instruction

____The importance of the instructor communicating with students with ease, sensitivity, and tact in an objective, factual manner is stressed

____Material encourages the use of a qualified classroom teacher for STD/HIV instruction as well as the use of carefully selected outside authorities only as supplemental speakers

____Material encourages schools to provide in-service education for people assigned to provide STD/HIV instruction

STD/HIV Instructional Activities

60. Learning Opportunities

____Learning opportunities provide maximum student participation, reflect theoretical behavior change models and the three learning domains, and emphasize health-enhancing behaviors

____Purpose, objective, and utilization procedures are included for learning opportunities

____Cognitive learning opportunities stress major health-enhancing concepts related to STD/HIV transmission and prevention

____Affective learning opportunities stress, for example, personal examination of attitudes, perceptions, confidence of self-efficacy, beliefs related to STD/HIV-related health behaviors and other issues

____Directions for utilization of affective learning opportunities suggest following standard procedures for values-related activities, including optional and anonymous student participation

---

Table 13-8 (*Continued*)

_____Skill-learning opportunities provide practice and simulation of STD/HIV prevention behaviors, such as decision making, problem solving, communication, resistance to negative peer pressure, finding help using the local health board and the Internet, and refusal skills

61. Learning Opportunities Worksheets
_____Any student worksheets required for the learning opportunities are included and are printed in a format that permits easy duplication

62. Student Content Supplement
_____Any material that may be determined too controversial for students (for example, directions for condom use) is given in a format which can be distributed to students based on local discretion

STD/HIV Education Evaluation

63. Classroom Test Questions
_____Several types of questions that evaluate cognitive learning are included
_____Questions that assess cognitive levels beyond memory are included

Source: Yarber, W. L. Standards for STD/HIV prevention curricula in secondary schools, *SIECUS Report,* 31, no. 1 (2002), 27–37.

HIV/AIDS Instructional Strategies

We have pointed out that education about HIV/AIDS is logically included as part of sexuality education which, in turn, should be a part of comprehensive health education. At the same time, we have recognized that the critical need for HIV/AIDS education often results in separate educational efforts. Because of this, we are including instructional strategies that might be helpful specifically as part of HIV/AIDS education.

You will notice that only a small fraction of the instructional activities relate to HIV/AIDS knowledge. This is no oversight. There is ample evidence that people have a good deal of information about AIDS (Adams & Hardy, 1991). Yet, they do not take action to prevent their risk of infection. For example, although the risk of AIDS to teenagers has been well documented (Kann, et al., 1991), only 40% of teenaged females reported using a condom during the last time they had sexual intercourse (Fishein, 1988). Furthermore, in spite of the "AIDS scare," college women are as active sexually as they were in 1975 (Booth, 1990). What is needed for people to protect themselves against HIV transmission is to learn skills such as resistance skills and communication skills, and to deal with their feelings concerning their relationships with others. That is the goal of the activities presented here.

HIV Case Study

Recall from Chapter 12 that case studies are complete stories which can then be analyzed and the actions of the people in the case critiqued. Here is a case study that is specific to an important issue pertaining to HIV/AIDS.

Paul was born a hemophiliac, which meant he periodically had to undergo kidney dialysis. Before more attention was paid to the danger that HIV might be transmitted during these dialysis procedures, Paul unfortunately became infected with HIV. That was several years ago and now Paul is a second grader in Winston Churchill Elementary School. A newspaper reporter was preparing an article about children who are HIV infected and the ways in which their lives are affected when he learned that Paul was one of those children. He approached Paul's parents, who agreed to have him interviewed, hoping it would have a positive influence on how children infected with HIV were treated. Little did they realize the controversy that would be generated.

As soon as the parents of the other children at Winston Churchill Elementary School and, in particular, in Paul's class, learned that he was infected with HIV, many wrote to the school principal insisting that Paul be removed from the school. They did not want their child to be infected by Paul. Other parents came to Paul's defense arguing that he was just as entitled to an education as were the other students at Winston Churchill Elementary School. The principal decided the best way to handle this controversy was to call a special meeting.

At the meeting, Mrs. Palmer spoke with emotion: "If anything happened to my Thomas I would be devastated. I feel for Paul, but my son's health is of most importance to me. I do not want him in the same building with anyone who is HIV positive much less in the same classroom." Then Mrs. Lopez spoke: "I love my Maria as much as Mrs. Palmer loves her Thomas. However, HIV is spread by sexual contact and that just won't happen in the classroom. There is nothing to fear."

The school decided to allow Paul to attend school but to train the teachers how to protect themselves and the other students from contracting the virus from Paul. The principal contacted the local health department and arranged for an expert to conduct the training for the school staff.

With which of the following do you agree (and why):

1. The principal's decision to allow Paul to stay in school

2. The principal's decision to have an expert from the local health department conduct training for the school staff

3. Mrs. Palmer's concerns about her son contracting HIV from Paul

4. Mrs. Lopez's argument that HIV cannot be transmitted to the other children in the school

5. The newspaper reporter's decision to write an article about children infected with HIV and to include Paul's name in the article

6. Paul's parents' decision to allow the reporter to include Paul's name in the article

This case study can be used to accomplish several objectives:

1. To provide program participants the opportunity to express feelings about being around someone who is HIV positive

2. To present accurate information regarding the means by which HIV is spread and the myths surrounding HIV transmission

3. To discuss the rights of people who are HIV positive compared with the rights of those who seek protection from the virus

You can even generate other objectives that can be achieved through the use of this case study. Try doing that now.

HIV Critical Incident

A critical incident is like a case study except that the ending is missing and the learners are asked to supply the ending that makes most sense to them. To change the case just presented into a critical incident, eliminate the paragraph that discusses the principal's decision to allow Paul to stay in school and to train the school staff. Then ask the program participants to agree about how the principal should decide this issue and upon what basis. The sexuality educator might ask the following questions to facilitate this discussion:

1. If you were a parent of a student in Paul's class, how would you react to learning he was HIV positive?

2. Would it make a difference if he actually had AIDS?

3. Assuming it was decided that Paul would remain in school, what precautions would you suggest be taken to ensure that other students and school personnel do not contract the virus from Paul?

The ensuing discussion will elicit fears about being around people who are HIV positive, will uncover myths about the transmission of HIV and counter those with fact, and identify means of finding out about HIV from accurate sources.

Scales and Questionnaires

One of the reasons magazines like *Cosmopolitan* are so popular is the use of scales and questionnaires. When an article in *Cosmo* is about self-esteem, a self-esteem scale will be included—or at least some questions designed to elicit readers' views of themselves—to make the contents of the article relevant to the reader. Sexuality educators can learn a lesson from this approach. An example of a scale that can be used to separate HIV/AIDS myths from facts appears in Insight 13-3.

Insight 13-3

Myths and Facts about HIV

DIRECTIONS: Read each statement carefully and respond in the space provided deciding whether it is a myth or a fact.

1. You can tell when people are HIV infected because they look unhealthy. _____

2. The human immune system usually protects you from disease. _____

3. HIV is spread through the sharing of IV needles or syringes and through sexual intercourse with a person who is infected with HIV. _____

4. People get HIV because they are gay. _____

5. You cannot become HIV infected by donating blood. _____

6. HIV is not transmitted by casual everyday contact such as hugging, sharing bathrooms, and clothing. _____

7. A blood test exists that can determine whether you will contract AIDS. _____

8. If a woman has sexual intercourse with just one man, her child cannot be born HIV infected. _____

(continued)

Insight 13-3 (*Continued*)

9. People with AIDS or people infected with HIV should be quarantined.
10. A man cannot become HIV infected if he has sexual intercourse only with women. _____
11. Blood, vaginal secretions, and semen pass HIV from one person to another. _____
12. Any person who has sexual intercourse can become infected with HIV. _____
13. HIV can be spread by sneezing and coughing. _____
14. Even with medical technology, there is no cure for AIDS. _____

Answer/Explanation Key:

1. MYTH: People infected with HIV may look healthy and may stay healthy; however, they are able to transmit HIV every time they have unprotected sexual intercourse or share IV drug needles or syringes. You cannot tell by looking at someone whether they have been infected with HIV. Many infected persons do not know they are infected.

2. FACT: One function of the immune system is to fight germs that enter the body. With HIV infection or AIDS, the immune system can break down until it is no longer able to fight off what are known as opportunistic infections. Opportunistic infections are infections that would normally not occur if the immune system were healthy and working.

3. FACT: In addition to being transmitted through sexual intercourse and the sharing of IV drug needles or syringes, the virus can also be passed from an infected mother to her unborn child. Before a blood test was developed, there was also the risk of contracting the virus through contaminated blood used during transfusions; however, there is now very little risk of this in the United States, because all blood supplies are now screened and any contaminated blood is discarded.

4. MYTH: HIV is transmitted primarily through sexual intercourse and IV drug use, including steroids. Therefore, anyone is able to acquire the virus. AIDS is not just a disease of homosexual men. HIV is found in heterosexuals, people of all races and colors, men, women, and children. People become HIV-infected because of what they do, not who they are. Homosexual and bisexual men have become HIV-infected by having sexual intercourse with infected partners, a high-risk behavior.

5. FACT: Only disposable needles are used at blood collection centers. These needles are never reused. Therefore, there is no risk in donating blood.

6. FACT: The human immunodeficiency virus (HIV) does not live or grow in the environment. It cannot be transmitted through casual, everyday contact. There have been no reported cases of transmission through such activities as sneezing, coughing, eating in restaurants, swimming in swimming pools, or using toilets.

7. MYTH: The blood test technique called the ELISA can detect the presence of antibody to HIV in people who look and feel well. A positive test result does not mean that a person has AIDS or will get AIDS in the near future. It means that the person became infected at some time with HIV and might infect others with whom he or she has sex or shares needles or syringes. The test is not a diagnosis of AIDS.

8. MYTH: If the man is infected, the mother may be infected by him, and the baby by her.

9. MYTH: Since HIV is not transmitted by casual contact—that is, through nonsexual, day-to-day interaction—there is no need to keep people with AIDS (or people who are infected with HIV) separate from the rest of the population.

10. MYTH: Women who are infected with HIV can transmit the virus to their male sexual partners.

11. FACT: HIV is transmitted primarily through sexual intercourse and IV drug use. Infected semen and vaginal secretions can transmit HIV from one person to another during sexual intercourse, and infected blood can be injected from one person to another during IV drug use.

12. FACT: Men and women, heterosexual or homosexual, can get HIV infection if they do not take such precautions as abstaining from IV drug use; having sexual intercourse only within marriage or a long-term, mutually faithful relationship when it is known that both partners are not infected; or practicing protected sex (using latex condoms) or abstaining from sexual intercourse.

13. MYTH: HIV is a very fragile virus. It cannot be transmitted through sneezing or coughing. There have been no reported cases of transmission through such activities as sneezing or coughing.

14. FACT: AIDS is a worldwide disease and medical researchers all over the world are searching for a cure. Unfortunately, a cure or a vaccine is probably many years away. Prevention is the only way to protect yourself against HIV infection.

Source: Valois, R. F. & Kammermann, S. *Your sexuality: A self assessment.* New York: McGraw Hill, 1992, 303–5.

HIV Sentence Completions

Sentence completions provide program participants a non-threatening manner in which to express points of view. The following sentence completions can be used when the topic of concern is HIV/AIDS:

1. The best way to prevent contracting HIV is to . . .

2. People with AIDS should be . . .

3. Society should manage people with AIDS by . . .

4. Homosexuals should be . . .

5. IV drug users should be . . .

6. School children who are HIV positive should be . . .

7. An HIV positive pregnant woman should . . .

8. Regarding the advertisement of condoms . . .

9. Abstinence education should . . .

10. The most common myths about HIV/AIDS are . . .

Role-Playing

An excellent way to allow program participants to vicariously experience what it is like to have AIDS or to be HIV positive is to use role-playing. An example of how role-playing can be used in this context follows:

Ask learners to agree to act out these roles:

1. A person who has contracted HIV but has not as yet developed AIDS

2. The parents of the HIV positive person

3. The friend of the HIV positive person

4. The family doctor of the HIV positive person

5. The boy/girlfriend of the HIV positive person

6. The brother or sister of the HIV positive person

The situation: There is a family holiday dinner being prepared. The parents want to make sure no one is exposed to HIV. They meet with the family doctor for advice. The other invited guests (the other role-players) wonder how to protect themselves from infection. We are privy to the conversations going on in their minds regarding this issue: their fears about contracting the virus, about offending the person who is HIV positive, about offending their host and hostess, and so on.

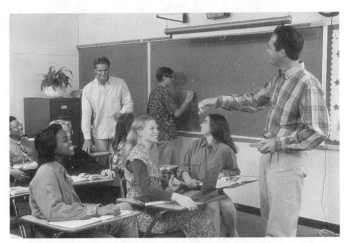

Role-playing can help learners identify their myths and fears about acquiring HIV/AIDS. Once uncovered, these myths and fears can be discussed and corrected.

The first role-play situation is the meeting with the family physician. The second role-play situation involves the conversations occurring in the minds of the invited guests. The third role-play situation is of a group meeting (all role-players except the physician) prior to the dinner to alleviate any concerns and agree to any precautions. That meeting is the major focus of the role-play activity.

Program participants should then discuss how they felt in their respective roles. What were their concerns? What were their thoughts? What were their fears? How were these different or similar to those experienced by real people in the situation in which they role-played?

Resistance Skill Training

Sexuality is but one area in which people need to learn how to resist pressure to do things they know are not in their best interest. Furthermore, it is not just teenagers who are influenced by peer pressure; all of us are. To help program participants be able to resist pressure to engage in HIV/AIDS high-risk behaviors, they can be taught **resistance skills.** One important goal of resistance skill training is to show people how to refrain from succumbing to pressure while still maintaining their personal relationships; that is, without offending the person pressuring them. One way to accomplish this goal is to begin the resisting remark with a positive point or one of agreement. For example, if Bill is pressuring Sam to use IV drugs with him, Sam can say, "Thanks for including me, but I don't want to place myself in that kind of danger. Perhaps you may not want to as well."

---

resistance skills   The ability to resist pressure to perform in ways that are unhealthy, while maintaining relationships and status in the group.

The following can be used with program participants to practice resisting pressure while not ruining their relationships:

1. Your girl/boyfriend says, "You're making me sexually frustrated. I'm going to have to go out with someone else or I'll explode."

2. Your girl/boyfriend says, "Don't you have any sexual feelings at all?"

3. Your girl/boyfriend says, "We'll just play around some. We can stop whenever we want."

4. Your girl/boyfriend says, "But I hate to use condoms. It takes all the fun out of it, and I lose the sensitivity."

5. Your girl/boyfriend says, "Let's try these drugs. We can share this needle, since it is the only one I have."

Assuming Responsibility

When people can engage in behaviors that place them at risk for contracting HIV, they are in need of accepting the responsibility that accompanies that freedom. The following activity is effective in raising this issue and of demonstrating the responsibility that is a concomitant to freedom.

Ask program participants to form teams of an equal number of learners and line up—in a straight line—behind their teammates. Instruct learners that they are competing against the other teams to see how long they can remain with their arms straight out to the side, elbows straight, palms down, with their feet together. As soon as any member of the team bends his or her elbows or lowers his or her arms, the whole team is disqualified. The last remaining team wins.

By the time the activity is over—approximately 1 minute—program participants will probably feel some physical discomfort. Their arms may hurt, their necks may feel stiff, and their shoulders may be in need of a good massage. The sexuality educator then conducts a discussion centering on why they participated in this activity to the extent that they allowed themselves to become uncomfortable. Soon someone will say that, although they were free to drop their arms at any time, they felt a sense of responsibility to their teammates who wanted to win.

The sexuality educator then concludes the activity by summarizing the importance of recognizing that with freedom comes the responsibility to use it well. With the freedom to engage in many different HIV/AIDS high-risk behaviors, comes the responsibility to limit the risk by not engaging in some behaviors (for example, choosing abstinence or refraining from anal intercourse) and adapting other behaviors in ways as to make them less dangerous (for example, using a condom when engaging in sexual intercourse and limiting the number of sexual partners).

Summary

The primary purpose of HIV/AIDS education is the prevention of HIV infection. Educational programs should address behaviors including avoiding sexual relationships with infected people or those whose HIV infection status is not known, using latex condoms, seeking treatment in cases of drug addiction, not sharing needles, and seeking HIV counseling and testing.

Educators must be prepared to answer many common questions about HIV/AIDS. Fortunately, many excellent sources of factual information are available.

When implementing HIV/AIDS education programs, it is important to maximize community support, ensure teacher competency, utilize resources, and defend students' rights to complete health information. Many issues needing attention go beyond the educational program.

There are special considerations when teaching about HIV/AIDS with learners of different ages and in different settings. Particular attention is needed, because today's adults (including educators) have not generally been well educated on the subject.

Many suggestions about handling sexuality education also apply to HIV/AIDS education; however, some additional ones apply specifically to HIV/AIDS education. For example, there is a delicate balance between fear and reassurance; there is a need to be nonjudgmental and avoid scare tactics, and there is a need to stress abstinence in a realistic manner.

References

Adams, P. F. and A. M. Hardy. AIDS knowledge and attitudes for July–September 1990: Provisional data from the National Health Interview Survey. *Advance Data*, no. 198 (April 1991), pp. 13–42.

Booth, W. College Women Surveyed About Sex. *The Washington Post* (March 22, 1990): A15.

Centers for Disease Control and Prevention. *HIV/AIDS Surveillance Report, 2001* 13(2) (2002).

Division of HIV/AIDS Prevention. *Young people at risk: HIV/AIDS among America's youth.* 2003. http://www.cdc.gov/hiv/pubs/facts/youth/htm.

Dorman, St. M., Collins M. E., and R. A. Brey. A professional preparation course on AIDS/HIV infection. *Journal of School Health* 60(6) (1990): 266–69.

Edwards, M. AIDS spread to millions worldwide signals urgent prevention needs. *SIECUS Report*, 31(1) (2002): 3.

Facilitator's guide for HIV/AIDS prevention workshop: Issues in teacher education. Rockville, MD: American College Health Association, 1991.

Fishein, J. Teenage girls know about AIDS, but don't act accordingly. *The Nation's Health* 18 (1988): 8.

Ford, K., Sohn, W., and J. Lepkowski. "Characteristics of adolescents' sexual partners and their association with use of condoms and other contraceptive methods. *Family Planning Perspectives* 33(3) (2001): 100–105, 132.

Greenberg, J. S., C. E. Bruess, and D. W. Haffner. *Exploring the Dimensions of Human Sexuality,* Second Edition Sudbury, MA: Jones and Bartlett, 2004.

Irwin, C. E. The theoretical concept of at-risk adolescents. In Strasburger, V. C. and D. E. Greydanus, Eds. *Adolescent medicine: The at-risk adolescents.* Philadelphia: Hanley & Belfus, 1990, 1–14.

Kann, L., J. E. Anderson, D. Holtzman, J. Ross, B. I. Truman, J. Collins, and L. J. Kolbe. HIV-related knowledge, beliefs, and behaviors among high school students in the United States: Results from a national survey. *Journal of School Health* 61 (1991): 397–401.

Laing, S. J. and W. Yarber. Sexually transmitted disease (STD) education. In Bruess, C. E. and J. S. Greenberg, *Sexuality education: Theory and practice, 3rd ed.* Dubuque, IA: Wm. C. Brown Communications, 1994, 321–223.

Lyons, C. The religious setting: A natural place for learning. In *The AIDS challenge: Prevention education for young people.* Edited by M. Quackenbush and M. Nelson. Santa Cruz, CA: Network Publications, 1988, 207–10.

Piccinio, L. J. and Mosher, W. D. Trends in contraceptive use in the United States: 1982–1995. *Family Planning Perspectives* 30(1) (1998): 4–10, 46.

Pickerel, C. AIDS education in religious settings—A Catholic response. In Quackenbush, M. and M. Nelson, Eds. *The AIDS challenge: Prevention education for young people.* Santa Cruz, CA: Network Publications, 1988, 211–18.

Rose, A. Educating for life: AIDS and teens in the Jewish community. In Quackenbush, M. and M. Nelson, Eds. *The AIDS challenge: Prevention education for young people.* Santa Cruz, CA: Network Publications, 1988, 219–26.

Simpson, K. M. Teaching about AIDS: Youth with sensory or physical disabilities. In Quackenbush, M. and Mary Nelson, Eds. *The AIDS challenge: Prevention education for young people.* Santa Cruz, CA: Network Publications, 1988, 419–27.

Smith, W. Politicians urged to rise above prejudices and embrace HIV/AIDS prevention strategies. *SIECUS Report* 31(1) (2002): 38–39.

Stiggall, L. AIDS education for individuals with developmental, learning or mental disabilities. In Quackenbush, M. and Mary Nelson, Eds. *The AIDS challenge: Prevention education for young people.* Santa Cruz, CA: Network Publications, 1988, 405–17.

Summers, T., J. Kates, and G. Murphy. The global impact of HIV/AIDS on young people. *SIECUS Report* 31(1) (2002): 14–19.

Turner, C. F., H. G. Miller, and L. E. Moses, Eds. *AIDS, sexual behavior, and intravenous drug use.* Washington, DC: National Academies Press, 1989.

UNAIDS. AIDS *epidemic update,* December 2001.

Watkins, S. A. Demographic shifts change national face of HIV/AIDS. *SIECUS Report* 31(1) (2002): 10–12.

Webster, C. L. AIDS: Contemporary challenge to protestant churches. In Quackenbush, M. and M. Nelson, Eds. *The AIDS challenge: Prevention education for young people.* Santa Cruz, CA: Network Publications, 1988, 227–36.

Yarber, W. L. *STDs and HIV: A guide for today's young adults.* Reston, VA: American Alliance for Health, Physical Education, Recreation, and Dance, 1993.

Yarber, W. L. Standards for STD/HIV prevention curricula in secondary schools. *SIECUS Report* 31(1) (2002): 27–37.

Suggested Readings

National survey of teens on HIV/AIDS: Public knowledge and attitudes about HIV/AIDS. Menlo Park, CA: The Henry J. Kaiser Family Foundation, 2000.

Maldonado, M. *HIV/AIDS: African Americans.* Washington, DC: National Minority AIDS Council, 1999.

———. *HIV/AIDS: Latinos.* Washington, DC: National Minority AIDS Council, 1999.

Someone at school has AIDS: A complete guide to education policies concerning HIV infection. Arlington, VA: National Association of State Boards of Education, 2001.

Ruiz, M. S., Gable, A. R., Kaplan, E. H., Soto, M. A., Fineberg, H. V. & Trussell, J., eds. *No time to lose: Getting more from HIV prevention.* Washington, DC: National Academies Press, 2001.

Trevor, C. Number of controversies decline as schools adopt conservative policies, *SIECUS Report* 30, no. 6 (2002), 4–19.

16 programs that combine pregnancy, STD, and HIV/AIDS prevention, *SIECUS Report* 31, no. 3 (2003), 18–27.

What Should Be Taught at Different Levels and in Different Settings?

CHAPTER 14

Key Concepts

1. Developmental characteristics of learners influence sexuality education content and activities.

2. Typical questions asked by learners can provide insight to the educator for curriculum development.

3. Sexuality education programs for school-aged learners should be comprehensive and sequential.

4. College-aged and adult learners also have sexuality education needs.

5. Sexuality education for older adults has been neglected until recently.

6. Sexuality education for those recovering from circulatory problems and for culturally varied groups is similar to other sexuality education, but some special considerations are needed.

What is included in a sexuality education program in any setting depends upon who makes the final decision. Various groups decide on their own programs based on criteria that are thought to be sound in their particular situations. Individuals may debate the exact placement of contents as well as the appropriateness of specific learning activities. This chapter, however, describes the foundation for a sexuality education program that may be relevant to many settings and groups.

One thing is certain: most of the content of present school sexuality education programs could be handled by learners in much earlier grades. The students will be well prepared for it if a good program is conducted from preschool through grade 12.

It is also increasingly obvious that parents of students (particularly in grades 7 to 12) support comprehensive sexuality education by a wide margin. There is a large gap between their specific wishes and what is actually taught. Parents reject abstinence-until-marriage programs by about a two-to-one ratio. Parents also want substantial amounts of time to be dedicated to sexuality education (What the latest surveys tell us, 2001).

Obviously, one of the early steps in the development of a program is to establish objectives. As noted earlier, there are many different ways in which sexuality education objectives can be approached and written. Most educators are aware of many informative sources that are helpful in writing good educational objectives. Here, we want to consider developmental characteristics and special needs of learners. Learners' typical questions will also aid in your development of objectives. After reviewing the first two concepts in this chapter, you should be able to get started on writing sexuality education objectives.

Developmental Characteristics of Learners

There are different age and grade groupings for preschool and school-aged children in educational systems around the country. We will use a grouping that can easily be adapted to any system. Preschool will include ages 3 to 5, early elementary will include grades K to 3, upper elementary will include grades 4 to 6, lower secondary will include grades 7 to 9, and upper secondary will include grades 10 to 12.

Preschool

Students participating in preschool education, ages 3 to 5, have experienced a gradual deceleration in their growth rate since their earlier years. During these years their bodies are in transition from the appearance of infancy to the appearance of young childhood. Since their internal organs are relatively large, it is common to see protruding abdomens.

Preschool learners have a short attention span. They really like "fun" activities, however, and will thrive on make-believe games, daydreams, and imaginary friends.

The play of preschool children is *parallel* rather than really social. They will play alongside other children but probably not *with* them. Peers are not too important at first, but they become more important near the end of the preschool period. The curriculum for preschool children is actually life itself. They learn and adapt through experiences.

Educators and parents should keep their information short and simple when dealing with preschool children. It is important to progressively tell stories with more content and information as the child gets older. If children are not given information about birth, they will make up their own explanations. Exploration of their own bodies and those of others is natural. At the same time, children need to learn that sexuality is an acceptable topic for conversation, even though children are also entitled to privacy. It is also suggested that when children tell parents of a sexual occurrence the parents should ask the child, "What was it like?" This gives children a chance to think for themselves and encourages reality as opposed to fantasy.

Early Elementary

Students in the early elementary grades are 5 to 8 years old. Their physical growth progresses at a slow and steady pace. In the earlier part of this period, children often have fears about school and other new experiences. Toward the end of this period, they are more aware of social aspects of life.

Children are very much interested in how various aspects of their bodies work. Body care is important because of rapid development and changes. Natural situations arise in classrooms that facilitate learning about bodies, emotions, reproduction, and the differences between males and females.

It is common for students to be given more responsibilities at home during this time. Family relationships can be explored, and the student needs assistance in understanding his or her contribution to the family.

Upper Elementary

Students in the upper elementary grades are 9 to 12 years old. Toward the end of this period, some students show a spurt of relatively rapid physical growth, while others continue their earlier slow and steady pace.

Curiosity about the body is evident, and many students show interest in the other sex as well as in their own. Students at this age feel the need to improve personal and social relationships through a better understanding of themselves and others.

It is common for both males and females to show affection for their peers, but they do not necessarily do this in the same way. For example, girls might put their arms around each other, while boys might punch or wrestle each other.

Learners have an increased curiosity about reproduction as they reach the ages of 10 and 11. There is a tendency toward self-consciousness about the other sex, but a real interest, nevertheless.

It is interesting to note that a large proportion of school personnel are doing little to prepare students in grades 5 and 6 for puberty, much less for dealing with pressures and decisions related to sexuality. Those who teach sexuality education often feel unsupported by the community, parents, or school administrators (Landry, Singh & Darroch, 2000).

Lower Secondary

Students in the lower secondary grades are 12 to 14 years old. A relatively rapid growth spurt associated with puberty is common at this age. Girls are likely to experience this spurt before boys, and both sexes have concerns related to rapid growth.

Physical changes in body size, body control, reproductive ability and menstruation, and general appearance may cause concerns that appear in various direct or incidental ways. Along with the development of secondary sex characteristics (such as hips, hair, breasts, and voice changes) and a concern for personal appearance comes an increased interest in sexual relationships with other people.

Independence is a key word for students in this age range. They have difficulty in achieving a balance between responsibility and privilege.

This is a time of turmoil because of the many physical and emotional changes students experience. Forces pull young teens in conflicting directions, and sexuality education is needed to help with personal and social adjustment.

Upper Secondary

Students in the upper secondary grades are 15 to 17 years old. Some may still be growing at a rapid rate, but most have settled down to a slow and steady pace. Because of varied changes associated with puberty, there will still be a great many obvious physical differences among students of the same age.

Most high school students have developed great interest in sexual topics and activities. Concerns about interpersonal relationships, families, reproduction, and various sexual activity patterns are common. A desire for social acceptance and a continuation of emotional difficulties that may have started several years earlier create the need for educators to deal with such topics as peer relationships and self-concepts.

Problems associated with dating need consideration. Subjects addressed at this time might include responsibility and moral behavior, effective communication, and problem-solving methods.

Typical Questions Asked by School-Aged Learners

Listening to questions asked by school-aged learners can be very enlightening for curriculum planners. While adults and college-aged students have learned to cover up their questions, young people will usually ask them quite openly. This may not be the case with preschool learners, however, since they do not seem to ask nearly as many questions related to sexuality education as do school-aged children. As pointed out earlier, their curriculum is actually life itself. In turn, their questions relate to something they see. For example, they might ask questions such as these:

1. What is that (with respect to their own or another person's body parts)?

2. What do mommies do? What do daddies do?

3. Where did the baby come from?

As will be seen, the items appropriate to teach preschool children are not keyed to their questions in the same way as is possible for school-aged children. For the curriculum planner, once learners reach school age, time spent on gathering questions can result in the basis for entire units or even a curriculum at a particular grade level. It is wise to gather questions from the population for which the program is designed, but chances are the questions would be similar to those that follow (Schulz & Williams, 1969; Byler, Lewis & Totman, 1969). Even though this outline is over 30 years old, basic questions have not changed much in that time (with the exception of questions about HIV/AIDS).

Typical early elementary questions:

1. How can you tell which is a cow or a bull?

2. Where was I before I was born?

3. Why does my mommy get a baby?

4. Did I come from an egg?

5. How do babies get born and how does it work?

6. My mother and father don't love each other any more. Which one should I love?

Typical upper elementary questions:

1. How does the reproductive system work?

2. How come I don't have any friends?

3. How does the sperm get into the egg?

4. Why do some girls have larger breasts than others?

5. Do boys menstruate?

6. Why do girls have periods?

7. How do we stay alive in our mother's stomach?

8. Why do I sometimes hate my friends?

9. Why can't I get along with my brother (or sister)?

10. Why don't some women have babies?

Typical lower secondary questions:

1. How do you overcome embarrassment?

2. How do you French kiss a girl?

3. Why do parents think it is so terrible for kids our age to make out?

4. Why do boys give girls the finger? Should I give it back?

5. How can you keep yourself looking attractive?

6. What if kids at a party are doing things you don't want to do?

7. Should your parents know if you're going steady?

8. Why does a boy's penis get hard and stiff sometimes?

9. Does a girl ever have a wet dream?

10. What does your personality include?

11. Is it bad to masturbate?

12. Why are some people homosexual?

13. Does sexual intercourse hurt?

14. What is real love?

15. Why are parents so stupid?

16. Why do adults quarrel so much?

17. Why do people get married?

Typical upper secondary questions:

1. Can premarital sexual relations be made clean?

2. How can I learn to cope with emotional problems?

3. What is prostitution?

4. What do girls really want in a good date?

5. How far should you go on a date?

6. How do you get along with people of your own age?

7. How can we understand our parents better?

8. How should sex be used?

9. What is the role of the unwed father?

10. Why don't parents answer kids' questions frankly?

11. Are sex relations habit forming?

12. Is it good to have sexual intercourse before marriage?

13. Are there any sure ways to prevent pregnancy?

14. Why do parents hide sex from their children?

15. Can rape ever result in a pregnancy?

16. Why is sex regarded as a dirty word?

In addition, Tepper (2001) pointed out that the following questions are also common among learners of this age:

1. How am I going to get a date if I can't drive?

2. Why won't so-and-so go out with me?

3. Is it okay to go all the way if so-and-so does?

4. Can someone with a disability participate in sexual activity?

5. How does sexual activity work if you have a disability?

Insight 14-1

Objectives for Different Ages

With what you know about school-aged learners, write down three objectives that would be appropriate for sexuality education at each of the following four levels.

Early elementary

1. _____
2. _____
3. _____

Upper elementary

1. _____
2. _____
3. _____

Lower secondary

1. _____
2. _____
3. _____

Upper secondary

1. _____
2. _____
3. _____

Now that we have given you a brief picture of some of the developmental characteristics of school-aged learners as well as their questions and concerns, you should be getting an idea of what might be taught at different levels. Let us check to see where your thinking is at this point. Insight 14-1 challenges you to use the information just presented to develop sexuality education objectives for students of different ages.

Certainly, there are no absolutely right or absolutely wrong ideas of what objectives ought to be included within sexuality education for the various age groups. However, you should be able to justify objectives based on characteristics learners possess and questions that learners have. Keep your objectives in mind as we look at some ideas for what should be included in a comprehensive and sequential sexuality education program.

Sexuality Education for Preschool and School-Aged Learners

The words *comprehensive* and *sequential* are fundamental to what should be taught in sexuality education. Too often sexuality education programs have been narrow. Some teachers believed they were implementing adequate sexuality education programs just because they talked about reproduction or discussed dating or presented information on STI. All of these topics are important, but a comprehensive program deals with the many aspects of sexuality that we have presented early in this book—the physical, psychological, social, and spiritual components.

It is not enough to have a one-sided view of sexuality. In curriculum planning, attention needs to be given to interpersonal relationships with parents and peers, moral questions, and social concerns, as well as to the obvious physical topics. To help learners develop a broad-based concept of human sexuality, a comprehensive program is essential.

At the same time, the program should be sequential. This simply means that there should be a logical order to the curriculum. It is still common to see curricular plans that are almost the same from year to year as well as plans that jump around so much it is amazing that learners can make any sense out of them. Sequence should be carefully planned—it will not happen by chance.

No one knows for certain what is right to teach at any given grade level. The suggestions that follow are based on our experience and research, but you will undoubtedly want to adapt them to your own needs. Remember that any curriculum may need to be adapted to meet particular needs.

Preschool

Among the stated benefits of preschool experiences, it is generally accepted that children should become more confident, more spontaneous, less inhibited, more independent, more self-reliant, and more interested in the world around them.

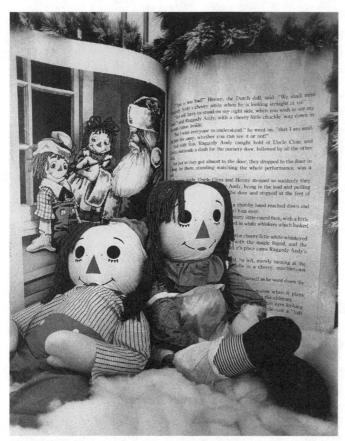

At what age should our young children be taught about the many decisions Raggedy Ann and Andy or themselves will have to make regarding sexuality and sexual behaviors?

It is then logical that preschool sexuality education should contribute to these benefits. Preschool sexuality education should include the following:

1. A recognition of the roles of family members
2. A recognition of the authority and concern of parents and others responsible for the care of preschool children
3. Emphasis on the development of a positive self-image
4. Opportunities to make friends with children of both sexes
5. Ways to cooperate with family members and others in work and play
6. An understanding that living things grow, may reproduce, and die
7. Consideration of the behavior of babies
8. An introduction to public and private behavior

Early Elementary Grades

Good elementary teachers have been providing sexuality education for their students for years, but often there has been no label attached to this education. The kind of foundation that will prepare learners for the rest of the program includes the following:

1. The basics of plant and animal (including human) reproduction
2. The similarities and differences between males and females
3. Growth and development (physical changes and emotional feelings)
4. Family roles and responsibilities
5. Discussions of individual feelings about oneself and other people
6. An introduction to HIV/AIDS
7. An exploration of basic social skills and a continuation of public and private behavior

Upper Elementary Grades

Assuming that the solid foundation has been laid in the early elementary grades, the emphasis in the upper elementary grades should be as follows:

1. Biological information in greater depth:
   a. The endocrine system
   b. Menstruation
   c. Birth and pregnancy
   d. Nocturnal emissions
   e. Masturbation
   f. Body-size differences (temporary and permanent)
   g. Response to sexual stimulation (contact, pictures, and reading)
   h. Birth control and abortion
   i. Physical abnormalities (this subject may seem peculiar, but at this age children are often hung up on the unusual rather than the usual)
   j. Appropriate facts about HIV/AIDS
2. Interpersonal relations:
   a. Heterosexual feelings
   b. Homosexual feelings
   c. How emotions affect body functions
   d. Changing family responsibilities and privileges
   e. The need to use different approaches with different people
   f. Different male and female feelings
   g. Why brothers and sisters (mothers and fathers) fight

3. Self-concept:

    a. How do people react to me?

    b. What kind of a person am I?

    c. How do I feel about myself?

    d. Why do people like me sometimes and not other times?

    e. Why do I hate people sometimes?

Lower Secondary Grades

Now that we have seen that young learners have the basics, let us look at what might be considered at the next level:

1. Overview of biological material (a review of what has previously been covered)

2. More detail on birth control:

    a. How various methods work

    b. Research in contraception

3. More about intimate sexual behavior:

    a. How far to go

    b. Why individuals feel the way they do

    c. Why people behave sexually the way they do

    d. Being responsible for personal behavior

4. Dating and interpersonal relationships:

    a. What to expect from a date (both the person and the experience)

    b. Why people date and why some do not date

5. Variations in sexual behavior:

    a. Homosexuality

    b. Voyeurism

    c. Transvestism

    d. Transsexualism

    e. Exhibitionism

6. The AIDS crisis:

    a. Facts and statistics

    b. Behavioral issues

    c. Prevention and control/treatment

Upper Secondary Grades

Issues to be covered include the following:

1. Birth control research and details:

    a. Population dynamics

    b. Abortion

2. Dating decisions:

    a. Dating standards and regulations

    b. Premarital sexual behavior

    c. Communication

3. Contemporary marriage patterns:

    a. Companionship and patriarchal structures

    b. Communes and group marriages

    c. Three-way marriages

    d. Living together

    e. Contract marriages

4. Sexual myths

5. Moral decisions

6. Control of sex drives and responsible sexual behavior

7. Parenthood:

    a. Childbirth

    b. Childrearing

    c. Sexuality education of children

8. Masculinity and femininity

9. Research in sexuality:

    a. Human sexual response

    b. Sexual dysfunction

    c. Sterility

    d. Pornography

    e. HIV/AIDS research

10. Sexuality and legality:

    a. Personal behavior

    b. Treatment and information

    c. Sexuality education

11. Historical and social factors affecting sexuality:

    a. Selected historical accounts related to sexuality

    b. Cultural aspects of sexuality

12. Sexuality and advertising

With the foundation students would have under this program, almost any issue could be effectively dealt with. Sexual myths and hang-ups would be virtually eliminated, and sophisticated discussion would be possible on a mature level.

For those skeptics who feel that these suggestions naively expect too much, we will hasten to point out that most of these suggestions have been and are still being used by many sexuality educators today. Teachers, students, administrators, and parents can handle this content if the program is properly planned, if appropriate public relations activities are utilized, and if skillful teaching is employed. To do this may be difficult, but an effective sexuality education program should be the result.

Two excellent examples of what should be taught at different levels are available. One of these, *Sexuality Education Within Comprehensive School Health Education* (1991), published by the American School Health Association, contains chapters on preschool and kindergarten, elementary school, middle/junior high school, and senior high school. Each chapter covers student characteristics, general teaching suggestions, concepts, content and activities, responding to student questions, and resources.

In the second resource, *Guidelines for Comprehensive Sexuality Education* (1996), published by the Sexuality Information and Education Council of the United States, concepts and topics in a comprehensive sexuality education program are organized into six categories as shown in Table 14-1. Developmental messages, which give guidelines for content to be covered, are included for four stages of development: (1) middle childhood (ages 5 to 8); (2) preadolescence (ages 9 to 12); (3) early adolescence (ages 12 to 15); and (4) adolescence (ages 15 to 18).

At all levels there has been an increase in sexuality education curricula that rely on fear and shame. These "abstinence-only" curricula typically omit important information, contain misinformation, include sexist and anti-choice bias, and often have a foundation in fundamentalist religious beliefs. These programs are in direct opposition to the goals of comprehensive sexuality education curricula. Sexuality educators need to be wary of fear-based curricula when planning programs.

Sexuality Education for College-Aged and Adult Learners

It is impossible to prescribe a standardized sexuality education program for college-aged learners because of the wide variety of programs available. It has been said that most sexuality education today is really remedial education. We are constantly trying to make up for education that should have occurred previously. Therefore, in practice most sexuality education programs for college-aged learners probably cover many of the topics we have listed for secondary-school students. As we have said to college students in sexuality education classes, if secondary schools were doing a good job of

---

Table 14-1 Key Concepts and Topics in a Sexuality Education Program

Key Concept 1: Human Development	**Key Concept 4: Sexual Behavior**
Reproductive Anatomy and Physiology	Sexuality Throughout Life
Reproduction	Masturbation
Puberty	Shared Sexual Behavior
Body Image	Sexual Abstinence
Sexual Identity and Orientation	Human Sexual Response
	Sexual Fantasy
Key Concept 2: Relationships	Sexual Dysfunction
Families	
Friendship	**Key Concept 5: Sexual Health**
Love	Contraception
Dating	Abortion
Marriage and Lifetime Commitments	Sexually Transmitted Diseases, Including HIV Infection
Raising Children	Sexual Abuse
	Reproductive Health
Key Concept 3: Personal Skills	
Values	**Key Concept 6: Society and Culture**
Decision Making	Sexuality and Society
Communication	Gender Roles
Assertiveness	Sexuality and the Law
Negotiation	Sexuality and Religion
Looking for Help	Diversity
	Sexuality and the Arts
	Sexuality and the Media

Source: Guidelines for comprehensive sexuality education. New York: Sexuality Information and Education Council of the United States, 1996.

sexuality education, college classes in human sexuality would either become unnecessary or would be far more sophisticated than anything available today.

Some people are surprised that sexuality education is still needed at the college level, but student ignorance is widespread. Fortunately, since institutions of higher education are relatively free from harassment from antisexuality education forces, they can approach sexuality education with honesty and thoroughness. There is no longer a need to avoid certain topics as there might have been in earlier years. Despite the fact that many good sexuality education courses exist in colleges and universities, it is still probably true that the major sources of sexuality information for college students are peers and reading materials.

College programs must do more than just inform students about sexuality. They need to help students integrate sexuality and life, relate responsibly as sexual beings to others, and help balance freedom and human values.

Table 14-2 Life Behaviors of a Sexually Healthy Adult

The *Guidelines* explain that the goal of a comprehensive sexuality education program is to facilitate sexual health. After learning the six key concepts and associated topics, subconcepts, and developmental messages, at an appropriate age, the student will demonstrate certain life behaviors.

A sexually healthy adult will:

Human Development

- Appreciate his or her own body.
- Seek further information about reproduction as needed.
- Affirm that human development includes sexual development that may or may not include reproduction or genital sexual experience.
- Interact with both genders in respectful and appropriate ways.
- Affirm his or her own sexual orientation and respect the sexual orientation of others.

Relationships

- View family as a valuable source of support.
- Express love and intimacy in appropriate ways.
- Develop and maintain meaningful relationships.
- Avoid exploitative or manipulative relationships.
- Make informed choices about family options and relationships.
- Exhibit skills that enhance personal relationships.
- Understand how cultural heritage affects ideas about family, interpersonal relationships, and ethics.

Personal Skills

- Identify and live according to his or her values.
- Take responsibility for his or her own behavior.
- Practice effective decision making.
- Communicate effectively with family, peers, and partners.

Sexual Behavior

- Enjoy and express his or her sexuality throughout life.
- Express his or her sexuality in ways that are congruent with his or her values.
- Enjoy sexual feelings without necessarily acting on them.

- Discriminate between life-enhancing sexual behaviors and those that are harmful to self and/or others.
- Express his or her sexuality while respecting the rights of others.
- Seek new information to enhance his or her sexuality.
- Engage in sexual relationships that are consensual, non-exploitative, honest, pleasurable, and protected against disease and unintended pregnancy.

Sexual Health

- Use contraception effectively to avoid unintended pregnancy.
- Prevent sexual abuse.
- Act consistent with his or her own values in dealing with an unintended pregnancy.
- Seek early prenatal care.
- Avoid contracting or transmitting an STD, including HIV.
- Practice health-promoting behaviors, such as regular check-ups, breast and testicular self-exam, and early identification of potential problems.

Society and Culture

- Demonstrate respect for people with different sexual values.
- Exercise democratic responsibility to influence legislation dealing with sexual issues.
- Assess the impact of family, cultural, religious, media, and societal messages on his or her thoughts, feelings, values, and behaviors related to sexuality.
- Promote the rights of all people to accurate sexuality information.
- Avoid behaviors that exhibit prejudice and bigotry.
- Reject stereotypes about the sexuality of diverse populations.
- Educate others about sexuality.

Source: Guidelines for comprehensive sexuality education. New York: Sexuality Information and Education Council of the United States, 1996.

As in the case of college-aged learners, sexuality education for adults cannot be adequately discussed without knowing what educational experiences have already occurred. Too often, not much has happened previously, but it would be an insult to adults if we assumed that they were ignorant about human sexuality. So at this point it is useful to consider the desired end product; educators can then assess each situation and determine what will need to be done to get there. There may be many similarities between sexuality education for adults and sexuality education in secondary and even primary schools.

An interesting way to view sexuality education for adults is to consider the life behaviors of a sexually healthy adult as shown in Table 14-2 (*Guidelines for Comprehensive Sexuality Education*, 1996). Since these behaviors represent what would be a result of sexuality education that occurred throughout life, there are many implications for goals and objectives of sexuality education for adults.

Adults who are parents have needs with regard to teaching their children about sexuality. Of course factual knowledge is needed, as it is for everyone, but education related to skill development and adult inhibitions is also needed. For example, parents must learn how to be better listeners, resolve problems, answer questions, and begin and maintain conversations about sexuality. A particularly strong need is for parents to feel more comfortable with their own sexuality and to better understand their values about sexuality (Alter, 1989).

One final consideration about sexuality education for adult learners is a reminder that those adults who choose to be sexuality educators in more formal educational settings need special preparation. Of course this is the main thrust of this entire book. The success of sexuality education efforts is closely tied to the attitudes of the educators. Successful programs depend on educators who are well trained in content areas, skillful in educational techniques, and comfortable with their sexuality. (Recall the qualifications for sexuality educators mentioned in Chapter 4.)

Sexuality Education for Older Adults

In Chapter 8 we discussed sexuality and aging and pointed out a number of myths about the sexuality of older people. One major problem, as we indicated, is that the entire subject has been completely neglected until recently. There are still many people who do not realize the importance of sexuality education for and about the elderly.

Sexuality education related to aging must be pointed in two directions at the same time. There is a need to help older persons with their sexual adjustment, but there is also a need to help younger persons develop more understanding about the sexual needs of the aged. Increasing numbers of our

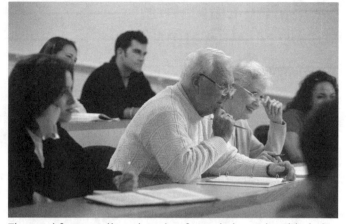

The need for sexuality education for and about the elderly is as great as ever.

population lead active lives well into their older years; we can no longer afford to ignore their sexual concerns.

We also know that for many older people, contrary to popular opinion, sexual activity remains an important part of their lives. For example, nearly half of all Americans aged 60 or older engage in sexual relations at least once a month, and 40% of them want to have sexual relations more frequently. The vast majority of sexually active men and women are as satisfied or even more satisfied with their sex lives than they were in their 40s. When older people are not sexually active, it is usually because they lack a partner or because they have a medical condition (Half of older Americans report they are sexually active; 4 in 10 want more sex, says new survey, 1998).

Again, many of the topics and approaches used in sexuality education for younger people are appropriate for older people, since many individuals still lack an overall background. However, a comprehensive program of sexuality education for older people should also include, at least, topics such as those included by the National Council on the Aging (New sexual education program launched for seniors, 1999). Topics in their *Love and Life* program include the following:

- Sex: A natural part of your life: Explores attitudes about sexuality and sexual practices

- Sexual challenges and solutions: Educates older adults about sexual dysfunction, chronic disease, and the aging process

- Talking to your doctor about sex: Designed to generate effective conversation between patients and physicians

- Health risk assessment profile: Self-guided survey for people to complete and bring to their physician for discussion

Sexuality Education for Special Groups

Coronary Patients

With continued medical advances, higher numbers of people are surviving heart attacks and resuming normal lives. Among the natural concerns of such people is sexual activity. Questions regarding what sexual difficulties develop after a heart attack, whether it is safe to participate in sexual activity soon after a heart attack, and how heart attacks affect sexual function are common concerns. Professionals working with coronary patients need to take the lead in addressing these questions and encourage patients to speak freely about their concerns. It is helpful to speak with the partner and the patient together if possible. The severity or type of heart attack has no correlation with the frequency, duration, or enjoyment of sexual activity in the period following illness. There appears to be no medical basis for implicating sexual activity, in a familiar and supportive relationship, as a hazard (Hackett, 1986).

Sexuality education for cardiac patients should address such issues as getting in touch again, feeling depressed, your body and sexuality, medications, and eating and drinking. With common sense and prudent living, the person who has had a heart attack can resume most, if not all, daily activities. This includes the most special function of the heart, the act of loving.

Culturally Varied Groups

While many of the basics remain the same, sexuality educators who work with people from a culture different from their own need to keep special considerations in mind. This is true with any culture, but here we consider examples related to the Latin American population, Native Americans, and Asians and Pacific Islanders. These are only examples, and sexuality educators working with culturally varied groups must learn a great deal about the individuals with whom they work.

Female Latin Americans (Latinas) commonly are more inclined to think of their family's health than of their own. Educators should stress Latinas' roles as mothers and caregivers and emphasize that by taking care of themselves they will also be taking care of their children and family. This is particularly true in the example of HIV/AIDS education. Also, the Latino (male Latin American) who exhibits bisexual behavior is found everywhere in Latin communities. Latinas know this, but are unlikely to admit it to strangers. In addition, there is a Latino mystique that the one who performs the penetration is the real male, while the one who is penetrated is not a real man (de la Vega, 1990).

When working with Native Americans, the sexuality educator must remember that a Native American's primary ethnic identity lies with his or her respective tribe. There is a mistaken view that Native Americans are all one people. Since they make up less than 1% of the U.S. population, many people have had little or no contact with them. Sexuality educators need to help all people realize that Native Americans have played an important role throughout history, not all of them reside on reservations, and there are many myths about this population. Because of stereotyping, Native Americans also have not been recognized as sexual beings in the same way as other people (Rowell, 1990).

Language problems can occur for sexuality educators working with Asians and Pacific Islanders. For example, the Chinese characters used to pronounce AIDS literally mean "love, disease, death"—and how will that be interpreted? In many Asian languages, the literal translation for homosexual is "deviant" (Lee & Fong, 1990). Unique aspects of traditional cultures must be known and appreciated in order to plan and implement effective sexuality education programs.

A Word of Caution

Throughout this chapter we have been emphasizing many positive aspects of sexuality that should be taught at different levels and in different settings. We would be remiss, however, not to point out also that there may be times or settings in which it might be wise *not* to teach purposely about something. For example, teaching techniques for sexual stimulation to fourth graders is probably not a wise choice. Not only is the information likely to be inappropriate for the learners, but the entire program might be placed in jeopardy because of the educator's poor judgment.

Likewise, it might not be wise to cover *all* sexuality topics with a group of adult learners that contains a number of people who are extremely uncomfortable with some topics. It might be possible to deal with these topics at a later time, but it makes little sense to "force" the learners to be exposed to the topics immediately. Doing so will only hinder the learning process.

As with all aspects of life, good judgment is necessary when conducting sexuality education programs. Sometimes this may mean *not* handling certain topics at a given time, but this good judgment will help strengthen the program in the long run.

Summary

Exactly what is included in a given sexuality education program depends on many factors, but preschool and school sexuality education programs designed for certain levels will probably have many similarities. Most existing school sexuality education programs could be cranked back several years and handled much earlier by learners.

There are many ways that sexuality education objectives can be approached and written, but they should be based on developmental characteristics of learners at the preschool, early elementary, upper elementary, lower secondary, and upper secondary levels.

Additional insight into sexuality education program development can be obtained through a look at typical questions asked by learners of different ages. Many apparently simple-sounding questions can open many possibilities for sexuality education.

Too often sexuality education programs have been narrow or fragmented. Programs should be comprehensive, giving attention to the physical, psychological, social, and spiritual aspects of people. In addition, there should be a logical sequence to the curriculum.

Just because learners have finished high school does not mean they have no further need for sexuality education. There is still a great deal of ignorance among college-aged students, and there is no justification for postponing education about any aspect of sexuality at this age.

Adults have many sexuality education needs. Because of the lack of good sexuality education programs, many of their needs are much the same as those of younger people. Adult programs need to be based on communication, self-awareness, and knowledge.

Sexuality education for older adults has received little attention until recently. There is a need to help older persons with their sexual adjustment, and there is also a need to help younger persons develop more understanding about the sexuality of the aged.

Sexuality education programs are needed for people of all ages. Careful planning can help meet the sexuality needs of all people.

Sexuality of those recovering from heart attacks and other circulatory problems, and those from diverse cultures, has generally not been considered. Recognizing the education needs of these people is the first step in providing sexuality education programs for them.

References

Alter, Judith. Sexuality education for parents, in *Sexuality education: A resource book*, Cassell, C. & Wilson, P. M., eds. 13–26. New York: Garland Publishing, 1989.

Byler, R., Lewis, G. & Totman, R. *Teach us what we want to know.* New York: Mental Health Materials Center, 1969.

de la Vega, E. Considerations for reaching the Latino population, *SIECUS Report*, 18, no. 3 (February/March 1990), 1–8.

Guidelines for comprehensive sexuality education. New York: Sexuality Information and Education Council of the United States, 1996.

Hackett, T. Men and sex after a heart attack, *Harvard Medical School Health Letter* (March 1986), 5–6.

Half of older Americans report they are sexually active; 4 in 10 want more sex, says new survey. National Council on the Aging (1998). Available: http://www.ncoa.org/news/archives/sexsurvey.htm.

Landry, D. J., Singh, S. & Darroch, J. E. Sexuality education in fifth and sixth grades in U. S. public schools, 1999, *Family Planning Perspectives*, 32, no. 5 (September/October 2000), 212–19.

Lee, D. A. & Fong, K. HIV/AIDS and the Asian and Pacific Islander community, *SIECUS Report*, 18, no. 3 (February/March 1990), 16–22.

New sexual education program launched for seniors. National Council on the Aging (1999). Available: http://www.ncoa.org/news/archives/new_sexual.htm.

Rowell, R. M. Native Americans, stereotypes, and HIV/AIDS, *SIECUS Report*, 18, no. 3 (February/March 1990), 9–15.

Schulz, E. D. & Williams, S. R. *Family life and sex education: Curriculum and instruction.* New York: Harcourt Brace & World, 1969.

Sexuality education within comprehensive school health education. Kent, OH: American School Health Association, 1991.

Tepper, M. S. Becoming sexually able: Education to help youth with disabilities, *SIECUS Report*, 29, no. 3 (February/March 2001), 5–13.

What the latest survey tells us, *Family Life Matters*, no. 42 (Winter 2001), 1, 6–7.

Suggested Readings

Human Sexuality: What children should know and when they should know it. Planned Parenthood Federation of America, 1998. Available: http://www.plannedparenthood.org/library/sexualityeducation/whatchildrenshould.htm.

McNab, W. L., and Henry, J. Answering questions students and adults ask about the wonderful world of sexuality. *American Journal of Health Education* 34, no. 2 (March/April 2003): 109–112.

Pope, E. When illness takes sex out of a relationship. *SIECUS Report* 27, no. 3 (February/March 1999): 8–11.

Price, J. H., Dake, J. A., Kirchofer, G., and Telljohann, S. Elementary school teachers' techniques of responding to student questions regarding sexuality issues. *Journal of School Health* 73, no. 1 (January 2003): 9–14.

Sanders, S. A. Midlife sexuality: The need to integrate biological, psychological, and social perspectives. *SIECUS Report* 27, no. 3 (February/March 1999): 3–7.

Ward, J. V., and McLean Taylor, J. Sexuality education for immigrant and minority students: Developing a culturally appropriate curriculum. In *Sexuality and the curriculum*, edited by J. T. Sears. New York: Teachers College Press, 1992.

The Educator and Sexual Counseling

CHAPTER 15

Key Concepts

1. Sexuality education is separate and distinct from sexual counseling.

2. Some situations are clearly within the domain of the sexual counselor.

3. The sexuality educator is often called upon to do some quasi-counseling.

4. Sexuality educators need to know when and where to refer learners who need sexual counseling.

In this chapter we attempt to differentiate between the roles of the sexuality educator and sexual counselor. We use the word *attempt*, because although there are some very specific situations for which either sexuality education or sexual counseling is most appropriate, there are also many gray areas. However, counselors and educators need to be specifically trained for their jobs, since these jobs are quite different from one another. Both require a high degree of skill, but the skills required of each are different.

Sexuality Education and Sexual Counseling

We can consider counseling to be a communication process between a trained, educated, or experienced person and individuals or groups seeking that person's advice and guidance. The advice and guidance address a greater understanding of the issue involved, its implications, possible solutions, arrangements to implement a solution, and evaluation of the solution selected with plans for adjustments if the solution is not satisfactory. As we shall soon see, different problems require different levels of counseling expertise. Consequently, for some sexuality issues, sexuality educators possess adequate knowledge and skills. For others, they do not and will need to refer the person or group seeking counseling to a more skilled counselor.

Generally, counseling involves a trained counselor working with a client to help that client improve an aspect of his or her life that is troublesome. According to the American Association of Sex Educators, Counselors, and Therapists (AASECT), sexual counselors perform the following function:

Counselors assist the client to realistically resolve concerns through the introduction of problem solving techniques of communication as well as providing accurate information and relevant suggestions of specific exercises and techniques in sexual expression. Sex counseling is generally short term and client centered, focusing on the immediate concern or problem. (AASECT certification, 2003)

The training of sexual counselors is different from the training of sexuality educators. Whereas educators are generally trained to aid people in preventing sexual problems, sexual counselors are trained to help people work through sexual problems once they exist. Sexuality education might be viewed as a sieve that filters sexual problems; the sexual counselor waits underneath the sieve to receive whatever gets through.

AASECT certifies sexuality educators, sexual counselors, and sexual therapists. For certification of an applicant as a sexual counselor, AASECT lists the following requirements (AASECT certification, 2003):

1. *Academic and counseling experience:*

   a. A minimum of a Bachelor's degree in a human service program

   b. A minimum duration of supervision by an AASECT certified sex therapist of at least 6 months

2. *General knowledge in the following core areas:*

   a. Sexual reproductive anatomy and physiology

   b. Developmental sexuality (from conception to old age) from a psychobiological perspective

   c. Dynamics of interpersonal relationships

   d. Sociocultural factors (ethnicity, religion, socioeconomic status) in sexual values and behavior

e. Medical factors that may influence sexuality including illness, disability, drugs, pregnancy and pregnancy termination, contraception and fertility

f. Knowledge of sexually transmitted infections and safer sex practices

g. Sexual abuse

h. Varieties of sexual orientation and gender identities

i. Atypical sexual behavior, hypersexuality, and sexual dysfunctions

j. Substance abuse and sexuality

k. History of the discipline of sexuality

3. *Sex counseling training:* A minimum of 60 clock hours of training in how to conduct counseling with patients/clients. At least 30 hours must be in sex counseling. Counseling training is to include the following:

   a. Theory and methods of personal counseling

   b. Theory and methods of sex counseling

   c. Theory and methods of approach to intervention in relationship systems

   d. Theory and methods of decision making concerning sexually related medical interventions

   e. Ethical issues in sex counseling

   f. Theory and practice of consultation, collaboration, and referral

4. *Attitudes and values training experience:* At least 12 hours of structural group experience consisting of process-oriented exploration of the applicant's feelings, attitudes, values, and beliefs regarding human sexuality and sexual behavior.

5. *Clinical, field work, or practicum training experience:* At least 100 hours of supervised sex counseling.

The initial certificate from AASECT is subject to renewal in 3 years and every 5 years after initial recertification.

This seems like a lot, doesn't it? Well, it should be. Counseling is a helping profession, one in which people's quality of living is at stake. It is nice to know, therefore, that although anyone can claim to be a sexual counselor, there is an organization that certifies sexual counselors and is stringent in its requirements. One of the sexuality educator's responsibilities is to encourage people who need sexual counseling to inquire about the qualifications of people claiming to be sexual counselors. The more people ask questions regarding sexual counselors' qualifications, the less

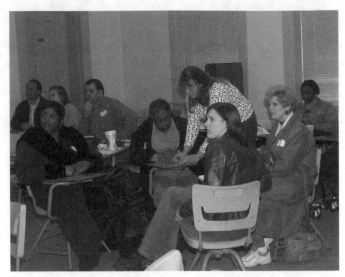

Professional sexual educators need extensive and very specific training and experience.

charlatans will be able to infest the field. Sexual counseling is fraught with unqualified, unethical charlatans out to make a fast buck from the sexual problems of others. What makes this situation complicated is the reluctance of people to report the "quacks." People in need of sexual counseling often hesitate to admit that they have sexual problems. Seeking counseling for these problems requires a great deal of courage. To report an unqualified counselor requires even more courage, for a patient would need to admit to authorities the existence of his or her sexual problems and, in addition, admit to having been conned by a charlatan. Consequently, people who know of charlatan sexual counselors do not often report them.

The Domain of the Sexual Counselor

What is the difference between a sexuality educator and a sexual counselor? Sexuality educators have a function in the informal counseling of learners. However, certain conditions and sexual problems are beyond the capabilities of the educator and are better responded to by a counselor. One category of such conditions is termed *sexual dysfunctions*. Although both males and females may on occasion find themselves unable to perform sexually (for example, after having ingested alcohol or when the interest is just not there), these situations are usually infrequent and temporary. Some people, however, have a chronic inability to respond satisfactorily sexually. These people experience a sexual dysfunction that may require treatment by a professional.

One of these sexual dysfunctions—experienced by males and females—is called *inhibited sexual desire* (ISD). ISD is a lack of interest in sexual activity. One of the difficulties regarding this sexual dysfunction relates to the varying degrees of interest in sexual activity that people possess. When is a low interest in sexual activity a sexual dysfunction? Therapists have decided that only when this lack of interest is a source of distress—personally or within a relationship—is it a problem. In addition, ISD must be accompanied by a lack of sexual dreams and fantasies, inattention to erotic material, and a disregard for attractive potential sexual partners. This lack of interest may be caused by physiological factors, such as hormone deficiencies, kidney failure, or some chronic illnesses, but is usually a result of psychological factors such as depression, shame regarding one's body, or some earlier traumatic sexual experience (for example, rape). Fortunately, sexual therapists are highly successful in treating ISD. Other sexual dysfunctions are described as follows.

Male Dysfunctions

Males experience sexual dysfunction predominantly from two conditions, premature ejaculation and erectile dysfunction.

Premature ejaculation is the inability of the male to "control his ejaculatory process for a sufficient length of time during intravaginal containment to satisfy his partner in at least 50 percent of their coital connections" (Masters & Johnson, 1970, 1992). Although premature ejaculation can be a result of surgery, trauma, or disease, it is usually caused by the inability of the mind to control the body's need to ejaculate. You may have heard that premature ejaculation occurs in males who masturbate frequently. This is not true.

There seems to be an increasing number of premature ejaculators. One possible reason for this is that with the use of the Pill, diaphragm, and intrauterine devices, males are using condoms less. Since use of the condom results in less stimulation than skin-to-skin contact, its decrease in use is resulting in greater male stimulation. Greater male stimulation is resulting in more inexperienced males being unable to control their ejaculation; consequently, there is an increase in adult male premature ejaculators.

Other explanations for what appear to be increasing numbers of premature ejaculators have been offered. Some experts argue that the women's movement has freed women to demand sexual satisfaction rather than sublimating their needs to the male's. More demands to satisfy the female, the argument continues, have created pressure on the male to perform well sexually. The fear of not performing well becomes a self-fulfilling prophecy, resulting in the inability to control ejaculation.

Others do not believe the incidence of premature ejaculation has increased at all. They argue that ever since premature ejaculation has been described as a sexual dysfunction not infrequently found in males, and since a method of treating this condition has been developed, it has been less threatening for males to seek treatment for this condition. In other words, the incidence of premature ejaculation is the same, but the number of those willing to admit to it has increased. The increased writing about premature ejaculation, this argument continues, has resulted also in more people recognizing the existence of the condition. The sum of these factors has led to the *impression* that there are proportionately more premature ejaculators now than in the past.

Regardless of its specific psychological cause, there is a highly effective method of treating premature ejaculation. This method is termed the *squeeze technique* and was described by Masters and Johnson (its developers) in their book *Human Sexual Inadequacy*. The squeeze technique requires the female to hold the penis between her thumb and first two fingers when the male achieves an erection and to squeeze with a fairly hard pressure for 3 to 4 seconds. As the partners learn this procedure, the squeeze can be timed to occur as the male feels ejaculation imminent, thereby preventing it. The squeeze technique has proven to be a vital ingredient of the sexual counselor's armamentarium for use with premature ejaculators.

Erectile dysfunction (previously known as impotence) is the other predominant male sexual performance problem. Erectile dysfunction is the inability of a man to attain or maintain an erection long enough to have sexual intercourse. (It should be stated here that different categorizations of sexual dysfunctions exist. Some authorities choose to consider premature ejaculation as a form of erectile dysfunction.) Masters and Johnson (1970) have described *primary* erectile dysfunction as existing when a man has never been able to achieve or maintain an erection long enough to have sexual intercourse, and *secondary* erectile dysfunction as existing "when a male only infrequently is able to achieve or maintain an erection long enough for sexual intercourse but has a history of having been coitally effective prior to the development of the secondary impotence." There are an estimated 15 million American men who have an erectile dysfunction (Potent solution: Treatments counter erection problems, 1990).

Erectile dysfunction is caused by a myriad of factors (Buvat, et al., 1990). Until recently it was thought that psychological factors accounted for the majority of the cases of erectile dysfunction. It is now thought that about 70% are at

---

premature ejaculation   The inability of a male to control his ejaculatory process for a sufficient length of time to satisfy his partner in at least 50% of their coital connections.

erectile dysfunction   The inability of a man to attain or maintain an erection long enough to have sexual intercourse.

least partially the result of physiological factors (Danoff & Katz, 1998). Erectile dysfunction can be caused by neurological or anatomical damage to the reproductive system, drug or alcohol abuse, deficiencies in hormonal secretions, problems with the circulatory system, old age, or physical exertion. Performance anxiety—the fear of not performing well during sexual intercourse—is the major psychological cause. What is believed to occur is that the fear of not performing well results in an inability to relax and, therefore, in an inability to perform well. As mentioned during the discussion regarding premature ejaculation, this is called a self-fulfilling prophecy. In addition to performance anxiety, guilt about one's masturbatory behavior, guilt regarding illicit sexual relations, feelings of inferiority, and viewing sex as "dirty" have all been cited as causes of erectile dysfunction.

Female Dysfunctions

Prevalent female sexual dysfunctions are orgasmic dysfunction, sexual unresponsiveness, dyspareunia, and vaginismus.

Orgasmic dysfunction is the consistent or frequent inability of a person to achieve orgasm (Greenberg, Bruess & Haffner, 2004). The inability to achieve orgasm is the most prevalent female sexual dysfunction.

Orgasmic dysfunction can be caused by several conditions, some within the female and some external to her. External factors include an inexperienced and ineffective sexual partner, an uncomfortable setting in which coitus occurs, or the use of depressant drugs (alcohol, for example). Orgasmic dysfunction can also be a result of internal factors such as pregnancy, self-consciousness regarding one's body or sexual behavior, or trying too hard to achieve orgasm (the self-fulfilling prophecy again). In addition, anatomical defects in the reproductive system, hormonal deficiency or imbalance, nervous system disorders, use of drugs, and factors associated with aging can all cause orgasmic dysfunction.

With the knowledge that communication between partners is usually at the heart of the problem, counseling for orgasmic dysfunction that is psychogenic in nature usually involves both sexual partners. Obviously, training is required for someone effectively to counsel couples in which the female experiences an inability to reach orgasm. This training is different from that usually experienced by the sex educator.

Sexual unresponsiveness is a condition in which the female experiences little or no erotic pleasure from sexually oriented stimulation (Haas & Haas, 1990). Sexual unresponsiveness was formerly called *frigidity*, but since women with this condition can be quite sensitive and feeling people, frigidity is no longer used by experts (although it is still commonly used by the lay public). Sexual unresponsiveness is difficult to treat, primarily because women with this condition usually manifest other personality disorders that precede the onset of the unresponsiveness. Although an initial reaction to rape may be short-lived sexual unresponsiveness, rape is not a major cause of this condition. Rather, it is caused by intrapsychic factors: shame, guilt, or fear relative to sex or males. However, a poor relationship in general can lead to unresponsiveness in the sexual aspects of the relationship, or an inexperienced, inept, hasty, or insensitive lover can contribute to the onset of this sexual dysfunction. In addition, situational factors can result in sexual unresponsiveness, although under these circumstances the unresponsiveness is usually only temporary. Examples of such situational factors are thoughts of a sick relative, offensive body odor emanating from the sexual partner, fear of pregnancy, and fear of being interrupted.

Dyspareunia is defined as painful intercourse. Although males may experience painful intercourse, dyspareunia is more common in females. As with the other sexual dysfunctions, many causes for this condition exist. Dyspareunia may result from contraceptive foams, creams, or jellys that irritate the vaginal walls. It can also be related to irritation by the glans of the penis, insufficient lubrication of the vagina, too frequent intercourse, or not enough sexual stimulation (thereby not enough vaginal lubrication) prior to the penis entering the vagina. Dyspareunia indicates the need for medical examination since this condition can often be easily corrected. The major concern with painful intercourse is that if it is left untreated, it might lead to orgasmic dysfunction or sexual unresponsiveness.

Vaginismus (a relatively rare condition) is an involuntary contraction of the muscles surrounding the vaginal entrance so that entry of the penis is prevented. As might be expected, women experiencing this condition are very often fearful of coitus. In addition, the following are related to the onset of vaginismus: sexual relations with a man who has erectile dysfunction, religious guilt, a traumatic sexual experience, or dyspareunia.

---

orgasmic dysfunction   The consistent or frequent inability of a person to achieve orgasm.

sexual unresponsiveness   A condition in which the female experiences little or no erotic pleasure from sexually oriented stimulation.

dyspareunia   Painful intercourse.

vaginismus   Involuntary contraction of the vaginal muscles so that entry of the penis is prevented.

Treatment

In the past few decades many highly effective therapeutic approaches to sexual dysfunction have emerged (although love and concern between partners is still an important ingredient). Masters and Johnson reported an average cure rate for all sexual dysfunctions of 80%, with a 5-year relapse rate of only 5% (Masters, Johnson & Kolodny, 1985). Even over 30 years ago, Helen Singer Kaplan (1974) reported that her treatment for vaginismus was almost 100% effective and that the vast majority of women with orgasmic dysfunction are treatable. The treatment for these conditions, however, requires a person with a great deal of specific training. Certainly, the sexuality educator is not trained for this function and should therefore refer learners experiencing sexual dysfunction to someone who is so trained.

One particular approach to sexual therapy was suggested by Jack Annon (1976). This approach is still advocated by AASECT (AASECT certification, 2003). Representing his four-level approach by the acronym PLISSIT, Annon's system goes from the simplest to the more advanced levels of treatment. The four levels of PLISSIT are permission (P), limited information (LI), specific suggestions (SS), and intensive therapy (IT). "Permission" refers to the therapist helping people accept their fantasies and desires and, where appropriate, even giving them permission *not* to engage in sexual intercourse. "Limited information" refers to the therapist providing the factual information that may help the client become more competent sexually, for example, information about penis size, clitoral sensitivity, or proper hygiene. "Specific suggestions" is the level of therapy where the therapist actually recommends activities for the client, for example, self-stimulation activities, sensate focus, and the squeeze technique. "Intensive therapy" is the level that is required when the client has problems that cannot be resolved in the short term. These clients need a longer period with the therapist and more intensive sessions.

Sex therapist Helen Singer Kaplan suggested a novel approach to couples who experience sexual dysfunction as a result of fear of contracting AIDS or some other sexually transmitted disease. She calls it "hot monogamy" (Lichenstein, 1991), that is, good, satisfying, exciting sex between monogamous partners. Kaplan recommended that therapists counsel clients on sexual technique to make their sexual relationship so exciting that they will refrain from seeking out other sexual partners. Kaplan also wrote books to help people overcome specific sexual dysfunctions, for example, *PE: How to Overcome Premature Ejaculation* (1989).

Other Problems

Not only are problems of sexual dysfunction beyond the scope of the sexuality educator's role, but so are some relationship problems. For example, much research has been conducted on the family, and a whole field of counselors and therapists have been trained to improve the functioning of families. For sexuality educators to take on the role of relationship therapist, when not specifically trained for it, would be inappropriate. In addition, a cadre of people are available who are called marriage counselors. Although some people use that term loosely, *trained* marriage counselors are the ones to whom people with marital problems should be referred. People who are not experiencing a sexual dysfunction per se but who seek to improve their sexual lives can be advised to seek help from a psychotherapist, a gynecologist, or a sexual counselor regarding techniques for sexual intercourse, methods of sexual stimulation, and so on.

The Sexual Educator and Quasi-Counseling

As stated earlier, where the sexuality educator's role ends and the sexual counselor's role begins is often a gray area, as Insight 15-1 demonstrates.

In addition to questions you posed in Insight 15-1 seeking more information about the nature of the conflicts dealt with by various kinds of therapists, at least one of your questions probably pertained to the relationship between you, your spouse, and the sexuality educator, or to the personality and characteristics of the educator. This is not surprising in view of what we know about effective counseling. It has long been known that the greatest constructive client gains or changes occur when a counselor exhibits the following characteristics (Carkhuff & Berenson, 1967):

1. *Empathy.* The counselor attempts to respond to the client's underlying feelings rather than just to the client's words. In other words, the counselor can tune in to the client's wavelength.

2. *Positive regard for the client.* The counselor respects the client's feelings and experiences. Communicating warmth and understanding seems to be related to the client's concluding that he or she is respected as a person by the counselor.

3. *Genuineness.* The counselor appears to be real and responds genuinely, rather than appearing to be applying a counseling technique or playing the therapeutic role.

4. *Concreteness.* The counselor shows specificity of expression. This dimension involves the fluent, direct, and complete expression of specific feelings and experiences, regardless of their emotional content.

Insight 15-1

Deciding Who to Consult

Imagine that you are married and that both you and your spouse are enrolled in an adult education course offered by your local school district entitled "Sexuality Education." During the course the instructor lectures about communication in marriage, particularly about how to resolve conflict effectively. You recognize that the way you and your spouse usually resolve conflict is ineffective. Further, both you and your spouse desire to improve your method of dealing with conflict.

Do you ask the sexuality educator (the course instructor) to work with both of you outside the class, perhaps prescribe certain assignments for the both of you to try at home, or perhaps recommend some further readings on the subject? Do you describe your problem in detail to the sexuality educator, expecting advice?

Or do you ask the educator for the name of a good marriage counselor from whom you could get the help you need, or a good psychologist to explore the causes underlying much of your conflict, or a good sexual therapist who could work with both of you to improve the sexual part of your marriage so as to eliminate conflicts in that area?

To decide what to do, you probably need more information. If you could ask three questions to clarify further the situation described above so as to be better able to decide to work with the educator, marriage counselor, psychologist, or sexual therapist, or perhaps even a family therapist, what would those three questions be? Write them down.

1. _____

2. _____

3. _____

---

5. *Other dimensions.* The counselor displays such characteristics as self-disclosure, confidence, spontaneity, intensity, openness and flexibility, and commitment to the client.

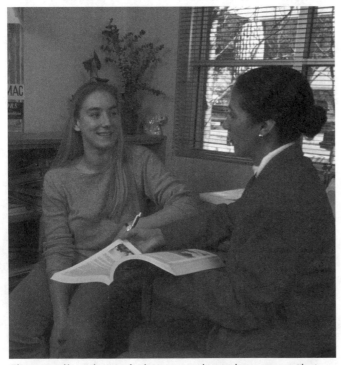

The sexuality educator's door must always be open so that students can seek help with their questions and sexual problems.

As can be noted, characteristics that result in effective counseling are not solely possessed by counselors. Many sexuality educators are empathetic, genuine, concrete, and have a positive regard for those whom they are charged with educating, for example. It follows that sexuality educators possessing the characteristics known to result in effective counseling might do a better job of counseling than trained counselors who do not possess these characteristics. All of us know some person who, because of his or her personal characteristics, is someone with whom we would feel comfortable discussing our problems. That person is probably understanding, a good listener, levelheaded, and caring. That person has probably not been trained to provide counseling, yet does an excellent job when asked for counsel.

Commitment entails time and energy. Often, counseling means extended conversations, repeated over time. If you are not prepared for such a commitment, some experts advise you to refer the student to a counseling professional from the outset.

While some specific situations are clearly within the domain of the counselor, some gray areas might best be handled by the sexuality educator *if* he or she possesses some of the characteristics just described. For example, if a learner approaches you after a sexuality education session (as many will do) and describes a problem that he or she is having with a parent, you can assume that being approached in this manner indicates that the learner thinks you can help. If you have established a good rapport with this learner, rather than recommend a family therapist you would do better to determine whether *you* could be of assistance. Since the problem may not be severe enough for the learner to speak to a stranger (counselor) about, since the learner might not be able to afford or qualify for counseling services, and since the learner feels comfortable discussing the problem with you and seeking help from you, the best bet for resolving this situation is probably for you to do the counseling. On the other hand, you may feel awkward in this role and need some guidance as to how to function—what to say, when to schedule meetings, with whom to meet, and so on. In this eventuality you would want to obtain some backup services. For example, you could consult with a counselor and seek his or her advice. Perhaps a counseling service or agency may be willing to assist you. In any case, help is available and should be employed when you are doubtful about how to function.

When in doubt about your ability to help a particular learner who needs counseling, you should discuss the desirability of referring the learner to a professionally trained sexual counselor. This discussion should include the learner, someone trained in counseling, and the sexuality educator. Generally, if you feel more uncomfortable as the session progresses, or if you grow more frustrated with your efforts to help, it may be time to refer the person seeking your help to a counselor.

Here are some recommendations of techniques to follow when and if you do become involved in counseling:

1. *Accept feelings.* You should accept the right of all people to feel any way they do. It is not appropriate to *behave* any way one wants, but it is all right to have any feeling. For example, feeling angry is fine, but beating up on someone is not.

2. *Reflect feelings.* Let the learner know that you understand the feelings behind the words and accept those feelings. For example, if a male student approaches you and says, "Girls think I'm stupid," it would be unwise to say, "Naw. I'm sure they don't really think you're stupid." This would be denying the learner's feelings rather than accepting them. A more appropriate response would be, "Gee, it must make you feel very sad to think that girls don't like you." Look for the feelings behind the words and reflect the feelings back to the learner.

3. *Gather data.* Ask questions of the learner and others to verify or refute the learner's perceptions of the situation.

4. *Analyze.* With the learner, study the situation to determine when it most often occurs, under what circumstances, what precedes and what follows the situation, what the symptoms are, what the causes are, and so on.

5. *Generate solutions.* Brainstorm ways of dealing with the situation or problem. Try to generate many possible solutions from which one or several can be chosen.

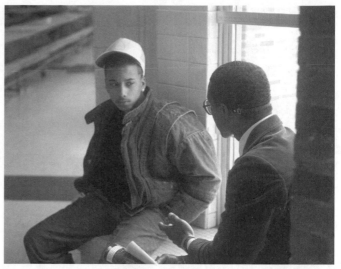

Part of the sexuality educator's role is to be available for individual consultation. However, the educator should refer students to those trained as professional counselors when appropriate.

6. *Choose a solution.* Explore each generated solution with the intention of the learner's choosing one or more to try. As part of this decision, consider resources available: people that can help, places to attend, qualities and characteristics of the learner, and so on.

7. *Try the solution.* Have the learner try the solution(s) chosen to see how it works. Designate a specific time period during which the solution will be tested.

8. *Evaluate the solution.* At the end of the trial period, evaluate the solution to determine whether it was effective. If not, repeat steps 5 through 8.

Although the use of counseling techniques requires training, those interested in acquiring further information regarding the counseling function of the sexuality educator may consult additional resources.

Referring Learners Who Need Sexual Counseling

When to refer learners to other more qualified professionals is often a difficult and very important question. As has been indicated in this chapter, there is no set answer. It is a decision involving competence and sensitivity. Simply put, however, a referral should be made when the problem is beyond the educator's level of skill, when a specialized or different type of assistance is needed, or when the problem presents a moral objection on the part of the sexuality educator.

As stated earlier, do not hesitate to get advice regarding the decision of whether to refer the learner to someone more qualified. In addition, the learner should be involved in this

---

Referral Sources

List 10 local counseling persons or agencies and the specific problems for which you think they are best suited to counsel. Make sure that they are sexuality-related persons or agencies.

Person or Organization

1. _____
2. _____
3. _____
4. _____
5. _____
6. _____
7. _____
8. _____
9. _____
10. _____

Sexuality-Related Problem

1. _____
2. _____
3. _____
4. _____
5. _____
6. _____
7. _____
8. _____
9. _____
10. _____

---

decision. The pros and cons of referral should be clearly delineated for the learner so that a rational decision can be made.

In order to decide where to refer a learner, you need to be familiar with what referral services and people are available. Certainly an important role the sexuality educator plays is one of resource person. He or she should be familiar with local resources (both human and institutional) that can be tapped. This requires a conscious effort on the part of the educator to be apprised of new services and facilities, new functions being served by existing facilities, payment mechanisms of various services, specialized services (like abortion clinics), and qualifications of personnel employed at the various counseling centers. Sexuality educators who are active in the community through participation in conferences and professional meetings, who serve as education resources for community agencies, and who are willing to serve in an informal and formal advisory capacity are probably those best able to identify referral resources.

A further consideration regarding referral is the educator's willingness to maintain a line of communication between the referral agency, the learner, and himself or herself. If a learner feels comfortable enough to raise a problem with you initially, it is conceivable that you might have a role in the counseling process even after referral is made. Perhaps you will be asked to observe and record certain aspects of the learner's behavior during instruction, or maybe you will be needed to provide the referral agency some anecdotal information prior to the first counseling session. In any case, do not assume that your responsibility to the learner and your involvement in the counseling process have ended just because a referral was made.

To get started in improving your ability to refer learners for counseling, complete Insight 15-2.

Summary

Sexuality educators are best trained to conduct sexuality education, and sexual counselors are best trained to provide sexual counseling. Sexual counselors are uniquely trained for the counseling role. Because of this specialized training, sexual counselors are clearly the ones to counsel people regarding problems of sexual dysfunction such as premature ejaculation, erectile dysfunction, orgasmic dysfunction, sexual unresponsiveness, dyspareunia, and vaginismus.

On the other hand, a rapport between learner and educator often requires that the sexuality educator be willing to provide the necessary counsel. Backup services should be employed by the educator when he or she is unsure regarding how to function as a counselor. Other counselors can be of great help on these occasions. However, a sexuality educator who is empathetic, genuine, concrete, fluent, direct, confident, spontaneous, intense, flexible, and willing to be self-disclosing and who has a positive regard for the learner will probably do a better job of counseling than a trained counselor lacking these characteristics.

Finally, the sexuality educator should know local referral resources well enough to know which ones learners should be referred to. Among other information, educators should know about the personnel employed by referral sources (qualifications, roles, and so on), means and amount of payment required, facilities available, and specialized services offered. Although there are no specific guidelines that the sexuality educator can apply to determine when to refer a learner to a more qualified counselor, referral should be made when the problem is beyond the sexuality educator's level of skill, when a specialized type of assistance is needed, or when the problem presents a moral objection on the part of the sexuality educator.

References

AASECT certification. American Association of Sex Educators, Counselors, and Therapists (2003). Available: http://www.aasect.org.

Annon, J. S. *The behavioral treatment of sexual problems: Brief therapy.* New York: Harper & Row, 1976.

Buvat, J., Buvat-Herbaut, M., Lemaire, A., Marcolin, G. & Quittelier, E. Recent developments in the clinical assessment and diagnosis of erectile dysfunction, in *Annual review of sex research,* vol. 1, Bancroft, J., Davis, C. M. & Weinstock, D., eds. 265–308. New York: Society for the Scientific Study of Sex Research, 1990.

Carkhuff, R. R. & Berenson, B. G. *Beyond counseling and therapy.* New York: Holt, Rinehart & Winston, 1967.

Danoff, D. S. & Katz, D. *The new miracle in male genital health.* 1998.

Greenberg, J. S., Bruess, C. E. & Haffner, D. W. *Exploring the dimensions of human sexuality.* Sudbury, MA: Jones and Bartlett, 2004.

Haas, A. & Haas, K. *Understanding sexuality.* St. Louis, MO: Times Mirror–Mosby, 1990.

Kaplan, H. S. *PE: How to overcome premature ejaculation.* New York: Brunner/Mazel, 1989.

Kaplan, H. S. *The new sex therapy.* New York: Brunner/Mazel, 1974.

Lichtenstein, G. Hot monogamy: A sex therapist's prescription for the '90s, *American Health* (May 1991), 18–20.

Masters, W. & Johnson, V. *Human sexual inadequacy.* Boston: Little, Brown, 1970.

Masters, W. H., Johnson, V. E. & Kolodny, R. C. *Human sexuality,* 2nd ed. Boston: Little, Brown, 1985.

Potent solution: Treatments counter erection problems, *American Health* (December 1990), 10.

Suggested Readings

AASECT code of ethics. American Association of Sex Educators, Counselors, and Therapists (2003). Available: http://www.aasect.org/codeofethics.cfm.

Bartoi, A. G. & Kinder, N. N. Effects of child and adult sexual abuse on adult sexuality, *Journal of Sex and Marital Therapy,* 24 (1998), 75–90.

Cooper, A. *Sex and the Internet: A guide book for clinicians.* New York: Brunner-Routledge, 2002.

Culley, S. *Integrative counseling skills in action.* Newbury Park, CA: Sage, 1991.

Egan, G. *The skilled helper: A systematic approach to effective helping.* Pacific Grove, CA: Brooks-Cole, 1990.

Fowler, C. J. The neurology of male sexual dysfunction and its investigation by clinical neurophysiological methods, *British Journal of Urology,* 81 (1998), 785–95.

Heiman, J. R., et al. Evaluating sexual dysfunction in women, *Clinical Obstetrics and Gynecology,* 40 (1997), 616–29.

Huber, C. H. & Backlund, B. A. *The twenty minute counselor: Transforming brief conversations into effective helping experiences.* New York: Continuum, 1991.

Cases for Part 4

The cases in this section are designed to use information included in Chapters 11, 12, 13, 14, and 15. Case 1 highlights the discussion of the need to effectively plan for sexuality education that appears in Chapters 11, 12, and 14. To answer the questions at the conclusion of Case 1 you must synthesize the information in these three chapters.

Case 2 requires you to recall, analyze, and synthesize information about planning for sexuality education, writing objectives, and deciding on placement of content in the sexuality education curriculum. Chapters 11, 12, 13, and 14 all contain discussions related to this case.

Case 3 draws on the differentiation made between sexuality education and sexual counseling described in Chapter 15. You are asked to apply the contents of Chapters 14 and 15 to a situation in which the question is whether sexuality education or sexual counseling is most appropriate.

Case 1

Being Ready: Planning for the First Sexuality Education Session

Sexuality educator Hank R. Chief knew that he still had several weeks prior to his sexuality education group's first meeting. Being conscientious and hard working, Mr. Chief decided that he would be exceptionally well prepared for that opening session. The group he was going to teach consisted of elderly citizens from the city and suburbs. Advertising was widespread, with ads in local newspapers, notices posted at senior citizens' centers, and letters to agencies serving this population. It was expected that 50 people would participate in the six-session sexuality education program (2 hours per session). The question now facing Hank R. Chief was what should he do at the opening session (and how could he now plan for that session) to make subsequent sessions more meaningful.

1. What information about the learners should Mr. Chief acquire at the opening session?

2. How should he obtain this information?

3. What should he do with this information once it is obtained?

4. What can Mr. Chief do prior to the opening session to help that session meet its objectives?

5. Whose help might Mr. Chief seek?

Case 2

Starting from Scratch: Developing a Sexuality Education Curriculum

Professor Will Counsill was hired by administrators of a local school district to help them develop a sexuality education curriculum for kindergarten through grade 12. Professor Counsill decided to establish a committee to help him with this task.

1. Who should be asked to serve on this committee?

2. What should be its purpose?

Professor Counsill's counsel was to pay particular attention to the rationale serving as the basis for the initiation of sexuality education in this school district. "What are the objectives of the program?" he asked. He was told it was hoped the program would result in students' acting more responsibly sexually.

1. Write three objectives for this purpose of the sexuality education curriculum. Make sure that these objectives are consistent with the criteria cited in Chapter 12.

2. Select the appropriate grade-level placement for each of the three objectives. Provide a rationale for these grade-level placements based on information cited in Chapters 13 and 14.

Case 3

Miss Advice: Sexuality Education versus Sexual Counseling

Connie Job is a sexuality educator working for a family planning organization. Her task is to serve as the first person seen by people seeking the organization's services and to provide them with necessary sexuality education or refer them to counseling or medical services personnel as appropriate. For the past several weeks, however, all the clients who came to the organization's offices have either needed counseling or medical services of some kind. None have needed sexuality education. Well, since she is beginning to feel like a secretary instead of a sexuality educator, Con Job decides that she will work with the next person approaching the organization no matter what the nature of the person's problems. No sooner has she made this decision than Mr. Upton Set enters.

Complaining of an inability to satisfy his wife sexually, Up Set asks for help. Con Job starts to counsel him.

1. Based on your reading of Chapter 15, make a list of sexual dysfunctions that might include Upton Set's problem.

2. What *should* Con Job have done when Up Set described his problem?

3. How might Up Set be able to decide whether to accept Con Job's counseling help?

4. Assuming that Con Job is fired and another sexuality educator is hired in her place, what guidelines should be given to this new employee so that he or she will know when to provide sexuality education services and when to refer the client to some other service personnel in the organization?

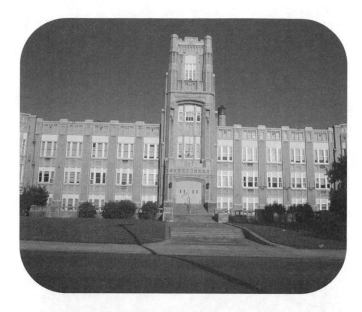

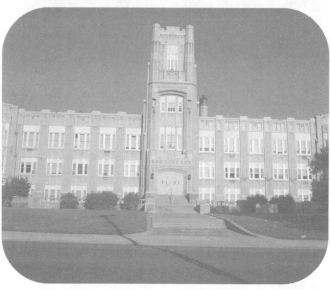

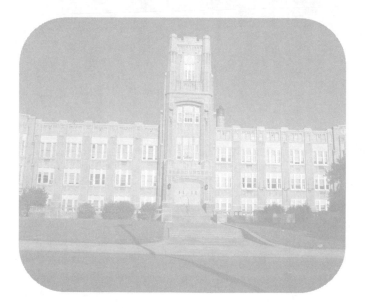

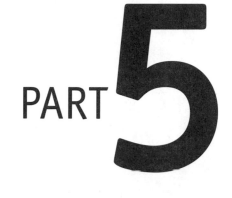

PART **5**

Program Implementation and Evaluation

Chapter 16
Implementing a Sexuality Education Program

Chapter 17
Evaluation of Sexuality Education

Chapter 18
Effectiveness of Sexuality Education and the Sexuality Educator

Implementing a Sexuality Education Program

Key Concepts

1. Certain steps can promote needed broad-based community and institutional support for a sexuality education program.

2. Sexuality educators need to be aware of basic ways to bring about change.

3. An understanding of group dynamics facilitates working with people in sexuality education program endeavors.

4. Attention must be paid to handling community concerns about sexuality education programs.

In implementing a sexuality education program, it is useful to think of "expanding" on aspects of the existing educational programs that relate to sexuality education. Depending on the setting and the current program, these expansions will vary a great deal, but you need to appreciate already present features that can be used as the basis of a program. Furthermore, it usually helps to have others realize that your program is an expansion of existing components rather than a whole new entity. People are more receptive to improving an existing program than to adding a radically new one with which they are unfamiliar. Before reading further, complete Insight 16-1.

Chances are you have already supported our contention that it makes sense to talk in terms of expanding rather than starting a sexuality education program. You probably noticed aspects of the present program that at least provide a beginning for sexuality education. It is with those aspects that your implementation should begin.

Achieving Support for a Sexuality Education Program

There are various ways to view the steps needed to achieve support for a sexuality education program. We will briefly look at three authors' interpretations of these steps. Note the similarities and differences among their approaches.

Haffner and de Mauro (1991) listed four main steps with activities needed within each step:

1. *Develop a community advisory committee.* The committee's tasks include assessing community and family values on different subjects; undertaking a needs assessment by conducting community-parent polls of perceived students' needs for information about different subjects; conducting a needs assessment based on state and community demographics (statistics on pregnancies, abortions, births, STI, etc.); outlining course goals and objectives; and setting standards so goals can be measured and evaluated. In addition, it is suggested that subcommittees of the community advisory committee be formed to carry out specific tasks. For example, there might be a curriculum advisory subcommittee, a community education and outreach subcommittee, and a media subcommittee, among others.

Insight 16-1

Assessing the Present Situation

You must know of a situation in a clinic, the community, or a school where there does not appear to be a sexuality education program at the present time but in which you feel there should be one.

Answer the following questions about that situation:

1. Remembering our total concept of human sexuality, what aspects of the present program have educational implications for dealing with sexuality (indicate subject-matter areas or perhaps entire units or courses)?

2. Among the present personnel, who has the training and ability to deal with sexuality education?

3. If there are written guidelines, units, or even a curriculum, where are there (or could there be) places where sexuality education fits?

---

2. *Involve parents.* This means keeping parents informed, having parents participate in curriculum design and evaluation, and having parents assist in the selection of resources and materials. It is wise to have parents meet and talk with teachers and administrators of the proposed program to help promote mutual trust and respect.

3. *Involve teachers.* Teachers should be involved from the very beginning. Ways to do this include surveying them on their perceived need for the program, asking if they would like to be considered to teach the program, presenting the proposed program at teachers' meetings, and gaining the support of local teachers' organizations.

4. *Involve community leaders.* This can be done by including community leaders on the community advisory committee, surveying community organizations for their support of the proposed program, holding meetings with key community leaders, developing collaborative relationships between school programs and community agencies, and asking the local clergy organization to issue a statement in support of the program. All of these steps can help reassure parents and others about the program.

Bensley (1991) listed 11 steps for implementation of a sexuality education program as follows:

1. *Study the feasibility of sexuality education.* Determine the needs, identify community support, determine needs and sources for financial support, determine inservice needs of teachers, assess community readiness, and review literature on sexual attitudes, morals, and behaviors in the community as well as in other areas.

2. *Establish goals and a definition of sexuality education.* The definition should be based on a program's goals and should be succinct and easy to understand.

3. *Obtain administrative approval.* This is more likely when a clear definition of sexuality education has been determined. Approval may involve input from parents, students, teachers, board members and administrators.

4. *Establish a community sexuality education advisory committee.* Members must have a willingness to serve, the respect of the community, communication skills, emotional stability and objectivity, and an interest in the learners. Parents, students, educators, administrators, and appropriate community leaders should be members of the committee.

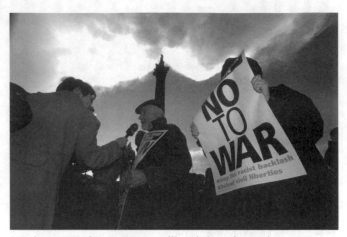
It takes more than a strong will to bring about change.

5. *Develop policies.* They will probably center on three areas: (1) tasks such as teacher selection, parental notification, evaluation, and public relations; (2) strategies for establishing teaching content and ways to answer student questions; and (3) policies concerning materials and resources as well as how to answer questions requiring content that is not part of the curriculum.

6. *Establish the curriculum.* Sexuality education should be part of a comprehensive school health education program.

7. *Establish qualifications of educators* (see Chapter 4).

8. *Establish a positive public relations program.* Meet with groups of allies in the education and health professions, encourage parents to play an active role in sexuality education programs, and work wisely with the media.

9. *Present the program to the public.* Inform parents through public presentations by the advisory committee.

10. *Present the program and recommendations to the board of education (or board of directors for a community agency or hospital).* A report, including proposed steps for establishing policy and implementing and evaluating the program, should be presented to the board.

11. *Evaluate the program.* Evaluation results are needed to strengthen the program, overcome limitations, and expand the program where needs are recognized (see Chapters 17 and 18).

As a result of a needs assessment of over 150 education and health leaders, the Sexuality Information and Education Council of the United States established a list of strategies to build broad-based support for sexuality education programs (Strategies to build support for HIV-prevention and sexuality education programs, 2000). The strategies are as follows:

- *Work with other groups.* Build coalitions, work together, and avoid duplicating efforts. Seek the involvement of local and state public education and health agencies.

- *Develop models.* Develop model programs, provide technical assistance for programs, develop appropriate policies, provide resources and materials, and provide training for educators.

- *Engage the media.* Mail press releases, have a staff person handle media requests, and make certain the local media is well acquainted with what you are doing.

- *Build community support.* Have community leaders attend training sessions, help program administrators work with others in the community, and make the community aware of the overall program.

- *Organize public meetings.* Have a skilled facilitator, anticipate differences of opinion, set time limits for speakers, and carefully plan the agenda to meet your needs and those of the audience.

- *Prepare for challenges.* Know the content of materials related to the program, do not make assumptions, meet with those who are resistant to the program, and practice conflict resolution skills.

- *Involve parents.* When dealing with children, it is important that parents understand the program. Serve as a resource for parents, conduct parent meetings, send parents newsletters, and conduct a parent education series.

All of the important steps might take several years or more to accomplish. Each takes more time than you might think. For example, it might take years to achieve administrative support. It could easily take 6 months to a year (or more) to convene a series of meetings to plan and carry out program evaluation. If you can implement a sound program more quickly, more power to you; however, patience and persistence are usually demanded.

When developing support for a sexuality education program, consideration should also be given to learners with special needs. Shapland (1999) developed a checklist for program planners (see Table 16-1), which summarizes the issues involved in meeting the needs of youth with disabilities.

Finally, there are many things *you* can do, or have others do, to show support for sexuality education. Some of them are listed here (Thirty things you can do to show support for sexuality education 2000):

1. Send letters of support to the editor of the local paper, and write opinion-editorial (op-ed) pieces for the local paper.

2. Invite speakers who support comprehensive programs to speak at community group meetings.

Table 16-1 Program Checklist

The following checklist for program planners summarizes the issues in meeting the needs of youth with disabilities.

_____Include youth with disabilities and their families in program development.

_____Include youth with disabilities, their families, and disability advocacy groups on the advisory board.

_____Identify all youth with disabilities who are in the program.

_____Emphasize strengths of individuals, accommodate and provide support for limitations.

_____Individualize programs, such as providing various formats to appeal to different learning styles and including experiential activities.

_____Support parents as the primary educators whenever possible.

_____Find community partners, including those from the disability community, to support and sustain the program.

_____Become informed about the various accommodation possibilities for youth with disabilities.

_____Provide developmentally and culturally appropriate information.

_____Assess accessibility of clinic and program facilities, including entrances, exam tables, and educational materials.

_____Provide self-advocacy by providing information that teens can understand and truly utilize.

_____Provide a sense of future.

Source: Sexuality issues for youth with disabilities and chronic health conditions. Institute for Child Health Policy (1999). Available: http://www.ichp.edu/hrtw/materials/930579144.html.

3. Encourage a group to place an ad in the local paper expressing support for comprehensive programs.

4. Wear buttons declaring "Just Say Know," or "Ignorance Kills," or "Ask Me About Comprehensive Sexuality Education."

5. Set up a table in a visible area and ask sexuality education supporters to sign petitions, sign up to volunteer, and take literature to distribute throughout the community.

6. Ask religious leaders who support sexuality education to be more vocal about their support.

7. Hold a sexuality education forum for parents and their children.

8. Develop a mailing list so you can get the word out about meetings, events, and issues on a timely basis.

9. Turn to national organizations for technical assistance, suggestions, materials, and other help.

Strategies for Change

For many years, Dale Carnegie has been well known for his book entitled *How to Win Friends and Influence People* (1936/1964). He listed nine ways to change people without giving offense or arousing resentment. As old as they are, they are still worth noting when implementing a sexuality education program. They are as follows:

Rule 1: Begin with praise and honest appreciation.

Rule 2: Call attention to people's mistakes indirectly.

Rule 3: Talk about your own mistakes before criticizing the other person.

Rule 4: Ask questions instead of giving direct orders.

Rule 5: Let the other man save his face. [We apologize for these sexist terms, but they were written many years ago and are Carnegie's words and not ours.]

Rule 6: Praise the slightest improvement and praise every improvement. Be "hearty in your approbation and lavish in your praise."

Rule 7: Give the other person a fine reputation to live up to.

Rule 8: Use encouragement. Make the fault seem easy to correct.

Rule 9: Make the other person happy about doing the things you suggest.

In recent years there has been a wealth of literature about change agents and change-agent strategies. It is our intent here to summarize this literature briefly with the hope that you will delve into it more deeply on your own. In order to implement a sexuality education program, you will need to operate as a change agent. *Implementation is change.*

There are several general ways to get other people to change. One way is through education. This involves showing people that it is in their best interest to change, helping them to understand why there should be change, and identifying new options. A second way to create change is through a unilateral action. In this instance, you indicate what you want, and people must do it. A third way, and usually the best way, to create change is through agreement or trade-off. This provides an incentive to change and is not really a compromise, because no one is giving up anything.

At each step of the change process, it is essential to brainstorm all possibilities. The possibility with the highest likelihood of working should be accepted. If none of the three ways works, it will probably be necessary to accept some givens that cannot be changed. Then you can concentrate on things you can change.

Sexuality educators need to understand that change is a process that requires time. Significant changes in people or groups do not occur in just a day or two. Although there are many differing theories on the change process, let us take a look at one example of the change process as presented in the form of a management model by Kurt Lewin (Albanese, 1975). His model involves three steps: unfreezing, moving or changing, then refreezing.

Unfreezing is needed before a person is willing to change. A recognition that behavior is inappropriate, irrelevant, or in some way inadequate can lead to an understanding that traditional ways of behaving are no longer effective. Once unfreezing occurs, it must be pointed out that alternative behaviors are available. It is one thing to know that the traditional ways are not effective, but it is another to know that realistic alternatives exist. Alternatives must be available in order for moving or changing to occur.

Refreezing of a new behavior means that the person accepts the new behavior as permanent. This occurs through experimentation and a realization that the behavior as learned is effective.

It can be helpful to understand that there are stages to the change process. One way to view the stages is summarized by Little (1997):

1. *Resistance.* All change is met with resistance. It is important to have a consistent message as to the need for the change, offer support and reassurance to people, create opportunities for people to be involved, make expectations clear, and be accepting and understanding of people's feelings.

2. *Confusion.* During change people may be distrustful and confused. It is important to show strong support for the change effort, answer questions and provide key information, set short-term achievable goals, create incentives for people to make the changes, and maintain standards to hold people accountable.

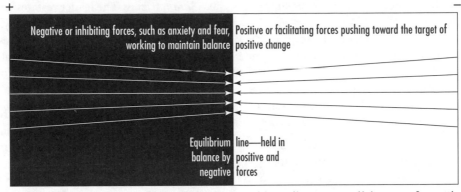

Figure 16-1   Analysis of forces facilitating and impeding accomplishment of a goal.

3. *Integration.* Feelings of optimism appear as a healing process begins. People may even focus on inherent possibilities (what is in it for me?). It is important to communicate effectively and repeatedly, recognize people's contributions, encourage people to work together, point out positive aspects of the change, and model integrity and expect it from others.

4. *Commitment.* People feel that things have finally gotten "back to normal." It is important to continue effective communication, recognize team and individual contributions, keep oriented towards future progress, and stimulate creativity.

One can also understand the process of change by considering the concept of **force-field analysis.** A force-field analysis is an analysis of the forces involved in a given situation to see which ones are present and which ones are most susceptible to change. If a situation is not changing, it is because forces moving in opposing directions are equal and the situation is stable. If there are more or stronger forces pushing in one direction, there will be change in that direction.

Figure 16-1 is a diagram of a force field. Note that the equilibrium line in the middle is held in balance by positive and negative forces. If these forces can be altered, the equilibrium line moves, and there is change in one direction or the other. The task of the change agent is to make the line move in the desired direction.

Fill out Insight 16-2 so you can more fully appreciate the idea. Although we do not usually arrange our thoughts in this way, this is really the process we go through whenever we try to change a situation. In order to implement or expand sexuality education programs, educators need to analyze the forces involved and then try to use the change process to attempt to move the equilibrium line in the "appropriate" direction.

Insight 16-2

Conducting a Force-Field Analysis

Think of a situation related to sexuality education that you would like to change. Perhaps it involves expansion of the program, increase of administrative support, or acceptance of curriculum ideas. With this situation in mind, refer again to Figure 16-1. Write in as many positive and negative forces as you can think of on the force field. Then do the following:

1. Determine what forces will influence movement toward the target. If you had a group to help you, this would actually be done through a brainstorming session. Be open-minded and identify as many forces in both directions as you can.

2. Evaluate the strength of the forces. Obviously, the overall strength of the positive and negative forces must be equal, but, within each group, what is the relative strength?

3. Determine which of the forces are the most likely to change. Remember: changes on either side (more force or less force) will result in a change in the position of the equilibrium line. Which forces are least likely to change?

When implementing a sexuality education program, it may be a good idea to utilize trade-offs from time to time. For example, you might agree not to discuss homosexuality, but in return be allowed to spend more time on contraceptives. This technique can be helpful in bringing about change more easily and quickly, and chances are, in the long run, your

force-field analysis   Analysis of the forces involved in a situation to see which ones are present and which ones are most susceptible to change.

entire program will be implemented anyway. As support grows, you can do more things.

When attempting to bring about change by implementing sexuality education programs, sometimes it may be necessary to pay attention to the politics of sexuality education. Here are some things that can be done to try to change the politics of sexuality education (Five easy things you can do to change the politics of sexuality education, 2003):

1. Contact your elected representatives and tell them what you believe young people need to know about sexuality and reproductive health issues to grow into healthy, responsible adults.

2. Vote for representatives that most closely hold your values and beliefs about sexuality and reproductive health issues.

3. Rally your friends and neighbors—make sexuality education a priority and a regular topic of conversation in your parent-teacher association meetings, school board meetings, social circles, and neighborhood gatherings.

4. Get involved in local politics. Change begins at home and if you can change your local school curriculum to a comprehensive sexuality education program from an abstinence-only-until-marriage program, you have made a difference!

5. Educate your own children about sexuality and reproductive health issues, including positive, nonjudgmental messages about gender, gays and lesbians, relationships, and disease prevention. If your local school board does not provide a comprehensive sexuality education program, you as a parent must do so for the health and future of your children.

Group Dynamics and Sexuality Education Program Endeavors

As is the case with change-agent strategies, the study of group dynamics is quite detailed; however, it is our desire to make sure that you are aware of some of the basics, so you can explore the topic further on your own. Since the implementation of sexuality education programs will always involve working with groups, let us take a look at some guidelines for leading and promoting positive group behaviors (Shaw, 1999):

- *Initiating.* The leader helps the group agree on a definition of the problem and ways to accomplish needed tasks.

- *Information seeking.* The leader asks specific group members to respond to questions, especially those who may be reluctant to contribute. Members of the group should ask each other questions to gather needed facts and opinions.

- *Summarizing.* The leader restates what the group has accomplished to check for accuracy. This also teases out any missing information and resolves disagreements that could cause problems later. The goal is to produce an effective summary, so the group can move forward to the next tasks.

- *Standard setting.* The leader helps the group reach consensus on the standards, including the number of meetings, the methods for sharing information, the number and types of subcommittees, the expected completion date, and how group progress will be appraised.

It is important for the leader to promote positive group roles. This can be done through expressing appreciation, emphasizing successes, and being a consistent role model.

Group Members Play Many Roles

There are many types of groups, but they all have two major functions. The first is to get the job done. The second is to provide for the socioemotional needs of its members. Few groups can average more than 50% of their focus on the task, and the group can actually lose members if it becomes only task oriented.

The person in charge of a group needs to be aware of these major functions to understand group dynamics and to help the group make progress. For example, it may be appropriate for the person in charge to crack a joke or be a harmonizer if the group's socioemotional needs demand it, or the leader may need to help the group return to its task from time to time.

Just as groups have functions, members within groups play roles related to those functions. There are many ways to identify the roles of group members; one is indicated in Table 16-2. Do you recognize any of these group members? Have you ever played any of these roles? At different times we all play different roles, depending on the overall situation.

Insight 16-3

Factors Influencing Roles in Groups

List five factors that influence the roles that we play in groups. (For example, members' ignorance of the group task may contribute to roles destructive to group maintenance.)

1. _____

2. _____

3. _____

4. _____

5. _____

Table 16-2 The Roles of Group Members

Types of Roles	Individuals
Roles that contribute to getting the task done in a positive way.	Orientor—strives for clarity and purpose to understand where the group is and why.
	Facilitator—interested in group process and wants to keep the group moving towards its goal.
Roles that maintain personal needs in a positive manner.	Encourager—asks for input and then listens and gives positive feedback.
	Harmonizer—attempts to blend conflicting feelings and objectives in the hope of "we-ness."
Task-destructive roles.	Blamer—accuses the group of doing the wrong thing or taking too long.
	Denier—when asked for help, answers "I don't have time" or "I don't know how."
	Censor—puts down any new idea because "it won't work."
	Saboteur—seems to be in favor of the task, but works behind the scenes to block it.
Roles destructive to group maintenance.	Dominator—seeks attention and controls group through wordiness and intimidation.
	Hand-clasper—deliberately agrees with others just to remain in favor.
	Sniper—hurls barbs at group members.
	Polarizer—points out differences to keep people apart.
	Sidetracker—wears the group out by bringing up a huge number of side issues.

Source: Smith, P. Members play variety of roles, in *San Diego County Mental Health Services Bulletin,* October 1978. San Diego, CA: Mental Health Services of the County of San Diego, 1978. Reprinted by permission.

The person interested in implementing a sexuality education program needs to be aware of the entire cast of characters in group situations. For example, if group members do not fill some of the necessary roles mentioned in Table 16-2, it may be necessary for the group leader to help play at least some of the roles.

Skillful group leaders and workers can successfully work with a whole cast of group roles and still see that both task and maintenance functions are successful. It is not easy, but it can and must be done—especially in a topical area such as sexuality, which also involves strong emotional feelings for some people. These feelings may make those playing the roles even more intense.

Resolving Conflict

Groups do not exist without conflict. Conflict is actually essential and healthy; in fact, if you do not have any, the group is probably dead. There are three general ways to resolve conflict. The first, collegial, is employed when two conflicting groups get together to work out a solution and come up with something better. This is probably the ideal model, but it only happens about 15% to 20% of the time (Shaw, 1999). The second way of resolving conflict, zero sum, exists when there is a winner

and a loser. Sometimes this is the necessary and best way, but it is not very common. The third way of resolving conflict, strategic, is what happens 75% of the time. In this method, each side comes in with a list of needs, and the conflict is worked out. This is a give-and-take situation, and each one gives a little.

Four rules for conflict resolution should be kept in mind when attempting to implement a sexuality education program (or for that matter in any group-conflict situation):

1. *Listen.* Write down the points if necessary to make sure you understand the feelings and arguments presented. Paraphrasing can be useful in highlighting listening difficulties and in developing listening skills (Greenberg, 1992). As an example, divide a class (or other group) into groups of three to four people each. Present a question, such as, "Why should there be sexuality education?" and have the small groups discuss it for approximately 20 minutes in the following manner: after one person comments, others must first paraphrase what was said by the previous speaker—to that speaker's satisfaction—before making their own comments. If the first speaker does not feel the paraphrase is accurate, the original comments are repeated, and the paraphraser must attempt a new

paraphrase. Chances are, it will quickly become obvious that careful listening is necessary in order to be able to paraphrase accurately.

2. *Repeat.* As indicated in the exercise just described, it is wise to indicate what the person has said in your own words. "Let me see if I understand what you've said . . ." is a good way to communicate what you have heard to check for accuracy.

3. *Indicate areas of agreement.* There are usually more points of agreement than at first seems to be the case. Pointing out areas of agreement can improve morale, settle some issues quickly, and allow the group to focus on any problem areas.

4. *Indicate areas of disagreement.* What are the specific problems? Stating them can save lots of energy that might otherwise be focused on issues that are not real problems.

Two techniques have been demonstrated to be of great value when identifying areas of agreement or disagreement (Greenberg, 1992):

The first technique requires the group to discuss the issue about which they are disagreeing—but before offering comments the student speaking must first cite those aspects of the previous speaker's comments with which he or she agrees. All speakers therefore begin their comments on a positive note: e.g., "I agree with you that . . . ," rather than immediately disagreeing with what has been stated. In addition, while listening to others speaking, the listener must be attuned to viewpoint ideas with which he or she and the speaker are in agreement rather than only those about which they differ.

The second technique allows students to develop an empathetic feeling for those with whom they disagree and a better understanding of opposing points of view. This activity requires that those in disagreement switch positions so that they are, in effect, arguing for the position with which they disagree. By way of example, if student A is opposed to legalization of marijuana and is arguing with student B who favors its legalization (or decriminalization), the teacher requests that for a short period of time student A argue for legalization and student B against it (just the opposite of their actual opinions). Having to think of cogent arguments for a position you disagree with results in a better understanding of that position and greater appreciation for those favoring that position.

Remembering that groups exist because of both tasks and socioemotional needs, certain knowledge and skills will make you more effective in a group. There are advantages to large groups as well as small groups. Large groups are more likely to contain lots of talent, to have more people available to advocate and help sell the desired program, and to be divisible into subgroups to focus on selected parts of a bigger

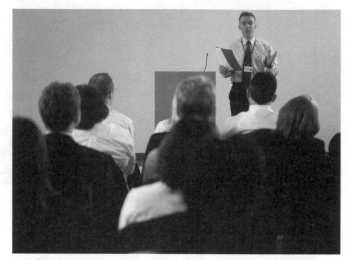

It takes a sensitive, knowledgeable, and skillful person to handle concerns that some people have about sexuality education programs.

problem. It is also likely, however, that only a few people will talk and therefore dominate, that many will feel secure by feeling anonymous, and that there will be little interchange among group members.

In small groups, certain people are less likely to dominate, there is greater opportunity for all members to verbalize, and varied opinions and hidden agendas are less likely to exist. It seems that the best group size for most tasks is between five and seven people. This group size is small enough that members feel they can talk and have a fair chance to express their ideas, but big enough that they do not feel like they have to be dominant in the group.

If you are in charge of setting up groups, you will need to determine the best size for the task. If your objective is to have a brainstorming session to get lots of ideas about something, it might be best to have a large group. On the other hand, a small group would make more sense if you are trying to write curriculum objectives or learning activities.

Most leaders seem to be stronger in either task or socioemotional skills. When you recognize your strength, it is a good idea to have someone working with you who has skills in the area in which you have less strength.

Conflict is sure to exist when a group discussion turns to sexuality education programs. Understanding a little about group dynamics as well as about conflict resolution can go a long way toward placing you in a position to make a real difference in the kind of program that will exist in your community or institution.

Handling Concerns about Sexuality Education Programs

So far we have talked about obtaining community support, change-agent strategies, group dynamics, and conflict resolution. We turn now to the issue of how to deal effectively with the concerns community members may have about sexuality education programs. In his discussion of interpersonal conflict in a business management situation, Albanese* (1975, 536–37) described five common approaches to resolving conflict that can be used when dealing with community members concerned about sexuality education programs: suppressing, smoothing, avoiding, splitting, and confronting.

Suppressing is the elimination of even the appearance of conflict. It represents a low concern for people and a high concern for getting on with the task. A suppressor might ignore the fact that many people are opposed to a sexuality education program and press for its implementation. Suppressing may appear to work in the short run, but in the long run it probably leads to more problems. Can you think of another example of suppressing in a sexuality education situation?

_____

_____

Smoothing involves attempting to convince people that things really are not as bad as they seem. This approach shows a high concern for people but little concern for the task. A smoother points out that things could really be a lot worse. If you were a smoother, what would you say if someone expressed concern about the increasing number of teenage pregnancies in your community?

_____

_____

Avoiding shows little concern for either the task or the people. It is obvious that this method of dealing with people's concerns does not work very well. What would the avoider say to someone who expressed concerns about implementing a sexuality education program in a community?

_____

_____

Splitting emphasizes both concern for people and for the task. In this method, the participants in a conflict situation are kept apart until a compromise can be found. An obvious effort is made to prevent direct confrontation because that might cause a win-lose situation. Can you give an example of splitting in a sexuality education controversy?

_____

_____

Confronting considers some conflict inevitable and as just something that must be managed. This approach shows

---

Insight 16-4

Resolving Conflict

What are examples of situations in which you think it would be best to use each approach?

1. Suppressing? _____

   _____

2. Smoothing? _____

   _____

3. Avoiding? _____

   _____

4. Splitting? _____

   _____

5. Confronting? _____

   _____

---

a high concern for both people and the task. It is designed to get conflict out in the open so it can be evaluated and resolved. Using your previous example, compare what might happen if you used confronting instead of splitting.

_____

_____

All of these approaches to handling concerns have merit in different situations. It is important to be aware of them and wisely choose the appropriate one in a given situation. There is no one approach that is always the best to use.

In Chapter 3 we discussed the controversy surrounding sexuality education. A number of typical reasons why some people are opposed to sexuality education programs were given along with suggestions on how to handle points of opposition. Many of the suggested ways of handling opposition are relevant to the present discussion. When thinking about handling concerns of community members about sexuality education programs, it is necessary to understand the opposition and to determine what facts can be used to respond to arguments against sexuality education. (See Table 16-3 for a case study about implementing a sexuality education program.)

Neutens (1992) indicated that there is often a state of moral confusion when attempts are made to implement

---

suppressing Ignoring or eliminating even the appearance of conflict.

smoothing Attempting to convince people that things are really not as bad as they seem.

avoiding Paying no attention to people's concerns in a conflict.

splitting Keeping participants in a conflict apart until a compromise can be found.

confronting Getting conflict out in the open so it can be evaluated and resolved.

Table 16-3 A Case Study about Implementing a Sexuality Education Program

The New Jersey Mandate and Essex County: A Study
—Paula R. Zaccone

For many school districts that survived the "battle of sex education" in the 1960s, the implementation of the New Jersey mandate meant dusting off old curricula to update content and producing evidence of newly-acquired community participation.

Districts that had abandoned the effort to teach family life topics almost twenty years earlier were confronted with decisions. In what grades will FLE be offered? What topics will be taught? By whom? For how long? In how much detail? With what materials? Existing programs called sex education, values clarification, human reproduction, drugs and alcohol education and decision making were renamed family life education.

Each school district's FLE program will eventually be monitored by a procedure established by the state department of education. Until the time-consuming task of visitations to all schools produces a more global assessment of the impact of the mandate, critics may point to isolated observations to substantiate their biases.

This study aimed to measure the impact the mandate has had in nineteen New Jersey public high schools. While the study and its results are limited in scope, it gives educators and others more than a clue as to what's happening in New Jersey.

Principals and superintendents of thirty-seven public high schools located in Essex County, New Jersey were asked to provide information and respond to a mail questionnaire. More than 50% returned the questionnaires.

All respondents agreed that a course outline, syllabus or curriculum guide for FLE was available at their school. Thus, all respondents are in compliance with the mandate.

More than half the respondents indicated that funds had been earmarked specifically for teaching FLE and that programs were being closely supervised by the director or supervisor of health and physical education.

The selection of grade levels in which a program is taught is left to local districts. Thus, programs in this survey did not exist in all grades or for equal amounts of time. Four high schools offered FLE only in the 12th grade. A respondent from one of these schools complained that the program "offered too little, too late." Of the schools that included grades 7–12, almost half provided FLE to all students. Other programs were arranged for alternating grades, mainly upperclasses, or excluded sophomores and juniors.

The time allocated to FLE ranged from 3 to 30 hours per month. Classes meeting for one semester or for 8–10 weeks were common.

All but two respondents indicated that students receive grades for their performance in FLE. All but three indicated that instruction is integrated into health education and that teachers are evaluated for their effectiveness.

In the majority of cases, programs are assessed by how effectively they promote responsible attitudes and values. Furthermore, a schedule and/or process for revising the program existed for most schools.

The mandate expects local school districts to provide inservice education to FLE teachers. The state department of education is to provide technical assistance to local districts for program development. Only three schools reported no inservice trainings. Twelve respondents felt that more teacher training in FLE topics would strengthen their programs. A number of respondents stated a need for workshops for health educators and continuing inservice programs for teachers.

While the development of curricula is the responsibility of the local school districts, the mandate clearly requires "appropriate consultation and participation of teachers, school administrators, parents and guardians, pupils in grades 9 through 12, community members, physicians, members of the clergy, and representative members of the community." Furthermore, it requires that the consultation process take place before beginning any program and continue as revisions are made.

Health educators contributed to the curricula in all but one school. Physical educators were involved in 84% of the schools. Sixty-eight percent of the respondents named school administrators. Almost 60% consulted school nurses, parents and teachers. Elementary teachers and clergy had input in slightly more than 50% of the schools. Physicians (32%), science/biology teachers (21%), psychology teachers (16%) and preschool teachers (11%) helped in many schools. In the majority of schools surveyed, health and physical education teachers were the primary FLE teachers. This responsibility was shared by the school nurse in two schools. Four schools employed health education specialists and one an FLE specialist.

Table 16-3 (*Continued*)

Seven schools held meetings so that parents could obtain information on FLE topics. Parents and students were involved in less than 60% of the schools surveyed. It might be concluded that much remains to be done to bridge the gap between FLE provided at home and at school. One school mailed FLE information to parents. Thirty-seven percent of the schools reported doing nothing about the requirement to seek community involvement.

Community controversy about teaching sexuality in the classroom has been a major concern of the school administrator. However, the educators surveyed reported little resistance to the programs in their schools. Two respondents reported resistance, and in both cases it came from the school principal. One respondent reported that a principal was opposed to "too much sex education." Another principal opposed the acquisition of a textbook.

Perhaps these findings suggest we have entered a new era of acceptance of FLE topics. There were no objections from parents or members of the community. The topic(s) named as the most sensitive or controversial were sex education, contraception, abortion and human sexual response.

Topics emphasized in the programs surveyed were birth control and human reproduction, family planning, drugs and alcohol, marriage, sexually transmissible diseases, human sexuality, personal relationships, sexual assault, child abuse, abortion, divorce, parenting, the family and nutrition.

This study attempted to determine how often the option for parents to excuse their child was used. In more than half the schools, no students were being excluded from classes. In approximately 25% of the schools, less than 2% of the student population were being excused.

The extent to which community-resource people were used to assist in teaching FLE was investigated. In the schools reporting, Planned Parenthood was most frequently listed as a community resource. Local and county law enforcement agencies were also popular. Physicians, Mothers and Students Against Drunk Driving, representatives from drug and alcohol rehabilitation centers and community health nurses were listed repeatedly.

Respondents were asked to make recommendations for improving programs. The following suggestions were submitted:

More inservice and workshops for teachers

More and better teaching materials

More comprehensive texts

Revision of program design to emphasize certain topics, including pregnancy prevention, was recommended. The need to increase time allotted to FLE was also mentioned. Other comments called for smaller classes and a room designated as the "health room." One respondent favored a standardized final test, and another preferred that the school nurse be invited to FLE classes.

This investigation suggests that in the New Jersey public schools surveyed, FLE programs have been operating smoothly. Teaching about birth control and abortion remain noticeably sensitive. Yet, most of the students (and their parents/guardians) opted to be included.

The requirement to involve the community in the development and revision of New Jersey FLE programs has been met by more than half the programs. None of the respondents reported this community involvement interfered with their program.

This investigation suggests there is a need for a thorough and expeditious procedure for monitoring FLE programs. Only then can it be determined which schools and to what extent there is compliance with the principles, rather than the print, of the mandate.

This research project was made possible by the cooperation of Dr. Elena S. Scambio, Essex County Superintendent of Schools, and Seton Hall University Faculty Research Council.
Paula R. Zaccone, EdD, is an Associate Professor of Health Education at Seton Hall University, South Orange, NJ.
Reprinted with permission from *Family Life Educator,* ETR Associates, Santa Cruz, CA. For information about other related materials, call 1-800-321-4407.
Source: Zaccone, P. R. The New Jersey mandate and Essex County: A study, *Family Life Educator,* 4, no. 3 (Spring 1986), 23–5.

sexuality education programs. He gave the following twelve recommendations to help avoid such confusion:

1. Educate yourself. Learn what sources or influences drive your community's opinions about human sexuality education and examine their backgrounds, motivations, and intentions. Read newspapers and magazines for trends as well as professional journals.

2. Make it clear what human sexuality education within comprehensive health education is—what many people are being told is erroneous.

3. When serving as an advocate, do not overstate goals and capabilities of a human sexuality education program.

4. Support a balanced, comprehensive program that reflects a pluralistic society, rather than a singular philosophy.

5. Examine events around you, such as homophobic messages, puritanical postures, or advertisements that make sexuality external such as the way you dress, rather than internal such as the way you feel.

6. Teach from a base that supports individual freedom and personal dignity.

7. Acquire the skills necessary to conduct human sexuality education within a restructured school system.

8. Support parents and family by involving them in your program.

9. Conduct research in human sexuality that goes beyond fertility behavior to concerns such as sequelae or benefits of early sexual behavior.

10. Develop political advocacy skills for public forums, community meetings, talk shows, letters to the editor, and position papers.

11. Write municipal officers and state and federal legislators expressing your opinion on human sexuality education in comprehensive school health programs for your community.

12. Work with local, state, and national organizations that support human sexuality education in comprehensive school health programs.

Even after a good sexuality education program is implemented, you cannot afford to sit back and congratulate yourself on your accomplishment. Support for the program must be maintained. There are several ways to do this (Haffner & de Mauro, 1991). For example, the advisory committee should meet at least twice a year to review and evaluate the program. Parents and community leaders should remain involved in the program. It should be clear how complaints or problems will be handled. The list of community organizations supporting the program should be updated regularly. (It would also be wise to thank community leaders for their support.)

Finally, educators must be supported. They might need periodic updates, inservice education programs, letters of support from administrators, and even public recognition for doing an outstanding job.

It is a challenging opportunity to implement a sexuality education program—in a school, clinic, community agency, or other organization. Many of the basics are the same regardless of the setting. However, the job is never done and the program needs constant attention.

Summary

In this chapter we have suggested that in implementing a sexuality education program you focus on expanding rather than starting a new one. In most situations, some parts of a program already exist. People are generally more receptive to expanding something that already exists than to starting something new. Steps needed to promote community support for a broad-based program include gaining support from the highest level of authority within the organization, forming an advisory committee, and using technical experts. Commonsense planning involves training, committee activities, and well-designed programs.

Implementing a sexuality education program involves change. Consequently, those in charge and working in the programs need basic knowledge about change-agent strategies. There are different ways to bring about change, but the process usually takes a great deal of time. Lewin's model for change involves unfreezing, moving or changing, and refreezing at a new level. The concept of a force-field analysis can be useful in attempting to implement a sexuality education program.

An understanding of group dynamics also facilitates sexuality education program activities. It is inevitable that we will need to deal with groups. The main functions of groups are accomplishing tasks and fulfilling socioemotional needs of members. This fact influences our ways of working with groups. We also need to understand that group members play many different roles.

Conflict is all around us, and educators are often found in the middle of an attempt to resolve it. There are several models of conflict resolution. There are also group membership skills such as initiating, opinion seeking, summarizing, standard setting, and meeting socioemotional needs, all of which help resolve conflict and place the educator in an influential position.

Concerns of the community about sexuality education programs must be handled. Methods used for handling such concerns include suppressing, smoothing, avoiding, splitting, and confronting. No one way is best in every situation. Group activities involving program implementation are logically related to previously discussed strategies for refuting opponents of sexuality education.

References

Albanese, R. *Management: Toward accountability for performance.* Homewood, IL: Richard D. Irwin, 1975.

Bensley, L. Steps for implementation, in *Sexuality education within comprehensive school health education.* Kent, OH: American School Health Association, 1991.

Carnegie, D. *How to win friends and influence people.* rev. ed. 217. New York: Pocket Books, 1936/1964.

Five easy things you can do to change the politics of sexuality education, *SIECUS Developments* (Winter/Spring 2003), 3.

Greenberg, J. S. *Health education: Learner centered strategies.* 2nd ed. Dubuque, IA: William C. Brown Communications, 1992.

Haffner, D. W. & de Mauro, D. *Winning the battle: Developing support for sexuality and HIV/AIDS education.* New York: Sexuality Information and Education Council of the United States, 1991.

Little, L. Stages of change, *Academic Leader,* 13, no. 10 (October 1997), 5–6.

Neutens, J. J. Sexuality education in comprehensive school health programs: Surviving the "moral smog." *Journal of School Health,* 62, no. 2 (February 1992), 74–75.

Shapland, C. Sexuality issues for youth with disabilities and chronic health conditions. Institute for Child Health Policy (1999). Available: http://www.ichp.edu/hrtw/materials/930579144 .html.

Shaw, K. A. *The successful president.* Phoenix, AZ: American Council on Education and Oryx Press, 1999.

Strategies to build support for HIV-prevention and sexuality education programs. Sexuality Information and Education Council of the United States (2000). Available: http://www.siecus.org/pubs/fact/fact0009.html.

Thirty things you can do to show support for sexuality education. Sexuality Information and Education Council of the United States (2000). Available: http://www.siecus.org/advocacy/kits0002.html.

Suggested Readings

Common questions about sexual health education. Sex Information and Education Council of Canada. Available: http://www.sieccan.org.

Hedgepeth, E. & Helmich, J. Effective sexuality and HIV education: What works and why, in *Teaching about sexuality and HIV.* New York: New York University Press, 1996.

Landry, D. J. Abstinence in promotion and the provision of information about contraception in public school district sexuality education policies, *Family Planning Perspectives,* 31, no. 6 (November/December 1999), 280–86.

McNab, W. L. Difficulties in implementing sexuality education— the Nevada experience, *Journal of School Health,* 51, no. 4 (April 1981), 295–99.

Online press kit. Sexuality Information and Education Council of the United States (2003). Available: http://www.siecus.org.

Evaluation of Sexuality Education

CHAPTER 17

Key Concepts

1. Evaluation is a key component in the continued improvement of the sexuality education program.

2. Evaluation should be applied to the educational process, the learners, and the sexuality educator.

3. Evaluation is dependent on well-stated objectives.

4. Evaluation can be a trap.

Evaluation and the Continued Improvement of the Sexuality Education Program

The story is told of a teacher who presented a lesson on the unhealthy effects of alcohol. The teacher demonstrated these effects by placing one worm in a glass of alcohol and another worm in a glass of water. When the worm in the alcohol died, the teacher asked the students what they would conclude from this experiment. Little Johnny, in the back of the classroom, was waving his hand so high and hard that the teacher just had to call on him. "What do you think we could conclude from this experiment, Johnny?" she asked. "Obviously," Johnny said with confidence, "if you don't want worms in your stomach, then drink a lot of alcohol."

This story demonstrates the important point that learners do not always learn what educators think they are teaching. Unless proper evaluation is an integral part of the educational process, sexuality educators can never really know whether their instruction is effective.

Several distinctions need to be made before a discussion of the need for evaluation of the instructional process

can take place. One of these is the difference between grading learners and the kind of evaluation being proposed here. Usually, when people talk about evaluating learners, they mean applying some process by which they can determine what grade to assign to each learner. This is one area in which school-based sexuality education programs differ from community-based ones. School-based sexuality educators are generally more concerned with measures of individual student growth. Community-based sexuality educators are generally more concerned with measures of program effectiveness. These differences stem from two major sources:

1. School sexuality education programs have a captive audience. Sometimes "captive" may be used in the most literal sense. Students are often required to pass a health education, health science, or home economics course in order to graduate from high school. Many times, sexuality education of some sort is a part of such a required course. The students have little if any choice whether to participate in sexuality education. Recognizing that students are there because they have to be rather than want to be, teachers believe they need some way of motivating students to be conscientious in their studies and to learn a minimum amount of human sexuality content. For this reason, student comprehension is evaluated; good grades then become a form of **extrinsic motivation.**

   Community sexuality education programs, on the other hand, involve people who voluntarily choose to participate. Motivation by grades is unnecessary, since their attendance indicates they are already motivated, and inappropriate, since they are probably not interested in receiving "credit" for attending (their interest is in what they might learn).

---

extrinsic motivation   Something, other than their own innate interest or need, that encourages people to want to do something or learn something.

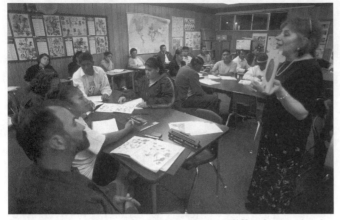

Community sexuality education programs differ from school sexuality programs in that schools have a captive audience whereas community-based programs have a need to recruit participants. Consequently, community programs often have an incentive to evaluate their programs so they can better meet participants' needs, thereby maintaining a steady stream of program participants.

2. Community sexuality education programs must compete for funding. Often, annual reports attesting to the effectiveness of community sexuality education programs are the basis for the continued funding of these programs. Many community sexuality education programs must be demonstrated to be effective in order to maintain their existence. Educators in these programs thus need to apply evaluation procedures that can assess effectiveness.

School sexuality education programs, however, are less dependent on demonstrations of effectiveness to maintain their existence. School educators are heard to argue that there often is a "lag time" between when education occurs and when the students apply what they have learned. Consequently, the effect of what is learned now upon how the student behaves after his or her schooling cannot be evaluated. Further, school sexuality educators state that their program is one of primary prevention; that is, it educates people who are not yet experiencing sexual problems in order to prevent future sexual dysfunction, irresponsible sexual behavior, and so on. Since it is impossible to determine how many sexual problems and irresponsible sexual behaviors the program prevents, the value of school sexuality education cannot be accurately determined. Consequently, school sexuality educators believe they can afford to be less concerned with evaluation of their programs than community sexuality educators.

What *is*, however, is not always what *ought* to be. Evaluation is necessary in order to determine what effect education has had. Remember the teacher who presented the alcohol lesson. Obviously, that teacher needs to revise some of the instruction on alcohol. Further, if subsequent learning experiences are dependent on students' understanding of the unhealthy effects of alcohol, these subsequent learning experiences will themselves be ineffective, since the prerequisite learning has not occurred. A teacher who does not evaluate will not know whether students have learned material on which subsequent learning experiences will be based.

A distinction needs to be made between measurement and evaluation. Kilander (1970, 146) differentiates between the two when he states, "Measurement may tell 'how much'; evaluation may tell 'how good.' We cannot say *how good* an educational program is without knowing *how much* it has achieved of certain objectives."

Therefore, the **evaluation process** becomes one of gathering as much information as possible and making an assessment with respect to some predetermined standard of effectiveness. Part of the information used in this evaluation process will be data obtained by the application of **measurement** devices, such as surveys, scales, tests, questionnaires, observations, and health records. Only after evaluation has occurred can meaningful and sensible decisions be made to improve the instructional process.

There are several different ways of categorizing evaluation. One of those ways is to consider formative and summative evaluation (Greenberg, 2004). When evaluation occurs in the midst of a program with the intent of using that information to revise the program as it is ongoing, that evaluation is called **formative evaluation.** When evaluation occurs at the completion of a program in order to determine its effectiveness in achieving program objectives, that evaluation is called **summative evaluation.** Both evaluations are valuable and should be employed by sexuality educators. In this way, programs can be revised immediately if necessary to be more responsive to their participants, and can be revised at their completion to be more effective for the next group of program participants.

---

evaluation process   The gathering of information with the purpose of making an assessment about something.

measurement   The acquiring of data through such means as surveys, scales, interviews, questionnaires, and other data generating methods.

formative evaluation   The gathering of information about a program and its objectives while it is ongoing; that is, before it is completed.

summative evaluation   The gathering of information about a program and its objectives at the conclusion of the program.

Applying Evaluation to the Educational Process, the Learners, and the Sexuality Educator

The next logical question to consider is, what should be evaluated? The three major components of the sexuality education program—the educational process, the learners, and the educator—should all be evaluated. However, regardless of the component of the program being evaluated, the evaluation should always be in terms of either an objective or a standard. Let us explore the evaluation of the educational process, the learners, and the sexuality educator.

Educational Process

When one is evaluating the educational process, the first task is to define what the **educational process** actually is. It may be obvious from the three categories above that the educational process includes all those factors and activities that relate directly to sexuality education, *excluding* the students and the educator. Specifically, the educational process includes the instructional objectives, sexuality content, learning strategies, and instructional materials, as well as the physical setting in which instruction occurs, the grading procedures, and the curriculum development process used. One way to evaluate all of these is to sit in a quiet room and contemplate subjectively whether they were **effective.** Even if you apply such a subjective evaluation, you still must have in mind a definition of *effective.* That definition, perhaps not even verbalized or formally conceptualized, is the standard against which you evaluate the various parts of the educational process. If something meets that standard, it is effective; if not, it is ineffective and must be revised or eliminated.

Let us use an example to demonstrate this concept: Suppose that you are evaluating the human sexuality content employed in your sexuality education program. If you did so subjectively, you might ask some pertinent questions: Is this content interesting to the learners? Is it relevant to their lives? Is it necessary for the learners to know this content in order to make sex-related decisions? What you have done by asking these questions is to establish a standard by which you will measure the appropriateness or lack of appropriateness of the content presently included in the sexuality education program. The standard you have established is that the content to be included in your program must be *interesting* to the learners, *relevant* to their lives, and *necessary* for them

to know in order to make sex-related decisions. Content not meeting these standards will not be included in the program or will be eliminated from the program if presently a part of it.

Such standards can be applied to the other components of the sexuality education process:

1. The instructional objectives should be stated in such a way that they can be evaluated (that is, behaviorally); should be appropriate to the learners (in terms of learners' ages, interests, and so on); and should be achievable given time, financial, and other constraints.

2. The learning strategies should involve the learner, convey the content, employ the most efficient way of teaching the content, and incorporate all we know about learning.

3. The instructional materials should include accurate information; should be presented in an interesting manner; should not be out-of-date; and should be able to be presented within the time, budget, and other limitations.

4. The physical setting in which the education for sexuality actually occurs should be conducive to learning. It should be well lighted and well ventilated, relatively quiet, and without many distractions, and it should provide ample space with adequate equipment (for example, movable desks and chairs) for varied instructional strategies.

5. The grading or evaluation procedures should be fair, not too time consuming, well understood by the learners, motivating to them, and used as feedback regarding learner progress for learners and others.

6. Curriculum development procedures should involve different groups of people (for example, learners, sexuality educators, obstetricians, and counselors), should be subjected to continual updating and revision, and should be supervised by someone with formal training in curriculum design and group process.

We are sure that you could add other standards for any of the categories of sexuality education considered so far. The point being made here, though, is that we do apply such standards whether or not we do so purposefully. Consequently, it makes sense for the sexuality educator to identify these standards, place them in writing, and then go about gathering as much information about them as possible. Only part of such a procedure would consist of the educator's sitting

---

educational process The instructional objectives, content, learning strategies, instructional materials, and other aspects of a program.
effective Achieving (a program's) objectives.

Insight 17-1

Evaluation Quiz

Before proceeding further, let us evaluate the effectiveness of this chapter up to this point. Match the *numbered* items with the *lettered* items that most pertain to them.

Correct Letter	Numbered Item	Lettered Item
_____	1. Grading	a. School sex education students
_____	2. Evaluation	b. Cost effectiveness
_____	3. Measurement	c. Student achievement
_____	4. Survey	d. Attempt at humor by authors
_____	5. Standard	e. Interval between learning and its application
_____	6. Alcohol joke	f. Type of measurement device
_____	7. Captive Learners	g. Cost benefit
_____	8. Lag time	h. Community sex education students
_____	9. Volunteer to participate	i. How much
		j. Research
		k. How good
		l. Predetermined cut-off point for goodness

The answers are: 1-c; 2-k; 3-i; 4-f; 5-l; 6-d; 7-a; 8-e; 9-h.

How did you do? If you answered at least seven correctly, you are ready to continue reading the remainder of this chapter. If you answered less than seven correctly, perhaps you should reread the beginning section of this chapter before proceeding further.

---

alone to subjectively apply these standards. In addition, learners should be questioned, media specialists queried, learning theorists consulted, visitations made, and whatever other activities conducted that would be deemed appropriate.

Learners

Evaluation of learners, the second major category of the sexuality education program we will be considering, should serve several purposes. First, it should provide a basis for applying grades in situations in which grades will be assigned. Second, it should provide the information needed to decide whether instruction can continue or whether a review is necessary. For programs that are sequential (one lesson building on the learning accomplished during prior lessons), learner evaluation is very important, for it is the basic tool for determining when to continue the sequence of lessons and when to backtrack. Third, learner evaluation should provide a basis for program revision. If learners are not satisfactorily achieving an objective, for example, the sexuality educator should study closely the content, learning experiences, and instructional materials. Perhaps adaptations in these areas may result in the accomplishment of the objective, or perhaps attention should be directed at the objective itself. (Is it appropriate? Is it well stated?)

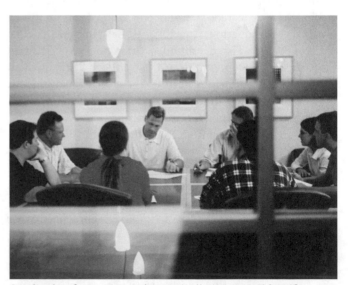

Conducting focus groups is an excellent way to identify effective and ineffective components of a sexuality education program.

Learners can be evaluated in terms of their sexuality knowledge, attitudes, or behaviors. Do they know more after sexuality education than before? Are their attitudes healthier after the program than before? Do they demonstrate more sexual responsibility in their sexual behaviors after sexuality education than before? Such an evaluation implies a knowledge of learners' entering knowledge, attitudes, and behavior. This baseline data can be acquired during the first instructional session by administering a measurement instrument; then a comparison with results obtained at the conclusion of the program can be made.

Sexuality Educator

Relative to the educator, evaluation should consider his or her knowledge of human sexuality content, instructional strategies, referral sources, and instructional materials and resources. Further, the attitudes of the educator might be important to evaluate. For example, is he or she able to nonjudgmentally accept different sexual lifestyles, religious beliefs, or moral and ethical points of view? Is he or she willing to present all sides of an issue? Does he or she consider each learner to be important? Does he or she believe that a sexuality educator needs continuing education to maintain accurate knowledge and educational skills? The sexuality educator's educational behavior is also important. For example, are instructional strategies varied (not lecturing all the time)? Is a rapport with learners established? Is time provided for private discussion after the instructional session at learners' requests? Does the sexuality educator enroll in continuing education courses or workshops, read professional journals, and in other ways maintain a current level of effectiveness?

Evaluation of the sexuality education program should be used to improve what presently exists. Deficiencies identified in the evaluation should be corrected and strong points reinforced. The purposes of evaluation are thus to (1) identify the present situation and (2) provide clues for subsequent program development. It is hoped that evaluation will be viewed as helpful rather than, as is too often the case, threatening.

The Importance of Well-Stated Objectives

Our experience indicates that sexuality education programs are inappropriately evaluated. An analogy that will make this criticism more understandable is one that involves suicide prevention hotlines. Many communities, concerned about the incidence of suicide, have established organizations with trained people (usually volunteers) to stand by telephones so that suicidal people may phone for help when in crisis. The intention is for the suicide prevention personnel to use counseling techniques (crisis intervention) to prevent the

caller from attempting to kill him- or herself. One might expect that such programs would be evaluated in terms of their intended outcome, namely, the number of suicides prevented. This would be possible by one of two methods:

1. Comparison could be made between the number of attempted (or successful) suicides the year prior to the establishment of the suicide hotline and the number during its first (or subsequent) year(s) of operation. This kind of analysis would assume that the year prior to the offering of the hotline service was similar to subsequent years—that is, that the socioeconomic nature, political nature, mental health, and physical health (or other variables that might affect suicide attempts) of the community remained constant.

2. Comparison could be made between two communities, one offering a suicide prevention hotline service and one without such a service, that are similar in terms of variables known to affect suicide rates. The expectation would be that the community with the suicide prevention service would experience fewer suicide attempts than the community without the service.

Both of these evaluation criteria are concerned with **outcome objectives** (the end result). Unfortunately, many suicide prevention hotline services have been evaluated in terms of **process objectives.** Such evaluations have considered:

1. The number of telephone callers

2. The number of volunteers offering to answer the telephones

3. The number of educational groups for whom lectures were given or tours of the organization's facilities were conducted

4. The amount of financial support acquired from local community sources

5. The testimonials of support from community leaders

These all evaluate *means* to an end; they do not evaluate the end itself. The end is to decrease the number of suicides, not to increase the number of telephone calls. Certainly, it is important to evaluate process objectives. Without financial and moral support from the community, without educating the community through lectures and tours, without obtaining volunteers, and so on, suicide prevention might be impossible. These functions must be evaluated so that they can be

---

outcome objectives　The end result a program seeks to achieve.

process objectives　The means by which a program's ends are sought to be met.

improved. This, though, is only one form of evaluation. The bottom line is, have suicide attempts decreased?

Relative to sexuality education, examples of process objectives often evaluated are as follows:

1. The number of learners who passed through the program

2. The number of inquiries or articles (newspapers, journals) about the program

3. The rapport developed with the learners

4. The support for the program from administrators, parents, and community leaders

5. The qualifications, training, and experience acquired by the staff

6. The number of learners who elect to participate in the program (if not required of them)

7. The number of requests to describe the program at professional meetings or mail requests for samples of materials used

8. The number of learners reporting that they like the program or think that it is valuable to them

All of these are means of achieving the outcome of sexuality education, namely, an increase in learners' sexual knowledge, attitudes, and behavior. As with the suicide prevention process objectives, these sexuality education process objectives should definitely be evaluated. However, that kind of evaluation is only a part of what a complete evaluation program should entail. The outcome objectives of sexuality education programs must also be evaluated. Examples of some outcome objectives are as follows:

1. To score 7% higher on a sexuality knowledge examination at the conclusion of the sexuality education program than at its beginning

---

Insight 17-2

A Sexuality Field Trip

To demonstrate the type of evaluation typical of sexuality education programs, try the following exercise. After reading this chapter and understanding what evaluation *should* entail, visit the site of a sexuality education program (either a school or community program). Arrange to interview an administrator, and ask for a description of how that program is evaluated. We suspect that the evaluation of the sexuality education program you visit will consist mainly of process objectives. Write down what standards and objectives you find. Share this information with others in your class.

---

2. To feel more comfortable discussing human sexuality at the conclusion of the sexuality education program than at its beginning

3. To behave more responsibly sexually at the conclusion of the program than at its beginning

As can be noted from these objectives, outcome objectives should state what the learner will be expected to do and how well the learner will be expected to do it at the end of the learning experience. Only with well-stated outcome objectives can the sexuality education program be adequately evaluated. For a more detailed discussion regarding the correct manner of writing objectives, refer to Chapter 12.

Evaluation Can Be a Trap

After having spent the major portion of this chapter describing the virtues of evaluation of sexuality education programs, how can we now suggest that evaluation may be a trap? Before we explain, take a few minutes to write down in Insight 17-3 two outcome objectives for each of the three areas with which sexuality educators are concerned: knowledge, attitude, and behavior.

We will come back to your objectives shortly. Now, imagine the predicament of school district X. This school district found that last year it had four high school girls who gave birth to babies out of wedlock. This rural community became alarmed and decided to do something about this problem. They remembered the following poem (*Healthways*, 1957):

Twas a dangerous cliff, as they freely confessed,
Though to walk near its crest was so pleasant;
But over its terrible edge there had slipped
A duke, and full many a peasant.

Insight 17-3

Sexuality Education Objectives

Write down two outcome objectives for each of the three areas of learning with which sexuality educators are concerned:

Knowledge

1. _____

2. _____

Attitude

1. _____

2. _____

Behavior

1. _____

2. _____

The people said something would have to be done,
But their projects did not at all tally.
Some said, "Put a fence 'round the edge of the cliff";
Some, "An ambulance down in the valley."

The lament of the crowd was profound and was loud,
As their hearts overflowed with their pity;
But the cry for the ambulance carried the day
As it spread through the neighboring city,

A collection was made to accumulate aid,
And the dwellers in highway and alley
Gave dollars or cents—not to finish a fence—
But an ambulance down in the valley.

The story looks queer as we've written it here,
But things oft occur that are stranger,
More humane, we assert, than to succor the hurt,
Is the plan of removing the danger.

The best possible course is to safeguard the source;
Attend to things rationally.
Yes, build up the fence, and let us dispense
With the ambulance down in the valley.

Not desiring to place an ambulance in the valley, the community decided on a preventive approach. They developed a sexuality education program to be presented to all high school students. Lo and behold, the following year saw five out-of-wedlock pregnancies! Many disappointed citizens decided that the sexuality education program had failed and should be scuttled.

Some might argue that the proponents of sexuality education in school district X should have originally educated parents, and others might assert that sexuality education should not be judged solely on its ability to reduce the incidence of out-of-wedlock pregnancies. Perhaps the incidence of sexually transmitted infections decreased, or its detection occurred more frequently at an early stage. Perhaps the incidence of abortion was affected. What about an accounting for "lag time" as discussed earlier in this chapter? The point is that programs with inappropriate or impossible objectives will, nevertheless, be evaluated against those objectives. Do not fall into the trap of accepting *any* objectives just to get a program started! Be sure that the expectations for the program are achievable, reasonable, and educationally sound and that these expectations (objectives) are articulated such that the community understands and accepts them and such that they can readily be evaluated.

On the other hand, if the objectives are valid and their achievement is reasonable to expect, you should be held accountable for them. Still, just because the outcome objectives are not achieved does not mean that you should "throw the baby out with the bath water." This is where your process objectives become important. Perhaps some instructional materials or strategies need revision, or perhaps the content is too difficult for the learners to comprehend. Maybe the sexuality educators need further training, or the place where the program is conducted needs changing. In any case, evaluation of the process objectives should provide clues for improvement of the program so the outcome objectives can be achieved.

Are the objectives you listed in Insight 17-3 achievable? Are they valid? Could they entrap you? If now you believe any of these objectives to be inappropriate, revise them so that they are acceptable.

Cost-Benefit/Cost-Effectiveness

Another consideration of evaluation is sexuality education's **cost-benefit** or **cost-effectiveness.** In the example of community X cited above, even if the program could result in zero out-of-wedlock pregnancies, would it be worth the cost? This is a difficult question to answer but one appropriate to our discussion of evaluation traps.

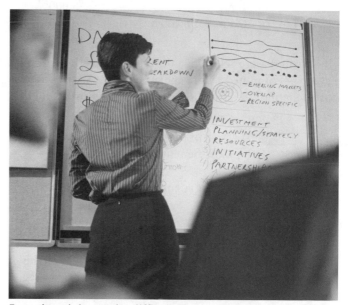

Even though it may be difficult to do and not as accurate as one would like, sexuality education programs should be evaluated based on their cost benefit and cost effectiveness. These variables are important considerations for administrators and those funding these programs.

---

cost-benefit   The cost of achieving the program's objectives.

cost-effectiveness   An assessment regarding whether the best use of resources was used to achieve a program's objectives.

Assume, for example, that the costs for a sexuality education program are as follows:

Two educators	$25,000
Instructional materials	3,000
Overhead (lighting, electricity, etc.)	1,000
Supplies (paper, duplicating, etc.)	2,000
Fringe benefits for educators (health insurance, etc.)	2,000
Total cost	$33,000

Of course, this $33,000 does not include the time that is lost from other curriculum areas or the cost of curriculum development, parent orientation, and other incidentals. If we were to determine the cost-effectiveness of a sexuality education program costing $33,000 designed to eliminate four out-of-wedlock pregnancies, we would calculate each pregnancy eliminated at $8,250. This would be a cost-effectiveness analysis. A cost-benefit analysis would then calculate the cost of each pregnancy prior to the sexuality education program. Such an analysis might look like this:

Hospital services	$900
Physician services	450
Social services (prior and subsequent to the birth):	
Aid to dependent children	4,000
Food stamps	5,000
Loss of income for mother	8,000
Total cost	$18,350

(If abortion were selected, a different cost estimate would have to be computed.) Using the simplified analysis above, the cost-benefit of the sexuality education program would be:

$73,400	($18,350 × 4 pregnancies)
−33,000	(cost of the program)
$40,400	Cost-benefit
or	
$10,100	savings per pregnancy eliminated

The problem with cost-effectiveness and cost-benefit analyses of sexuality education programs is the impossibility of assigning a cost value to personal experiences. In our example, for instance, we cannot assign a cost value to such things as the social stigma experienced by the teenaged pregnant girl; the interruption of schooling; the psychological experience and effect of abortion; the tendency for teenaged mothers to give birth to low-birth-weight babies with a greater incidence of birth defects; the effect of the pregnancy on the relationship between the girl and her boyfriend; or the lost opportunities for the young mother as a result of having to care for a baby (in particular, if the mother has not yet completed her schooling).

Because there are so many human and other factors for which we are unable to estimate a cost, do not get caught in the trap of trying to justify or evaluate sexuality education

based on its cost-benefit. How much are people worth—their comfort, their appreciation of their sexual selves, their ability to function as citizens expected to participate in societal decisions of a sexual nature (for example, abortion legislation)? A cost analysis will inevitably neglect these very important benefits of a sexuality education program.

Summary

Without evaluation, it is impossible to continually improve a sexuality education program's effectiveness. Evaluation, however, is something other than grading or measurement. The grading of a student is an estimate of the student's progress and may involve factors beyond the instructional setting (such as the student's family, background, or outside job). Measurement tells us "how much." That is, measurement gives us a point of reference with which we can make comparisons. Evaluation, however, tells us "how good." We use the results of measurements as input into our decision about the effectiveness of a program. Evaluation should be formative (occur as the program is occurring in order to make adjustments to better achieve program objectives) and summative (occur at the conclusion of the program to determine how effective it was).

Evaluation also involves value judgments that are applied to the results of measurement. These value judgments, however, should be specified in terms of objectives of the program. What are we trying to achieve by offering this sexuality education program? Objectives can be divided into process objectives and outcome objectives. Process objectives refer to the means by which we attempt to achieve the end results. The results we are attempting to achieve are the outcome objectives. Both should be evaluated so as to provide the basis for further program development. These objectives should pertain to the learners, the sexuality educator, and the educational process itself, and they should be stated behaviorally so that they can be evaluated.

Finally, sexuality educators interested in evaluation might find themselves in various traps. One of these involves accepting objectives for a program that are inappropriate. These objectives might be unreasonably shortsighted; that is, they may relate to changes in some specific behavior and ignore other outcomes of the program. In addition, it may be unrealistic to expect certain objectives to be achieved given the financial resources, time allocation, and personnel assigned to the program. To evaluate a program in terms of such objectives will certainly lead to the conclusion that the sexuality education program is ineffective. However, the problem would be in the objectives and the evaluation, not the program.

Another trap is evaluating a sexuality education program using a cost-effectiveness or cost-benefit analysis. Although some aspects of a program and its outcomes can be assigned a monetary value, it is impossible to assign a dollar figure to some very significant psychological and sociological consequences of sexuality education. Consequently, such an analysis should be recognized as incomplete and should not be the sole basis for the continuation or elimination of a program.

References

Greenberg, J. S. *Health education and health promotion: Learner-centered instructional strategies.* 5th ed. Boston: WCB/McGraw-Hill, 2004.

Healthways, 12 (1957). Reprinted by permission.

Kilander, H. F. *Sex education in the schools.* Toronto: Macmillan, 1970. Excerpt reprinted by permission.

Suggested Readings

Henry, P., Freeman, H. E. & Lipsey, M. W. *Evaluation: A systematic approach.* Thousand Oaks, CA: Sage Publications, 1998.

Linn, R. L. & Gronlund, N. E. *Measurement and assessment in teaching.* Englewood Cliffs, NJ: Prentice Hall, 1999.

Neal, J. A. *Effective phrases for performance appraisals: A guide to successful evaluations.* Toronto: Neal Publications, 2003.

Patton, M. Q. *Qualitative research and evaluation methods.* Thousand Oaks, CA: Sage Publications, 2001.

Posavac, E. J. & Carey, R. G. *Program evaluation: Methods and case studies.* Upper Saddle River, NJ: Pearson Education, 2002.

Effectiveness of Sexuality Education and the Sexuality Educator

CHAPTER 18

Key Concepts

1. Sexuality education research is fraught with difficulty.

2. Many sexuality education research findings are encouraging.

3. To be unsure of your capacity to be an effective sexuality educator is an encouraging sign.

As this is the last chapter of this book, you will soon be "released" to conduct sexuality education courses, workshops, and programs. Although previous chapters presented information derived from research studies, we recognized sexuality education to be as much an art as a science. Now we will describe the reasons for this conclusion by citing the limitations of sexuality education research. Within these limitations, however, we will mention some selected research findings that can be used to justify and plan sexuality education. Once that task is accomplished, we will leave you with a word of encouragement and a pat on the back. The rest will be up to you.

First, let us pause to consider why research on the effectiveness of sexuality education is so important. Perhaps the main reason is because sexuality educators are often asked to "prove" that their courses work, whereas educators in other subjects are not held to the same standard (Yarber, 1992). In addition, many officials are concerned about providing learners with an appropriate sexuality education program. Educators want programs that validate the sexual thoughts, feelings, and concerns of young people, but can at the same time withstand close scrutiny by parents, conservative community members, and those generally opposed to sexuality education programs (Young, Core-Gebhart & Marx, 1992).

It is a tall order to ask sexuality education programs to cure problems related to such topics as pregnancy, drug use, school drop-out rates, and contraceptive use; however, that is often what is expected. Given the current social and educational climate, it makes sense to continue to learn more about the effectiveness of sexuality education programs.

The Difficulty of Sexuality Education Research

The evaluation of sexuality education is troublesome. The broad concept of a healthy sexuality is difficult to measure, many studies are limited in methodology such as lacking a longitudinal component, and social constraints often prohibit access to young subjects. Yet, we must be careful to make any evaluation of sexuality education as realistic and methodologically sound as possible, remembering that sexuality education is only one part of a societal solution toward enhancing responsible sexual behavior (Yarber, 1992).

As complicated as research is when conducted in the basic sciences (such as physics, biology, and chemistry), it is not nearly as complex as research in the social sciences (such as sociology and psychology). The reason for this is that relevant variables are much easier to control in the basic sciences. A chemist, for example, knows exactly how much of each chemical is added to a solution and can accurately measure its effects. To study this new solution, the chemist might have 1,000 caged mice whose food intake is kept constant, whose activity is restricted, and who will later be dissected to identify effects of the new solution. In other words, the *only* differences between the mice will be that 500 of them will be administered the new solution (the experimental group) and the other 500 will not (the control group). If the experimental group of mice differ from the control group of mice, since the only variable manipulated was the administration of the new solution, this difference can be identified as resulting from the new solution.

The problem in the behavioral or social sciences is that there are just too many variables that cannot be controlled that can affect the results of research involving human beings. To expect to be able to research the effects of a particular sexuality education program and to then know how to conduct sexuality education programs elsewhere or with different people is unrealistic. The chemist in our example knows exactly what his or her new solution consists of. The chemist knows, for example, that water is two parts hydrogen to one part oxygen. The sexuality educator, on the other hand, does not know exactly what his or her sexuality education program comprises, since situations arise during instruction for which no plans were made and that need an artful response. Sexuality education consists of ever-changing variables that, even if able to be held constant, *interact* with many other variables. Whereas the chemist can keep mice in a cage to control these variables, the sexuality educator obviously cannot do the same. Whereas the chemist can dissect his or her subjects to identify the results of the experiment, the sexuality educator must rely on reports from the learners themselves or from written tests that at best involve some degree of error.

The variables involved in sexuality education that may differ from one educational situation to another include the learners, learning environment, educational strategy, sexuality educators, content, evaluation, and permission to conduct research. Remember, not only may each of these differ but they also interact with each other in different ways from one sexuality education program or session to another.

Learners

No one learner or one group of learners is ever exactly like any other. They may differ by sex (male, female); by education level; by socioeconomic level; by age; by religion; by ability; or by their sexuality knowledge, attitudes, and behaviors. Again, though any one of these may differ from one group to another, imagine how they interact to produce diverse groups of learners. Therefore, to study sexuality education as it is conducted with one group of learners and generalize the results of this study to other groups of learners is difficult at best.

Learning Environment

Sexuality education is conducted in many different settings. Some sexuality education is offered in schools, some in facilities of community agencies, and some in hospitals, for example. If we choose even one of these settings, for example schools, we still find many differences within that category. For example, some schools are traditional, others are more progressive. Some schools are junior high schools, others are middle schools. Some schools conduct coeducational sexuality education classes, others isolate boys and girls for sexuality education. Some schools have adequate lighting, ventilation, brightly colored walls, and so on; others do not.

With sexuality education conducted in affiliation with community organizations or hospitals, other differences can be described. Such variables as the time devoted, funding allocated, and instructional materials available for sexuality education are all significant factors in the effectiveness of a program, and these may vary dramatically from program to program.

Educational Strategy

We have looked at the many educational strategies available to the sexuality educator, which include case studies, critical incidents, values clarification activities, and gaming. Different sexuality education programs may involve a different mix of these strategies and thereby manifest different philosophies. To compare a program with a particular mix to another with a different mix is like comparing apples to oranges.

Sexuality Educators

Just as learners may differ on a range of variables, so may sexuality educators. They may differ by age, sex, religion, education level, and other factors. In addition, they may differ in teaching skill, sexuality knowledge, values, morals, personality, conscientiousness, and experience in conducting sexuality education. It is reasonable to expect these latter variables to have a significant impact on the effectiveness of sexuality education. It seems evident that attempts at generalizing results of a sexuality education program conducted by a particular sexuality educator to other programs conducted by other sexuality educators is an exercise in futility.

Content

Some sexuality programs are specifically prohibited from including consideration of abortion; others are not. Some sexuality education programs emphasize contraception; others emphasize other content. It would be difficult, if not impossible, to locate two sexuality education programs that include the same content and devote the same amount of time to each content area. Since the emphasis on the topics differs, sexuality education programs naturally differ. The question then becomes, how can different programs be compared? Our answer is that they cannot be compared.

Evaluation

Sexuality educators must often rely on learners' honesty and abilities to evaluate the effectiveness of a program. For example, if a program seeks to encourage more responsible sexual behavior and one way chosen to demonstrate this behavior is by using some means of contraception during sexual intercourse, the sexuality educator can ask prior to and after the program whether learners use a means of contraception during sexual intercourse. If more learners report that they use contraceptives after the program than reported before the program, sexuality education may be considered effective. However, if the learners were dishonest in their answers (and the very nature of sexuality education topics may, because of embarrassment or guilt, lead them to be dishonest), then the evaluation of the program is inaccurate. Such self-report data are always suspect.

Permission to Conduct Research

Since sexuality education is often controversial, administrators of these programs want as little publicity and attention as possible. *Don't rock the boat* is the predominant theme. They prefer to leave well enough alone. Consequently, when researchers seek permission to conduct research with ongoing sexuality education programs, permission is often denied.

The result of this situation is that much-needed evaluation of existing programs is most often nonexistent.

Sometimes this state of affairs borders on the absurd. When one of your authors sought permission to evaluate the results of an instructional unit on homosexuality in a public high school, the principal of the school objected to one part of the unit that called for a visit by homosexuals to the class. To accommodate this principal (so as to be able to conduct the study), it was suggested that a speech by the homosexuals be videotaped and later played back for the students. The principal stated that the videotape was not acceptable but that an audiotaped interview could be played for the students. In other words, homosexuals could be heard but not seen. What made this situation even more ridiculous was that the only parental objection received about the unit was from a father who suggested that, next time, homosexuals

---

Insight 18-1

Permission to Conduct Research on Sexuality Education

As with many other aspects of sexuality education, there are a variety of feelings about whether research on sexuality education should be conducted in certain settings—particularly schools. Conduct a minisurvey with the questions listed below. Ask the questions of school superintendents, school principals, elementary and secondary school teachers, religious leaders, parents, students of different ages, and community leaders.

1. How do you feel about research on the effects of sexuality education being conducted in our local schools? How about in local churches? How about in community agencies such as the teen club, the 4-H club, or other youth organizations? _____

   _____

2. Do you think there is a need for sexuality education in the organizations listed in question number 1? _____

3. What kinds of results (effects) should we expect from sexuality education programs? _____

   _____

4. How should we determine if the desired results are achieved? _____

   _____

5. Whose permission should we get in order to do research on the effects of sexuality education? _____

   _____

6. How should research on the effects of sexuality education programs be conducted? _____

   _____

7. What could you do to assist with research on the effects of sexuality education programs? _____

   _____

What conclusions can you draw as a result of your minisurvey?

1. _____

2. _____

3. _____

4. _____

be asked to visit the class so as to be able to answer student questions. As this incident illustrates, obtaining permission to conduct research studies in sexuality education programs is often a difficult task. What occurs, then, is that findings from research that is conducted can only be generalized and applied to the few select programs open and secure enough to allow investigators to study them. These findings should not be applied to other programs.

We must conclude that research applied to some vague concept of sexuality education, conducted with ill-defined learners by differing sexuality educators, cannot be expected to result in meaningful data. What you find about your program will probably not be applicable to others. What does make sense is that each of us should evaluate his or her *own* program, since at least the sexuality educator will remain constant, and probably the learners, learning environment, educational strategy, and content will not vary significantly. With each of us evaluating our own programs and making improvements based on these evaluations, sexuality education all over will be improved. Recognizing, then, that research or evaluation of individual programs is a useful endeavor, let us briefly describe the results of such studies.

Encouraging Findings in Sexuality Education Research

One of the arguments that people opposed to sexuality education have voiced is that sexuality education encourages sexual behavior, in particular premarital sexual intercourse. A number of researchers have looked at this issue for a long time and have concluded that sexuality education does not encourage sexual behavior. As far back as 1969, Wiechmann and Ellis studied the effects of sexuality education on 545 undergraduate college students and found that students receiving sexuality education did not differ from students not receiving sexuality education on premarital petting or coital experience.

Two more recent summary statements help put the issue of sexuality education's influence on sexual behavior into proper perspective. Fisher (1990) concluded that research findings clearly indicate that relevant sexuality education only directs ongoing sexual behaviors along more careful lines and does not encourage such behaviors. Haffner and de Mauro (1991) pointed out that there has been a great deal of research to determine if sexuality education courses increase teen involvement in sexual intercourse—and the vast majority of studies clearly say "no!"

Kirby (2000) summarized research results on this issue. He pointed out that sexuality education programs do not increase adolescent sexual intercourse, do not hasten the onset of intercourse, do not increase the frequency of intercourse, and do not increase the number of sexual partners.

So much for what sexuality education does not do. Now, what positive effects have been demonstrated? These effects have generally been categorized into changes in knowledge, attitudes, and behavior. Since around 1989, however, studies have become more comprehensive—perhaps because of increased concern about HIV/AIDS, teen pregnancies, contraception, and abstinence.

Therefore, we have organized our information about the effects of sexuality education into five categories: (1) examples of studies in the 1960s, 1970s, and 1980s; (2) examples of studies since 1987; (3) considerations of results that cannot be evaluated; (4) common characteristics of effective programs; and (5) implications for conducting sound sexuality education programs.

Examples of Studies in the 1960s, 1970s, and 1980s.

Many studies showed that sexuality education improves sexual knowledge. For example, when teachers participated in a sexuality education workshop, their sexual knowledge increased (Fretz & Johnson, 1971). When undergraduate students participated in a marriage and family course, they reported that they had developed a more adequate understanding of sexuality and human reproduction (Olson & Gravatt, 1968). Similarly, sexual knowledge scores of college students increased significantly as a result of a one-semester sexuality education course (Vincent, Bartley & Clearie, 1985).

Numerous studies designed to measure the impact of sexuality education courses on the knowledge of students of various ages in school indicated that sexuality education does increase knowledge of sexuality (Adame, 1985). It has even been shown that such a knowledge gain is retained for as long as two years (Thomas, et al., 1985).

Even medical students who experienced sexuality education improved their knowledge significantly (Garrard, Vaitkus & Chilgren, 1972; Hadorn & Grant, 1976). Other groups of people, such as nurses and the visually impaired, also scored knowledge gains from sexuality education (Mims, Yeaworth & Hornstein, 1974; Karpen & Lipke, 1974).

Attitude change has resulted from sexuality education as well. Machen (1970) reported that sexuality education for adult males reduced learners' anxiety regarding sexual concepts. Sexuality education also contributed to psychological adjustment (McCary, 1982). In general, more positive attitudes toward human sexual behavior and more tolerance of other people's choices of sexual lifestyle developed as a result of sexuality education. Whether with medical students (Hadorn & Grant, 1976; Marcotte & Kilpatrick, 1974), high school students (Hoch, 1968), 10- and 11-year-olds (Carton & Carton, 1971), or college undergraduate students (Olson & Gravatt, 1968), positive attitudinal changes have been associated with sexuality education.

As a result of school sexuality education programs, attitudes about premarital sexual behavior did not become more conservative or more liberal. However, programs did help students clarify their attitudes and make their behavior more consistent with their attitudes (Sex education programs confirm, don't change attitudes: New study, 1983).

As with knowledge and attitudes, behavioral changes and improvements in health resulted from sexuality education. Levine (1970), for example, found sexuality education to be effective in reducing the incidence of unwanted pregnancy and STI (including a reduced incidence of gonorrhea by 50% in 1 year). Zapka and Mazur (1977) studied a peer sexuality education program that was part of a multifaceted sexuality component of a university health service and found positive effects on STI awareness and incidence as well as on the use of contraceptive services. A church-affiliated sexuality education program for 10- and 11-year-old children and their parents resulted in improvements in parent–child communication (Carton & Carton, 1971).

It must be noted, however, that most sexuality education programs did not have much effect on sexual activity. Kirby (1980) pointed out that studies of college classes indicated that they did not affect sexual behavior. He said, "If college classes which are more permissive, exhaustive and explicit do not increase sexual behavior, then high school classes which are more limited probably do not affect behavior either."

Examples of Studies Since 1987.

One of the few studies designed specifically to reduce unintended adolescent pregnancy, and probably one of the more sophisticated studies designed to assess the effects of sexuality education, was reported by Vincent, Clearie, and Schluchter (1987). For 5 years, intervention messages targeted parents, teachers, ministers and church representatives, community leaders, and children in public schools. The messages emphasized the development of decision-making and communication skills, the enhancement of self-esteem, and the understanding of human reproduction and contraception. The number of pregnancies declined significantly (a 54% decrease) as compared to similar geographic areas without the intervention.

Stout and Rivara (1989) reviewed sexuality education literature and concluded that sexuality education programs have little positive or negative impact on sexual behavior of any type. Wang, Taylor-Nicholson, and Adame (1989) explored relationships between contraceptive education and the contraceptive behavior and attitudes of adolescents in a national survey. Those with the greatest exposure to contraceptive education reported the highest percentage of contraceptive use at first intercourse, the highest percentage of continued effective contraception, and the highest percentage of discussing contraception with partners.

Mudd and West (1989) reported that a 3-year evaluation of a family centered program for adolescents and their parents indicated improved sexual knowledge, self-esteem, and communication between parents and teens. In addition, 90%

of the teens and 97% of the parents were "very pleased" or "somewhat pleased" with the program.

Eisen, Zellman, and McAlister (1990) went beyond standard sexuality programs and included social learning theory (they included role playing and discussions of sexual risk and explorations of feelings, values, and emotions). Among their findings were (1) adolescent males who had not had sexual intercourse at the beginning of the study were less likely than those in standard courses to have initiated coitus even 1 year after the study started (surprisingly, there was no such difference in females); (2) greater sexual knowledge led to improved contraceptive use or continued abstinence for a longer time; (3) sexuality education programs as brief as 8 to 12 hours appeared to help participants increase their sexual and contraceptive knowledge, initiate and maintain relatively high levels of effective contraceptive use, and facilitate modest improvements in the use of effective contraceptive methods for both sexes.

Girls Incorporated (Girls' group urges increased sexuality-related information, 1991) conducted a 3-year research project with 750 girls aged 12 to 17 who were at high risk of unintended pregnancy compared to the general teen population. The programs used were designed to help build assertiveness, decision-making and communication skills, and provide information on health services and responsible sexual behavior. Girls who completed the programs were only about half as likely to have sexual intercourse for the first time in that 3-year period as girls who did not participate. Those who did participate in sexual intercourse were only about half as likely to have sexual intercourse without using contraception as those who were not in the programs.

The Alan Guttmacher Institute (Teenage sexual and reproductive behavior, 1991) reported that nearly all junior and senior high school teachers said their schools offered sexuality education, but that most thought it was often provided too late and too little time was spent on the subject. The Institute also indicated that studies have found no conclusive evidence that sexuality education causes teenagers to become sexually active earlier or later. In-depth studies of a few specific programs have shown that some approaches contributed to a greater delay in teenagers' becoming sexually active. Programs have effectively provided information about reproduction and contraception and thus increased teenagers' knowledge about these subjects.

Kirby and colleagues (1991) reported the impact of a curriculum entitled *Reducing the Risk* which is based on social learning theory and social inoculation theory. There was a significant increase in knowledge and parent–child communication about abstinence and contraception. Among students who had not had intercourse at the beginning of the study, the curriculum significantly reduced the likelihood that they would have intercourse within the 18 months following the program. It did not significantly affect the frequency of sexual intercourse or use of birth control among sexually experienced students. Overall, unprotected intercourse was reduced either by delaying the onset of intercourse or by increasing the use of effective contraceptives.

In summarizing research on sexuality education programs, Balog (2003) similarly indicated that programs delay the onset of intercourse and reduce the frequency of intercourse. In addition, they decrease the number of partners and increase condom or other contraceptive use.

In the early 1990s there seemed to be increased emphasis on abstinence-oriented sexuality education. The effects of one such curriculum (*Living Smart*) was reported by Young, Core-Gebhart, and Marx (1992). The curriculum helped delay the initiation of sexual intercourse as well as increase student knowledge about sexuality issues and parent–child communication about abstinence and contraception.

Given the increasing emphasis on (and even requirements for) abstinence-oriented curricula, however, it is important that the sexuality educator carefully analyze each of them just as carefully and critically as any other curriculum. It may be the result of an abstinence bandwagon forming in your community. For example, one such curriculum (*Sex Respect*) has been found to have a number of educational problems. Trudell and Whatley (1991) reported that it substitutes biased opinion for fact, conveys insufficient and inaccurate information, relies on scare tactics, ignores realities of life for many students, reinforces gender stereotypes, lacks respect for cultural and economic differences, presents only one side of controversial issues, fails to meaningfully involve parents, and is marketed by using inadequate evaluations.

In addition to *Sex Respect,* many other fear-based education programs have been identified. They go by such innocent sounding names as *Teen-AID, AANCHOR, Challenge Program,* and *You Are Unique.* They rely on scare tactics, inaccurate and biased information, gender stereotypes, outdated portrayals of the American family, and antichoice, homophobic, and sexist values. In addition, they withhold needed information about prenatal care, contraception, sexual orientation, and abortion from young people. They lack respect for cultural and economic differences and present only one side of controversial issues (Haffner, 1992).

While a growing number of U.S. public school districts have made abstinence education a part of their curriculum, one school district in three forbids dissemination of any positive information about contraception, regardless of whether their students are sexually active or at risk of pregnancy or disease (Landry, Kaeser & Richards, 1999). This occurs in spite of the fact that there does not currently exist any evidence that abstinence-only programs have actually delayed the onset of sexual intercourse or reduced any other measure of sexual intercourse. Their impact upon sexual behavior is simply unknown (Kirby & Coyle, 1997).

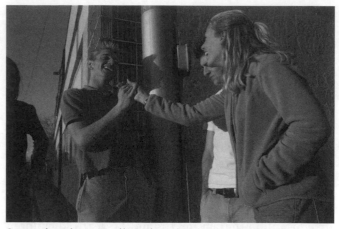

Comprehensive sexuality education programs that are properly carried out have shown many positive results. The results of abstinence-only programs, on the other hand, have not been as promising.

In summarizing research on abstinence-only programs, Balog (2003) concluded that no studies have found a consistent or significant impact on the initiation of sexual behavior as a result of these programs. In addition, no studies have found a consistent or significant impact on delaying the onset of sexual intercourse, and no programs have decreased or increased condom or other contraceptive use.

Haffner and Goldfarb (1996) reported that research indicates that quality sexuality education programs increase knowledge, clarify values, increase parent–child communication, help young people delay the initiation of sexual intercourse, and increase the use of contraception and condoms. However, they do not encourage young people to begin intercourse and do not increase the frequency of intercourse. In addition, they pointed out that effective programs target specific behaviors; rely on theoretical models for behavior change; provide information about the risk of unprotected sexual intercourse and how to reduce risk; provide students with opportunities to discuss situations that they find meaningful and realistic; address the influence of the media, peers, and culture on sexual behaviors and decisions; develop and reinforce beliefs and values among students that support their decisions to be abstinent or to otherwise protect themselves; and include opportunities for students to practice communication and negotiation skills.

Kirby and Coyle (1997) synthesized evaluations of 35 school-based programs. In summarizing the effects of the programs, they reported that some of the programs showed a reduction of sexual risk-taking behaviors by delaying the onset of intercourse, by reducing the frequency of intercourse, by reducing the number of sexual partners, or by increasing the use of condoms or other forms of contraception. None of the studies showed an increase in any measure of sexual activity, as is often feared.

Grunseit and colleagues (1997) examined 68 reports on sexuality education in 10 countries. The review indicated that quality sexuality education programs have been successful in helping to delay the onset of sexual activity and in protecting sexually-active youth from STIs and pregnancy. The results also supported the idea that responsible sexual behavior can be learned and that education is best started prior to the initiation of sexual activity. Sexuality education did not increase sexual activity.

Kirby (1999) examined 24 studies conducted in the United States and Canada that targeted adolescents aged 14 to 18 years old. The studies' conclusions included (1) sexuality and HIV education programs do not increase sexual activity; (2) sexuality and HIV education programs can delay the onset of intercourse, reduce the frequency of intercourse, and decrease the number of sexual partners; and (3) some programs increase condom use or contraceptive use.

Blake and colleagues (2001) evaluated the effects of sexuality education enhanced by five homework assignments designed to be completed by middle school students with their parents. Their results showed that the students had greater self-efficacy for refusing high-risk behaviors, less intention to have sexual intercourse before finishing high school, and more frequent parent–child communication about prevention and sexual consequences.

Another unique and interesting study was reported on by Murphy (2003). She looked at faith-based sexuality education programs that deliver comprehensive information about every aspect of human sexuality while stressing responsible decision making. One strong conclusion drawn was that teens—particularly girls—with strong religious views are less likely to have sexual intercourse, largely because their religious views lead them to perceive the consequences of having sexual intercourse negatively. Religious institutions can educate young people in a way that public schools cannot, because they can talk about and emphasize particular values.

Considerations of Results That Cannot Be Evaluated.

Brick (1999) pointed out that research efforts designed to provide statistical evidence about personal behaviors are important, but they should not come to define sexuality education. Life changes occur during sexuality education that will never be measured statistically. For example, people learn to be more comfortable with their bodies, they learn that their own questions and concerns are common to others, they learn about sexual communication, they learn how to better relate to others about sexual issues, and they become more understanding of the importance of human sexuality in their lives.

Relatedly, Haffner and Goldfarb (1996) pointed out that other important behaviors might be measured as we develop effective measurement techniques. Possibilities include appreciating one's own body; communicating effectively with parents, peers, and partners; practicing

effective decision making; identifying and living according to one's values; and interacting with both genders in respectful and appropriate ways.

Common Characteristics of Effective Programs.

After an extensive review of evaluations of both sexuality and HIV education programs, the National Campaign to Prevent Teen Pregnancy concluded that skills-based sexuality curricula delay the onset of intercourse, reduce the frequency of intercourse, reduce the number of sexual partners, and increase condom or other contraceptive use (Kirby, 1997). The report also identified nine common characteristics of effective curricula:

- Programs focused clearly on reducing one or more sexual behaviors that lead to unintended pregnancy or HIV/STI.

- The behavioral goals, teaching methods, and materials were appropriate to the age, sexual experience, and culture of the students.

- Programs were based on theoretical approaches demonstrated to be effective in influencing other health-related risky behaviors.

- Programs lasted a sufficient length of time.

- Programs employed a variety of teaching methods designed to involve the participants and have them personalize information.

- Programs provided basic, accurate information about the risks of unprotected intercourse and methods of avoiding unprotected intercourse.

- Programs included activities that address social pressures on sexual behaviors.

- Programs provided modeling and practice of communication, negotiation, and refusal skills.

- Programs selected teachers or peers who believed in the program they were implementing and then provided training for those individuals.

Implications for Conducting Sound Sexuality Education Programs.

Now we need to go out on a limb at least a little. Given the present state of the art, what can be learned from research about the effectiveness of sexuality education programs? Here is our reading of the situation:

1. The basic reasons for sound sexuality education programs have not changed; however, perhaps due to HIV/AIDS and concerns about teen pregnancy, there is a significant emphasis on prevention of sexual activity, pregnancy, and disease. This is not necessarily a problem as long as the reasons for comprehensive sexuality education (Chapter 2) are remembered.

2. Sexuality education programs can help teenagers delay involvement in sexual intercourse, but only if they are begun before teenagers experiment with steady dating and intimate behaviors (Haffner & de Mauro, 1991). The old concern about "too little, too late" remains true today. Therefore, programs that promote delaying sexual intercourse must begin in late elementary school and junior high/middle school if they are to be effective.

3. Young people (and those who are older as well) need support to resist the many pressures to become involved in sexual intercourse. This support can be furnished by teaching techniques for resisting peer pressure ("social inoculation"), involving parents in education programs, providing supportive services in the community, and using education techniques involving peers as well as groups of older teens.

4. Sexuality education programs can help decrease the number of pregnancies and STIs, but not alone. Related to number 3, programs must be comprehensive, skill-based, and linked with community efforts. For example, they can help learners identify origins of pressures for certain behaviors, examine the motives behind the pressures, and develop skills to respond effectively.

5. To decrease pregnancies and STIs, people in general (particularly teenagers) must be able to accept that they are sexual beings and have sexual feelings and desires; make decisions for themselves; know about alternatives to intercourse and methods and sources of contraception; talk about sexual limit-setting and contraception with a partner; and know how to say "no" and mean it.

6. Sexuality education programs which are purely moralistic are not effective.

7. Talking about abstinence is not at all incompatible with talking about contraception. They both relate to responsible sexual decisions.

8. "Information only" programs are not effective. Combination programs (with characteristics mentioned in numbers 3 through 5) can be very effective.

9. None of the research findings reduces the importance of the qualifications of the sexuality educator. The person handling the education program along with the characteristics of the program are the keys to success.

As would be expected, it is important to match programs and goals and not expect all things from all programs. For example, if the goal is to increase knowledge, almost any good program will work. However, if the goal is to increase parent–child communication, a parent–child program is also needed. If the goal is to reduce unintended pregnancies, an education/clinic combination is needed and can probably be successful.

The bottom line is that sexuality education has been demonstrated to affect positively sexual knowledge, attitudes, and behaviors in *some* programs. Your job will be to obtain these desirable outcomes for the sexuality education that you conduct.

As has been seen, evaluation of sexuality education programs is not easy. If you are in a position to plan or participate in a program evaluation, the following recommendations may be helpful (Improving evaluations of sexuality education, 2000):

- Doing no evaluation is better than doing a bad evaluation.

- Rigorous outcome evaluations are appropriate only after a program is successfully implemented for a period of years.

- Evaluations must be consistent with the expressed goals of the program and the course content.

- Evaluations of comprehensive sexuality education should go beyond measuring changes in whether young people are having intercourse or whether they are using a contraceptive method.

- Evaluations of *school-based sexuality education* should focus on changes in knowledge, attitudes, and skills. Be cautious about measuring outcomes outside the classroom.

- Simple programs should be evaluated by simple measures; complex outcome measures on behavior change should be reserved for multi-year, intensive strategies.

- There is a need for new instruments to measure sexual health objectives.

- Qualitative methods are an important supplement to quantitative methods.

Feeling Unsure: An Encouraging Sign

As you finish this book, you might still be doubting your ability to conduct an effective sexuality education program. As a matter of fact, we hope that you have such doubt. Doubt may be beneficial as stress can be beneficial. You might ask, how can any kind of stress be helpful? Well, imagine someone who must present a speech. If that person experiences little or no stress prior to the speech, perhaps he or she will not prepare for it very well. Another person experiencing stress prior to a

Insight 18-2

Personal Doubts and Remedies

Take a few moments to consider specifically any insecurities you may feel regarding your preparedness to teach sexuality education and to consider remedies for these insecurities. We have provided an example for you. Complete the chart yourself.

1.   Lack of sexuality information.

2.   _____
     _____
     _____

3.   _____
     _____

4.   _____
     _____
     _____

1.   Will subscribe to the *Journal of Sex Research* and read one book a month concerned with human sexuality.

2.   _____
     _____
     _____

3.   _____
     _____

4.   _____
     _____

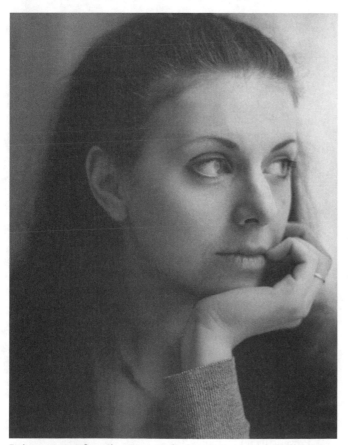

It is common for educators to feel unsure about whether or not they are fully prepared to be sexuality educators. This can be a positive sign.

speech would, because of the stress, prepare extra well, and the result might be an excellent speech. Similarly, doubt can be to sexuality education what stress is to the speaker. Without such doubt, your approach to sexuality education might be too casual and result in a lackadaisical, pedestrian program.

Concerns regarding your ability to conduct sexuality education can be positive forces you can use to do an even better job than you would have been able to do otherwise. However, to make the most of these doubts, you must plan to eliminate or diminish them. By doing so you will be taking charge of your own professional growth. Remember that new knowledge is uncovered each day, new instructional strategies are constantly being developed, and new instructional materials are continually being marketed. Keeping up with this ever-changing sexuality education scene necessitates conscientious, caring sexuality educators taking charge of their professional growth. Are you such a person?

Summary

The difficulties accompanying research in sexuality education include the inability to apply generalizations from one sexuality education program to other programs. The problem of such generalizations stems from the following variables:

1. Learners' varied ages, sexes, socioeconomic statuses, religions, knowledge, attitudes, and behaviors

2. Differences in the learning environment including school, community, or hospital settings

3. Varied use of instructional strategies and manifestations of sexuality education philosophies

4. Differences in sexuality educators themselves, such as different ages, sexes, religions, teaching skills, sexuality knowledge, values, morals, and personality

5. Varied emphases on content, as well as the exclusion of some topical areas from some sexuality education programs

6. Problems associated with the validity of self-report data often used to evaluate the effectiveness of sexuality education

7. Difficulty in obtaining permission to conduct research of ongoing sexuality education programs

In spite of these research limitations, evaluation of sexuality education has resulted in some programs demonstrating significant positive changes in sexual knowledge, attitudes, and behaviors. In addition, researchers have found that the concern that sexuality education would lead to increased premarital petting and coitus are unfounded. The positive attitudinal changes most often associated with sexuality education are increased tolerance of differing sexual lifestyles and a more positive attitude toward human sexual behavior in general. Regarding behavioral and health changes, researchers have found that sexuality education results in improved parent–child communication if that skill is taught in the program. Most programs will not have much influence on the direction of sexual values. Regarding changes in sexual behavior, traditional programs (such as lectures and fact-giving) have not had much effect. However, more recent studies seem to indicate that use of effective contraceptives can be increased and sexual behavior can be delayed if sound programs are started early and involve learning techniques that deal with peer pressure, involve parents in educational programs, provide supportive community services, and use peer education techniques. If the goal is to reduce unintended pregnancies, it is probably necessary to provide family planning services as part of the educational program. It is important to match programs and goals and to have realistic expectations.

Finally, we encourage you to make use of any doubts you still have regarding your ability to conduct effective sexuality education. Work to eliminate or diminish such doubts, thereby offering even better sexuality education than might otherwise be the case.

References

Adame, D. D. On the effects of sex education: A response to those who would say it promotes teenage pregnancy, *Health Education* (October/November 1985), 8–10.

Balog, J. E. The ethics of a school-based condom availability program. Presented at the American Association for Health Education national convention, Philadelphia, 2003.

Blake, S. M., Simkin, L., Ledsky, R., Perkins, C. & Calabrese, J. M. Effects of a parent-child communications intervention on young adolescents, *Family Planning Perspectives*, 33, no. 2 (March/April, 2001), 52–61.

Brick, P. Success stories: What statistics don't tell about sexuality education, *SIECUS Report*, 27, no. 6 (August/September 1999), 15–21.

Carton, J. & Carton, J. Evaluation of a sex education program for children and their parents: Attitude and interactional changes, *Family Coordinator* (October 1971), 377–86.

Eisen, M., Zellman, G. L. & McAlister, A. L. Evaluating the impact of a theory-based sexuality and contraceptive education program, *Family Planning Perspectives*, 22, no. 6 (November/December 1990), 261–71.

Fisher, W. A. All together now: An integrated approach to preventing adolescent pregnancy and STD/HIV infection, *SIECUS Report*, 18, no. 4 (April/May 1990), 1–11.

Fretz, B. R. & Johnson, W. R. Influence of intensive workshop on teachers' sex information and attitudes toward sex education, *The Research Quarterly*, 42 (1971), 156–63.

Garrard, J., Vaitkus, A. & Chilgren, R. A. Evaluation of a course in human sexuality, *Journal of Medical Education*, 47 (1972), 772–78.

Girls' group urges increased sexuality-related information, *Health Education Reports*, 13, no. 20 (October 24, 1991), 6.

Grunseit, A., Kippax, S., Aggleton, P., Baldo, M. & Slutkin, G. Sexuality education and young people's sexual behaviour: A review of studies, *Journal of Adolescent Research*, 12, no. 4 (1997), 421–53.

Hadorn, D. & Grant, I. Evaluation of a sex education workshop, *Medical Education*, 10 (1976), 378–81.

Haffner, D. W. Sexual backlash, *SIECUS Report*, 20, no. 4 (April/May 1992), 20–21.

———— & de Mauro, D. *Winning the battle.* New York: Sexuality Information and Education Council of the United States, 1991.

———— & Goldfarb, E. S. But does it work? Improving evaluations of sexuality education. Sexuality Information and Education Council of the United States (1996). Available: http://www.siecus.org/pubs/evals/eval0000.html.

Hoch, L. L. Attitude change as a function of sex education in a high school general biology class. PhD diss., Indiana University, 1968.

Improving evaluations of sexuality education. Sexuality Information and Education Council of the United States (2000). Available: http://www.siecus.org/pubs/evals/eval0004.html.

Karpen, M. L. & Lipke, L. A. Sex education as a part of an agency's four-week summer workshop for visually impaired young people, *New Outlook for the Blind*, 68 (1974), 260–67.

Kirby, D. *No easy answers: Research findings on programs to reduce teen pregnancy.* Washington, DC: National Campaign to Prevent Teen Pregnancy, 1997.

———— & Coyle, K. School-based programs to reduce sexual risk-taking behavior, *Children and Youth Services Review*, 19, nos. 5–6 (1997), 415–36.

———. Reducing adolescent pregnancy: Approaches that work. *Contemporary Pediatrics* (January 1, 1999). Available: http://cp.pdr.net/cp/static.htm.

———, Barth, R. P., Leland, N. & Fetro, J. Reducing the risk: Impact of a new curriculum on sexual risk-taking, *Family Planning Perspectives*, 23, no. 6 (November/December 1991), 253–63.

———. The effects of school sex education programs: A review of the literature, *Journal of School Health*, 50, no. 10 (December 1980), 559–63.

———. What does the research say about sexuality education? *Educational Leadership*, 58, no. 2 (2000), 72–76.

Landry, D. J., Kaeser, L. & Richards, C. L. Abstinence promotion and the provision of information about contraception in public school district sexuality education policies, *Family Planning Perspectives*, 31, no. 6 (November/December 1999), 280–86.

Levine, M. I. Sex education in the public elementary and high school curriculum, in *Human sexual development*, Taylor, D. L., ed. Philadelphia: F. A. Davis, 1970.

Machen, R. B. The effect of ten hours of instruction in sex education on anxiety related to sex concepts. PhD diss., American University, 1970.

Marcotte, D. B. & Kilpatrick, D. G. Preliminary evaluation of a sex education course, *Journal of Medical Education*, 49 (1974), 703–5.

McCary, J. L. *Human sexuality.* 4th ed. Belmont, CA: Wadsworth Publishing, 1982.

Mims, F., Yeaworth, R. & Hornstein, S. Effectiveness of an interdisciplinary course in human sexuality, *Nursing Research*, 23 (1974), 248–53.

Mudd, H. P. & West, E. N. Family centered sexuality education, in *Sexuality education: A resource book*, Cassel, C. & Wilson, P. M., eds. 307–17. New York: Garland Publishing, 1989.

Murphy, C. Programs help sort out sex, morality issues, *Washington Post* (April 6, 2003), C01.

Olson, D. H. & Gravatt, A. E. Attitude change in a functional marriage course, *Family Coordinator* (April 1968), 99–104.

Sex education programs confirm, don't change attitudes: New study, *Sexuality Today*, 6, no. 37 (July 4, 1983), 1–2.

Stout, J. W. & Rivara, F. P. Schools and sex education: Does it work? *Pediatrics*, 83 (1989), 375–79.

Teenage sexual and reproductive behavior, in *Facts in Brief.* New York: The Alan Guttmacher Institute, 1991.

Thomas, L. L., Long, S. E., Whitten, K., Hamilton, B., Fraser, J. & Askins, R. V. High school students' long-term retention of sex education information, *Journal of School Health*, 55, no. 7 (September 1985), 274–78.

Trudell, B. & Whatley, M. Sex respect: A problematic public school sexuality curriculum, *Journal of Sex Education and Therapy*, 17, no. 2 (1991), 125–40.

Vincent, M. L., Bartley, G. L. & Clearie, A. F. Attitude and knowledge change in response to sexuality education training, *Family Life Educator*, 3, no. 4 (Fall 1985), 23–25.

———, Clearie, A. F. & Schluchter, M. D. Reducing adolescent pregnancy through school and community-based education, *Journal of the American Medical Association*, 257, no. 24 (June 26, 1987), 3382–86.

Wang, M., Taylor-Nicholson, M. E. & Adame, D. E. The effects of sex education on adolescent contraceptive behavior, *Eta Sigma Gamman*, 21, no. 1 (Fall 1989), 28–32.

Wiechmann, G. H. & Ellis, A. L. A study of the effects of "sex education" on premarital petting and coital behavior, *Family Coordinator* (July 1969), 231–34.

Yarber, W. L. While we stood by . . . The limiting of sexual information to our youth. American Association for the Advancement of Health Education scholar presentation, Indianapolis, IN, April 9, 1992.

Young, M., Core-Gebhart, P. & Marx, D. Abstinence-oriented sexuality education, *Family Life Educator*, 10, no. 4 (Summer 1992), 4–8.

Zapka, J. M. & Mazur, R. M. Peer sex education training and evaluation, *American Journal of Public Health*, 67 (1977), 450–54.

Suggested Readings

Common questions about sexual health education. Sex Information and Education Council of Canada (1999). Available: http://www.sieccan.org/page32.html.

DeCarlo, P. Does sex education work? Center for Aids Prevention Studies at the University of California, San Francisco (1996). Available: http://www.caps.ucsf.edu/sexedtext.html.

Further funding for abstinence-only-until-marriage programs. Sexuality Information and Education Council of the United States (2000). Available: http://www.siecus.org/policy/PUpdates/pdate0011.html.

Issues and answers: Fact sheet on sexuality education, *SIECUS Report*, 29, no. 6 (August/September 2001), 30–36.

Kirby, D. *Emerging answers: Research findings on programs to reduce teen pregnancy.* Washington, DC: National Campaign to Prevent Teen Pregnancy, 2001.

Research into sexual health education, in *Canadian Guidelines for Sexual Health Education*, Health Canada (1997). Available: http://www.hc-sc.gc.ca/main/lcdc/web/publicat/sheguide/app3_e.html.

What is the impact of making condoms easily available to teenagers? Sex Information and Education Council of Canada (1999). Available: http://www.sieccan.org/page33.html.

Cases for Part 5

The cases in this section are designed to use the information included in Chapters 16, 17, and 18.

Case 1 deals with planning a sexuality education program, including the establishment of objectives. Chapter 16 gives most of the information needed to deal with this case, but a check back to Chapter 2 should be helpful.

Case 2 helps you consider an important part of school sexuality education programs—accompanying programs for parents. While information from Chapter 3 will be helpful with this case, most information should be found in Chapter 16.

Case 3 explores the relationship of evaluation to both the rationale for instituting sexuality education and the determination of its continuance. As described in Chapter 17, evaluation can be used as a positive force or a negative force. Consideration of this point is necessary to appreciate the implications included in Case 3.

Case 4 asks you not only to use the information on sexuality education research appearing in Chapter 18 but to go beyond this information to create a sexuality education research study of your own.

Case 5 serves to help you conclude this book by exploring apprehensions you may have regarding your ability to conduct sexuality education. A discussion pertaining to this topic appears in Chapter 18. Case 5 is designed to summarize this discussion as well as to reinforce the need for you to continue to pay attention to your professional development and growth.

Case 1

Planning Programs for Professionals: Planning a Sexuality Education Program for Nurses

Dr. Bea A. Planner, the dean of the Nursing School, is finally interested in making sure that all nurses who go through professional training in her program are educated in matters related to human sexuality. At the present time, there are no courses in the nursing curriculum that specifically relate to human sexuality. Dr. Planner does not expect the graduates of the nursing program to be certified counselors or educators, but she would like them to be aware of the way sexuality relates to nursing as practiced in a variety of situations.

1. What should be the objectives of the sexuality education component of the nursing curriculum?

2. What steps should be followed in planning the program?

3. What aspects of the present program are likely to be useful in the expanded program?

4. Why should the steps in number 2 be followed?

Case 2

Planning Programs for Parents: Educating Parents and Helping Them to Be Educators

Mr. Ed U. Cater, the curriculum coordinator for the Duitrite School District, believes that it is important to involve parents in school programs. He particularly feels that this is a good idea in relation to sexuality education. However, he is unsure of what should be included in a parent program.

1. What should be the objectives of the program?

2. What should be done to stimulate parent participation?

3. What major points should be covered during meetings with parents?

Case 3

Entering by the Wrong Door: Evaluation of Sexuality Education

The Board of Education is alarmed. They have just been presented the data regarding last year's incidence of teenage STI in their community. The health commissioner presenting this information chides the Board of Education for not doing its part in preventing STI among the school-aged population. Not wanting to be irresponsible, the board selects the school district's coordinator of health education to develop a sexuality education program that will decrease the community's incidence of teenage STI.

1. What evaluation trap might the coordinator of health education experience?

2. What should be evaluated after the first year of the sexuality education program? What about after 5 years?

3. List five process objectives and five outcome objectives that could be written for this sexuality education program.

4. Describe how you would evaluate each of the five process objectives and five outcome objectives.

5. How should the Board of Education decide whether to continue funding the sexuality education program after its first year? How about after subsequent years?

Case 4

What Works? Research of Sexuality Education

Ann Nomer teaches sexuality education to four different but similar groups of learners. She is very interested in three quite different methods of sexuality education: lecture, group interaction, and use of audiovisual instructional materials. Deciding to study each of these approaches to sexuality education, Miss Nomer begins organizing a research study whereby she can determine which, if any, is most effective.

1. Describe a study Miss Nomer can conduct to answer her question. Be sure to include details regarding the assignment of learners to the three approaches, methods of collecting data, what will be done with the data once collected, and how to determine whether any of the three approaches is better than offering no sexuality education at all (in terms of the money needed to conduct the program).

2. What limitations and problems regarding this study should Miss Nomer expect?

3. Based on the summary of sexuality education research appearing in Chapter 18, what would you guess the results of Miss Nomer's study would be?

Case 5

Who Me? Uncertainties Regarding Your Ability to Conduct Sexuality Education

The sexuality education course was over, and now F. Ective was expected to be able to conduct sexuality education. However, he was very unsure of his ability to do so. Seeking help, he approached Professor Conrad Fident with his apprehensions. Con Fident explained that being unsure of one's ability to conduct sexuality education is not unusual.

1. List five reasons Con Fident gave for students' being unsure about their abilities to conduct sexuality education.

2. Professor Fident continued by stating that, as a matter of fact, being unsure is a good sign. List five reasons Con Fident gave that being unsure of one's ability to conduct sexuality education is a good sign.

3. The professor did offer F. Ective suggestions for relieving some of these uncertainties. List five suggestions Professor Con Fident may have offered.

The National Coalition to Support Sexuality Education

 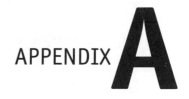

The National Coalition to Support Sexuality Education consists of over 135 national nonprofit organizations which are role models in promoting health, education, and social concerns for American youth. Coalition members are committed to the mission of assuring that comprehensive sexuality education is provided for all children and youth in the United States.

These organizations represent a broad constituency of child development specialists, educators, health care professionals, parents, physicians, religious leaders, and social workers whose combined work reaches more than 30 million young people.

The Coalition's goals are to:

- Advocate for sexuality education at the national and state level.

- Assist national organizations concerned with youth to establish policies and programs on sexuality education.

- Develop strategies for facilitating national and local implementation of sexuality education initiatives and efforts.

- Develop proactive strategies to address the activities of those who oppose providing children with comprehensive sexuality education.

- Provide an opportunity for networking, resource sharing, and collaborating on a national level.

- Develop joint goals and objectives into the 21st century.

- Hold semi-annual meetings to discuss progress made toward achieving its mission.

Coalition Members

- Advocates for Youth
- AIDS Action Council
- AIDS Alliance for Children, Youth and Families
- The Alan Guttmacher Institute
- American Academy of Child and Adolescent Psychiatry
- American Academy of Pediatrics
- American Association for Health Education
- American Association for Marriage and Family Therapy
- American Association of Family & Consumer Sciences
- American Association of School Administrators
- American Association of Sex Educators, Counselors and Therapists
- American Association of University Women
- American Association on Mental Retardation
- American Civil Liberties Union, Reproductive Freedom Project
- American College Health Association
- American College of Nurses-Midwives
- American College of Obstetricians and Gynecologists
- American College of Sexologists

Source: The National Coalition to Support Sexuality Education. Sexuality Information and Education Council of the United States (2003). Available: http://www.siecus.org/pubs/fact/fact0005.html.

- American Counseling Association
- American Federation of Teachers
- American Jewish Congress
- American Library Association
- American Medical Association
- American Medical Student Association
- American Medical Women's Association
- American Nurses Association
- American Orthopsychiatric Association
- American Psychiatric Association
- American Psychological Association
- American Public Health Association
- American School Health Association
- American Social Health Association
- Association for Sexuality Education and Training
- Association of Reproductive Health Professionals
- Association of State and Territorial Directors of Health Promotion and Public Health Education
- Association of State and Territorial Health Officials
- ASTRAEA National Lesbian Action Foundation
- Balm in Gilead
- Blacks Educating Blacks About Sexual Health Issues
- Bridge for Adolescent Pregnancy, Parenting and Sexuality
- Catholics for a Free Choice
- Center for Law and Social Policy
- Center for Policy Alternatives
- Center for Reproductive Health Policy Research
- Center for Reproductive Rights
- Center for Sexuality and Religion
- Center for Women Policy Studies
- Child Welfare League of America
- Choice USA
- Coalition on Sexuality and Disability, Inc.
- Education Development Center, Inc.
- EngenderHealth
- Equal Partners in Faith

- ETR Associates
- Exodus Trust Archives of Erotology
- Federation of Behavioral Psychological and Cognitive Sciences
- Feminist Majority Foundation
- Gay and Lesbian Medical Association
- Gay, Lesbian and Straight Education Network
- Gay Men's Health Crisis
- Gender Public Advocacy Coalition
- Girls Incorporated
- Hetrick-Martin Institute
- Human Rights Campaign
- The Institute for Advanced Study of Human Sexuality Alumni Association
- International Center for Research on Women
- Jewish Women International
- The Kinsey Institute for Research in Sex, Gender and Reproduction
- Lambda Legal Defense and Education Fund, Inc.
- The Mautner Project
- Midwest School Social Work Council
- Ms. Foundation for Women
- NARAL Pro-Choice America
- National Abortion Federation
- National Alliance of State and Territorial AIDS Directors
- National Asian Women's Health Organization
- National Assembly on School-Based Health Care
- National Association for Equal Opportunity in Higher Education
- National Association of Counties
- National Association of County and City Health Officials
- National Association of People with AIDS
- National Association of School Psychologists
- National Black Women's Health Project
- National Center for Health Education
- National Coalition of Abortion Providers

- National Coalition Against Censorship
- National Coalition of Advocates for Students
- National Coalition of STD Directors
- National Committee for Public Education and Religious Liberty
- National Council of Churches, Committee on Family Ministries and Human Sexuality
- National Council of Jewish Women
- National Council of La Raza
- National Council of Negro Women
- National Council of State Consultants for School Social Work Services
- National Council on Family Relations
- National Education Association Health Information Network
- National Family Planning and Reproductive Health Association
- National Gay and Lesbian Task Force
- National Information Center for Children & Youth with Disabilities
- National Latina Health Organization
- National Latina/o Lesbian, Gay, Bisexual & Transgender Organization (LLEGO)
- National Lesbian and Gay Health Association
- National Medical Association
- National Mental Health Association
- National Minority AIDS Council
- National Native American AIDS Prevention Center
- National Network for Youth
- National Organization on Adolescent Pregnancy, Parenting and Prevention
- National Partnership for Women and Families
- National Resource Center for Youth Services
- National School Boards Association
- National Urban League
- National Women's Health Network
- National Women's Law Center
- National Youth Advocacy Coalition
- Network for Family Life Education
- New York State Department of Health, Bureau of STD Control
- Our Bodies Ourselves (formerly Boston Women's Health Book Collective)
- Parents Families and Friends of Lesbians and Gays
- People for the American Way
- Physicians for Reproductive Choice and Health
- Planned Parenthood Federation of America
- Population Communications International
- Population Connection
- Presbyterians Affirming Reproductive Options
- Religious Coalition for Reproductive Choice
- Religious Institute on Sexual Morality, Justice, and Healing
- Sexual Minority Youth Assistance League
- Sexuality Information and Education Council of the United States
- Shield Institute
- Society for Adolescent Medicine
- Society for Public Health Education
- Society for the Scientific Study of Sexuality
- Unitarian Universalist Association
- United Church of Christ, Justice and Witness Ministries
- United States Conference of Mayors
- United States Student Association
- University of Pennsylvania, Graduate School of Education
- Women of Reform Judaism
- YAI/National Institute for People with Disabilities
- The Young Women's Project
- YWCA of the U.S.A.

State Policies in Brief

 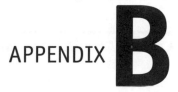

Sexuality Education

BACKGROUND: The advent of AIDS in the 1980s spurred states to reevaluate their sexuality education policies and, in some cases, expand their requirements. Currently, education on HIV/AIDS and other STDs is mandated in 38 states, although only 22 states require broader sexuality education. Even in states that have mandates, local policymakers generally have wide latitude in crafting their own policies. What substantive guidance states provide is heavily weighted toward stressing abstinence; while many states allow or require that contraception be covered, none requires that it be stressed. Further affecting whether students receive instruction on sexuality or HIV/STDs are parental consent requirements or the more frequent "opt-out" clauses, which allow parents to remove students from instruction the parents find objectionable.

Statewide Requirement to Teach

HIV/STD or sexuality education

HIV/STD and Sexuality Education		Only HIV/STD Education	
22 + DC		**17**	
Alaska	Minnesota	Alabama	New York
Delaware	Nevada	California	North Dakota
District of Columbia	New Jersey	Connecticut	Ohio
Florida	North Carolina	Idaho	Oklahoma
Georgia	Rhode Island	Indiana	Oregon
Hawaii	South Carolina	Michigan	Pennsylvania
Illinois	Tennessee	Missouri	Washington
Iowa	Utah	New Hampshire	Wisconsin
Kansas	Vermont	New Mexico	
Kentucky	West Virginia		
Maine	Wyoming		
Maryland			

Source: State Policies in Brief. New York: The Alan Guttmacher Institute, 2003.

Content Requirements, if Taught

State	**Abstinence** must be covered/stressed in		**Contraception** must be covered/stressed in	
	STD Education	Sex Education	STD Education	Sex Education
Alabama	stressed	stressed	covered	covered
Alaska				
Arizona	stressed	stressed		
Arkansas	stressed	stressed		
California	stressed	stressed	covered	covered
Colorado				
Connecticut		covered		
Delaware	covered	covered	covered	covered
Dist of Columbia				covered
Florida		covered		
Georgia	covered	covered	*	*
Hawaii	stressed	stressed	covered	covered
Idaho				
Illinois	stressed	stressed	covered	
Indiana	stressed	stressed		
Iowa				
Kansas				
Kentucky	covered	covered		
Louisiana	stressed	stressed		
Maine	stressed	stressed	covered	covered
Maryland	stressed	stressed	covered	covered
Massachusetts				
Michigan	covered	covered		
Minnesota				
Mississippi†	stressed	stressed	*	*
Missouri	stressed	stressed	covered	covered
Montana				
Nebraska				
Nevada				
New Hampshire				
New Jersey	stressed	stressed	*	*
New Mexico	stressed		covered	
New York	stressed		covered	
North Carolina	stressed	stressed	*	*
North Dakota				
Ohio	stressed			
Oklahoma	covered	stressed	covered	
Oregon	stressed	stressed	covered	covered
Pennsylvania	stressed		covered	
Rhode Island	stressed	stressed	covered	covered
South Carolina	stressed	stressed	covered	covered

	Abstinence must be covered/stressed in		Contraception must be covered/stressed in	
State	**STD Education**	**Sex Education**	**STD Education**	**Sex Education**
South Dakota‡				
Tennessee	stressed	stressed		
Texas	stressed	stressed	*	*
Utah	stressed	stressed	§	§
Vermont	covered	covered	covered	covered
Virginia	covered	covered	covered	covered
Washington	stressed		covered	
West Virginia	stressed	stressed	covered	covered
Wisconsin				
Wyoming				
Total	**7 covered, 26 stressed**	**8 covered, 22 stressed**	**19 covered**	**14 covered**

*State specifically authorizes localities to teach about contraception, but in MS, NC, NJ, and TX, if taught, it must include failure rates or effectiveness and failure rates among adolescents.
†State law allows localities to override the state's requirements for which topics must be taught, including abstinence; however, the law states that "no program or instruction may include anything that contradicts the excluded components."
‡Abstinence is taught within character education.
§Prohibits "the advocacy or encouragement of the use of contraceptive methods or devices" and prohibits teachers from responding to students' spontaneous questions in ways that conflict with this and the law's other requirements.

Parental Involvement

in a student's participation in HIV/STD or sexuality education

Parents May Opt to Remove students from HIV/STD or sexuality education			**Parental Consent Is Required** for students to engage in HIV/STD or sexuality education
34 + DC			**3**
Alabama*	Maine	Oregon	Arizona††
Arizona†	Maryland	Pennsylvania*,†	Nevada
California‡	Massachusetts*	Rhode Island	Utah
Connecticut	Michigan	South Carolina	
Dist of Columbia	Minnesota§	Tennessee	
Florida	Mississippi	Texas	
Georgia	Missouri	Vermont*	
Idaho	Montana†	Virginia	
Illinois	New Jersey*	Washington	
Iowa	New York†,**	West Virginia	
Kansas	North Carolina	Wisconsin	
Louisiana	Oklahoma		

*Removal of student must be based on religious or moral beliefs.
†Applies to HIV/STD education only.
‡Localities may require parental consent for HIV/STD education, but not for sexuality education.
§Requires an "alternative curriculum" to be offered to students whose parents have opted to remove them from sexuality or HIV/STD education.
**Parents who opt to remove their child must assure the school "that the pupil will receive such instruction at home."
††Applies to sexuality education only; for HIV/STD education, parents may opt to remove students.

Teaching Strategies for Sexuality Education

The following teaching strategies are presented as an aid to the sexuality educator. We have taken some of the more effective learning strategies and described one lesson that can be taught employing that strategy. The reader is encouraged to develop other lessons using these same strategies, thereby making these strategies more appropriate to the particular learners and the learning situation. Each strategy—or learning activity—is designed to achieve an educational objective by involving the learner in the learning process. It should be noted that many of these teaching strategies can be adapted to various age groups and various human sexuality content areas.

1 Case Study Lesson

- *Purpose:* To demonstrate the nature of sex-role stereotyping.

- *Procedure:* The following story is distributed on a handout and learners are asked to answer the questions at the conclusion:

A father and his son were involved in a car accident in which the father was killed and the son was seriously injured. The father was pronounced dead at the scene of the accident and his body taken to a local mortuary. The son was taken by ambulance to a local hospital and was imme-diately wheeled into an operating room. A surgeon was called. Upon seeing the patient, the attending surgeon exclaimed, "Oh, my God, it's my son!" Can you explain this? (Keep in mind the father who was killed in the acci-dent is not a stepfather, nor is the attending physician the boy's stepfather.)

- *Results:* Usually, learners will not be able to figure out that the surgeon was the boy's mother. A discussion regarding the following questions should then be conducted:

1. Why are women viewed as nurses and men as physicians?

2. Is sex-role assignment a function of biology or of our society?

3. Which of your sex roles have you adopted without thought?

4. Which sex role have you assigned to someone of the opposite sex without thought?

5. How will this activity change your behavior?

2 Brainstorming Lesson

- *Purpose:* To study the nature and logic of society's reaction to homosexuals.

- *Procedure:* The sexuality educator should ask the learners to develop a list of all possible effects that could result from the hiring of a homosexual as a school teacher. Learners should be given these instructions:

1. Both beneficial and harmful effects should be listed.

2. Comments on the merits of any item on the list should be saved for later in the activity.

3. Whatever comes to mind should be verbalized and included on the list.

4. Even though you do not believe what comes to mind, if someone else is likely to believe it, add it to the list.

Once the list is of sufficient length (there should be at least 20 items on the list) each item should be reexamined and its validity determined. If the likelihood of any item on the list occurring is less than 10%, eliminate that item from the list. The remaining items should be judged as either "likely," "unlikely," or "don't know."

- *Results:* The learners should discuss the "probable" outcomes of employing homosexual school teachers. They should then write one paragraph stating whether or not they believe homosexuals should be hired as school teachers and present justifications for their conclusions.

3   Role-Playing Lesson

- *Purpose:* To understand the functioning of the reproductive system.

- *Procedure:* Learners are divided into two groups. Group A will be the male reproductive system and Group B will be the female reproductive system. The cast of characters comprising Group A will be as follows:

Scrotum	Penis foreskin
Testes	Cowper's gland
Prostate gland	Urethra
Penis	Ejaculatory duct
Prostate gland secretion	Sperm
Epididymis	Cowper's gland secretion
Ampulla	Seminal vesicle

These role-players must develop a skit to act out a male orgasm.

Group B actors will play these roles:

Vagina	Labia minora
Uterus	Vaginal lubricant
Hymen	Cervix
Clitoris	Labia majora

These role-players must develop a skit to act out a female orgasm.

- *Results:* The result of this activity will be a much better understanding of some of the anatomy and physiology of the male and female reproductive systems.

4   Buzz Group Lesson

- *Purpose:* To better understand one's family.

- *Procedure:* The learners are divided into small groups of eight members each. Each person is then asked to draw a picture of his or her family engaged in some activity. Next, the drawings are collected by the buzz group leader who shuffles them and distributes one at random to each member. The learners are instructed to look at each drawing and identify something interesting about the family, any of its members, or the family dynamics. This insight is written on the back of the drawing, and then group members exchange drawings until every person has written a comment on every drawing. Learners should be cautioned not to look at the comments written on the back of the drawings until the comment he or she will write is determined. In this manner, earlier comments will not influence those made later.

- *Result:* When the drawings contain comments from each group participant, its drawers reclaim them and read the comments. Based on the comments, the drawer should answer the following questions:

1. What generalities appear in the comments relative to your family? a family member? your family's interactions or dynamics?

2. What have you learned about your family life?

3. How can you help improve your family life?

5   Values Clarification Lesson

- *Purpose:* To determine which sexual roles are valued most.

- *Procedure:* Learners are asked to place six different sexual roles they play on six index cards. Some examples of roles they may include are as follows:

Boyfriend	Teaser
Husband	Male chauvinist
Lover	Virgin
Feminist	Hedonist
Exploiter	Macho
Girlfriend	Cutesy
Wife	Son
Daughter	Grandchild

Next, each person's index cards are taped to his or her clothing. Learners are then instructed to wander about reading the index cards of others. After 10 minutes of this wandering about, 20 minutes is provided for trading of index cards. The rules for the trading are as follows:

1. Trade away those roles you value least.

2. Trade for those roles you value most.

3. You *must* trade at least two of your roles away.

- *Results:* The discussion following this activity should pertain to the following questions:

1. Why did you give away the roles you traded?

2. Why did you obtain the roles you traded for?

3. Which roles did you want but were not able to get?

4. Do you have sexual roles in your actual life which you would like to eliminate?

5. Are there sexual roles that you do not play but would like to?

6. How will you change as a result of this activity?

6 Sentence Completion Lesson

- *Purpose:* To begin discussions in sexuality education.

- *Procedure:* Below are examples of sentence stems which learners can be asked to complete. Not all of these should be used in one lesson. Remember, it is important to provide time for learners to discuss the reasons they completed these sentences the way they did.

1. My body . . .
2. Sex . . .
3. Love feels . . .
4. Mothers are . . .
5. Fathers act . . .
6. The thing I love most about my family is . . .
7. I hate it when a grandparent of mine . . .
8. I think penis envy is . . .
9. Love at first sight . . .
10. I've used sex to . . .
11. Pregnancy can . . .
12. I'm jealous when . . .
13. I love people who . . .
14. Sexual responsibility is . . .
15. I think marriage . . .
16. My sexuality . . .
17. Boyfriends/girlfriends usually . . .
18. When I see a homosexual I . . .
19. Masturbation . . .
20. I think that oral–genital sexual behavior is . . .
21. I get "goose-bumps" when . . .
22. Sex-role stereotyping limits me by . . .
23. When I was younger, sexuality . . .
24. Sexual desire . . .
25. The opposite sex . . .

- Results: Sentence completions provide a database for learners to process. Interesting and educationally meaningful discussions often result from sentence completion lessons.

7 Fishbowl Lesson

- *Purpose:* To study the implications of premarital sexual intercourse.

- *Procedure:* Learners are asked to rate their feelings about premarital sexual intercourse: -10 is strongly opposed, $+10$ is strongly in favor, and scores in between are scaled accordingly. Each person's rating is written on a sheet of paper in large enough numbers so that it is easily visible. The instructor asks students to hold up their rankings so that four people can be chosen to debate the value or harm associated with premarital sexual intercourse. Two students with "plus" ratings and two with "minus" ratings are selected. These four learners are seated in a circle with an empty chair also in this circle. The remaining learners form a circle around this inner circle of debaters.

  Debaters then begin a discussion arguing their points of view. If a participant in the outer circle wants to say something regarding the discussion, he or she must sit in the empty chair and wait to be recognized by the four debaters. Once recognized, he or she makes the statement and then returns to the outer circle. The inner circle debaters can ignore the statement made or react to it.

- *Results:* Since the inner circle consists of people with differing points of view, a lively discussion will result. At the conclusion of this discussion the total group should be asked to list five harmful and five beneficial results of premarital sexual intercourse.

Glossary

abstinence-only-until-marriage An approach to sexuality education that restricts instruction to encouraging abstinence from sexual intercourse until one is in a marital relationship, thereby ignoring the educational needs of those who choose not to refrain from sexual intercourse.

active listening Listening to a communication and then paraphrasing it when responding, also called reflective listening.

aggressiveness Expressing oneself and getting what one is entitled to but at the expense of someone else's rights.

AIDS An incurable disease caused by the human immuno-deficiency virus that compromises the effectiveness of the immunological system, which can result in death.

amniocentesis Extraction of amniotic fluid to determine whether birth defects are present in a fetus.

assertiveness Expressing oneself and getting what one is entitled to without violating anyone else's rights.

avoiding Paying no attention to people's concerns in a conflict.

bestiality Sexual contact with animals.

biological dimension of sexuality Involves physical appearance, responses to sexual stimulation, reproduction, and general growth and development.

bisexual (ambisexual) Person who enjoys sexual relationships with members of both sexes.

body image One's view of one's body; may be positive or negative.

brainstorming A method of generating multiple solutions or ideas.

breech birth When a fetus is positioned with the buttocks, not the head, being the body part nearest the cervix during birth.

buzz groups Small groups of learners charged with discussing a topic.

calendar method A natural family planning method of contraception that entails recording the shortest and longest menstrual cycles over a period of time to determine a woman's infertile period.

case study A story with a beginning, middle, and end that can be analyzed to elicit learning.

certification Designation by some overseeing group of an applicant's having met the minimum requirements to perform a job.

cervical cap A shallow cap that covers the cervix more snuggly than does the diaphragm, thereby preventing sperm from entering the vagina during sexual intercourse.

chorionic villi sampling Extraction of pieces of the thin tissue protruding from the chorion to determine whether birth defects are present in a fetus.

clitoris A highly sensitive structure of the external genitalia of females, which is homologous to the male penis.

cluster marriage Cooperative relationship among a group of individual families. There is no common economic base, possessions are generally privately owned, and the families meet periodically.

cohabitation Living together with someone with whom a romantic involvement exists.

commune Larger numbers of people unite around a common idea or objective (such as a shared religious principle). There are many types of communes.

comprehensive sexuality education Sexuality education programs that are sequential and broad in scope. Subsequent learning builds upon previous learning.

condom A sheath that covers the penis, thereby preventing sperm from entering the vagina during sexual intercourse.

confronting Getting conflict out in the open so it can be evaluated and resolved.

congenital A trait or condition that is not transferred from one generation to another.

contraception Methods designed to prevent conception (pregnancy).

contraceptive sponge (spermicidal sponge) A sponge, filled with spermicides, that is placed in front of the cervix to prevent conception.

contract marriage A written agreement spelling out aspects of a marriage. It may relate to details of the relationship, what happens if the marriage is severed, or periodic renewals of the contractual relationship.

cost-benefit The cost of achieving the program's objectives.

cost-effectiveness An assessment regarding whether the best use of resources was used to achieve a program's objectives.

Cowper's gland   A small gland that secretes a lubricant and neutralizes any acidity in the urethra.

critical incident   A story, similar to a case study, but one without an ending provided that can be used to elicit learning.

cultural dimension of sexuality   Sum of the cultural influences that affect our thoughts and actions, both historical and contemporary.

cunnilingus   Oral contact with a female's genital area.

Depo-Provera   A synthetic chemical (a form of progestin) used to prevent conception.

diaphragm   A shallow cap that covers the cervix, thereby preventing sperm from entering the vagina during sexual intercourse.

dyspareunia   Painful intercourse.

educational process   The instructional objectives, content, learning strategies, instructional materials, and other aspects of a program.

effective   Achieving (a program's) objectives.

ejaculation   The expulsion of semen from the penis as a result of muscular contractions.

emergency contraception   The use of oral contraception in a prescribed manner after sexual intercourse has occurred to prevent pregnancy.

epididymis   The place in the testes where sperm are stored and where nutrients help the sperm further develop.

erectile dysfunction   The inability of a man to attain or maintain an erection long enough to have sexual intercourse.

estrogen   A female sex hormone.

ethical dimension of sexuality   Includes questions of right-and-wrong, should-I-or-shouldn't-I, yes-or-no related to decisions about sexuality.

ethics   The rationale behind decisions regarding morality; the use of guiding principles.

ethnicity   Designation of a subgroup of people having a common cultural heritage consisting of customs, characteristics, language, or common history.

evaluation process   The gathering of information with the purpose of making an assessment about something.

exhibitionism   Achievement of sexual gratification by exhibiting the genitals to observers.

extended family   Family members other than a married couple and their children.

extrinsic motivation   Something, other than their own innate interest or need, that encourages people to want to do something or learn something.

fallopian tubes   Tubes through which ova travel down, sperm travel up, and fertilization takes place.

fellatio   Oral contact with a male's genital area.

fertility cult   A group (usually in ancient times) that regards the act of sexual intercourse as an act of worship.

fetishism   Sexual fixation on some object other than another human being.

fishbowl   Learners organized into an inner group and an outer group as a way to elicit learning.

force-field analysis   Analysis of the forces involved in a situation to see which ones are present and which ones are most susceptible to change.

formative evaluation   The gathering of information about a program and its objectives while it is ongoing; that is, before it is completed.

freedom   The ability to make free choices and decisions.

frottage   Act of obtaining sexual pleasure from rubbing or pressing against another person.

gender   Traits associated with acting, behaving, and feeling like a female or a male.

graafian follicle   The area of the ovary from where an egg ruptures.

group marriage   Several people are married to each other and there is a communal living arrangement.

hemophilia   A blood clotting disorder that often requires regular dialysis.

HIV   The human immunodeficiency virus, which causes AIDS, thereby decreasing the effectiveness of the immunological system.

homosexual   One whose primary erotic, romantic, and affectional attraction is toward members of one's own sex.

hormonal implants   Matchstick-sized capsules containing hormones that release slowly over time to prevent conception.

human chorionic gonadotropin (HCG)   A hormone produced by the placenta and whose presence in urine is tested to determine whether a woman is pregnant.

hymen   A thin connective tissue that covers the vaginal opening to protect the vagina from infection.

identity diffusion   The state of confusion when one does not have a clear sense of one's strengths, values, and other important components of one's makeup.

incest   Sexual behavior between relatives who are too closely related to be legally married.

induced abortion   The forced termination of a pregnancy.

IUDs   Small devices that are placed within the uterus to prevent conception.

labia majora   Outer folds of skin surrounding the labia minora.

labia minora   Inner folds of skin lying inside the labia majora.

latency   An alleged period of development when sexual development and interest in sexuality are supposedly nonexistent.

latency period   A time described by Freud that lasts through the elementary school years during which it was thought little sexual development occurred, although we now know much development does occur at this time.

learner-centered activities   Instructional strategies that actively involve students in the learning process.

lesson plan   Outline of a particular class session.

license   The ability to make any decisions regardless of their effects on other people or society in general.

masochism   Sexual gratification from experiencing pain.

masturbation   Self-stimulation of the genitals for the purpose of sexual pleasure.

measurement   The acquiring of data through such means as surveys, scales, interviews, questionnaires, and other data generating methods.

menopause   The cessation of menstruation.

menstruation   The cyclical sloughing off of blood from the vaginal opening.

morality   A designation of what is right or good (moral) or what is wrong or bad (immoral).

natural family planning   Methods of contraception that use "natural" means to prevent the sperm-egg union.

necrophilia   Sexual relations with a dead person.

nocturnal emission   Emission of semen while asleep.

nonassertiveness   Not expressing oneself and, therefore, not getting what one is entitled to because of concern regarding someone else's rights.

nonverbal communication   Actions and body posture that send a message.

nuclear family   A married couple and their children.

nymphomania   Extremely high sex drive in women.

obscene telephone caller   Receives sexual gratification from calling people and making obscene remarks related to meeting for sexual relations.

open marriage   May be defined in different ways—usually refers to a relationship in which the partners are committed to their own and to each other's growth. This probably includes partners allowing each other to have intimate and emotional relationships with others.

orgasmic dysfunction   The consistent or frequent inability of a person to achieve orgasm.

outcome objectives   The ends a program seeks to achieve.

ova   Eggs that can be fertilized by sperm.

ovaries   The part of the female reproductive system in which ova are housed before traveling down the fallopian tubes.

ovulation method   A natural family planning method of contraception that entails determining a woman's infertile period by monitoring her temperature.

pedophilia   Sexual behavior that demands a child as the sexual object.

postpartum depression   Feelings of depression (sadness, fatigue) that occur after a woman has given birth.

premature ejaculation   The inability of a male to control his ejaculatory process for a sufficient length of time to satisfy his partner in at least 50% of their coital connections.

process objectives   The means by which a program's ends are sought to be met.

progesterone   A female sex hormone.

prostate gland   A gland through which the urethra passes that secretes a substance that prolongs sperm life.

psychological dimension of sexuality   Learned attitudes and feelings toward ourselves and other people related to sexuality.

race   Designation of a subgroup of people distinguished by physical traits (such as hair, eyes, skin, color), blood types, genetic code pattern, and unique inherited traits. Primary divisions are Caucasoid, Negroid, and Mongoloid.

rape   Forcible sexual intercourse with a person who does not give consent.

resistance skills   The ability to resist pressure to perform in ways that are unhealthy, while maintaining relationships and status in the group.

role-playing   Students acting out a scenario as a way to elicit learning.

RU-486   A chemical that can terminate a pregnancy.

rule ethics   Guiding principles that are applicable to all situations.

sadism   Sexual gratification from inflicting pain.

satyriasis   Extremely high sex drive in men.

scrotum   A sac that contains and protects the testes.

self-esteem   How highly or positively you regard yourself.

seminiferous tubules   The area in the testes that produces sperm.

serial monogamy   The practice of marriage to one partner at any one time, but repeated divorces and remarriages.

sex-role stereotyping   Categorizing men and women according to highly defined traits and abilities.

sexual harassment   Unwelcome verbal, physical, or sexual conduct that has the effect of creating an intimidating, hostile, or offensive environment.

sexual unresponsiveness   A condition in which the female experiences little or no erotic pleasure from sexually oriented stimulation.

sexuality   A natural and healthy part of who we are. It is not only about taking part in sexual behaviors. It is an integral part of everyone's personality and includes cultural, psychological, ethical, and biological dimensions.

sexuality education   A lifelong process of acquiring information and forming attitudes, beliefs, and values about identity, relationships, and intimacy. It encompasses sexual development, reproductive health, interpersonal relationships, affection, intimacy, body image, and gender roles. It addresses the biological, sociological, psychological and spiritual dimensions of sexuality.

situation ethics   Guiding principles that are applicable to individual situations and circumstances, no one set of rules applies to all situations.

smoothing   Attempting to convince people that things are really not as bad as they seem.

Social Learning Theory   A theory of human behavior that states societal rewards and punishments shape attitudes and behaviors.

societal mores   A set of practices deemed to be acceptable and others deemed to be unacceptable by a large group of people or a society.

sodomy   Anal intercourse. The term is also used in legal language to refer to various sexual behaviors other than sexual intercourse.

spermicide   A chemical that kills sperm on contact and is used as a method of contraception.

splitting   Keeping participants in a conflict apart until a compromise can be found.

spontaneous abortion   A natural cessation of pregnancy, also called a miscarriage.

sterilization   A means of contraception involving either cutting, plugging, or clipping the fallopian tubes or the vas deferens to prevent the union of egg and sperm.

summative evaluation   The gathering of information about a program and its objectives at the conclusion of the program.

suppressing   Ignoring or eliminating even the appearance of conflict.

swinging   Swapping mates for sexual activities.

sympto-thermal method   A natural family planning method of contraception that entails monitoring temperature and cervical secretions to determine a woman's infertile period.

teachable moment   A time when learners are interested in a topic and motivated to learn about that topic.

testosterone   Male sex hormone.

theoretical effectiveness   The ability of a method of contraception to prevent conception when used under laboratory controlled circumstances.

transsexualism   Belief of person that he or she is trapped in a body of the wrong gender.

transvestism   Achievement of sexual gratification by wearing clothes of the other sex.

troilism   Having sexual relations with another person while a third person watches.

tubal ligation   A means of female sterilization involving blocking the fallopian tubes.

unit plan   Outline of a major portion of study, or unit, from which lesson plans can be derived.

user effectiveness   The ability of a method of contraception to prevent conception when used by people in a real-life setting.

vagina   A hollow, tunnel-like structure of the female reproductive system that receives the penis during coitus.

vaginismus   Involuntary contraction of the vaginal muscles so that entry of the penis is prevented.

values   An estimation of the worth ascribed to something.

values clarification   A set of instructional activities designed to assist learners in identifying their values.

voyeurism (scopophilia)   Achievement of sexual pleasure by watching people undressing or engaging in sexual behaviors.

zygote   A fertilized egg.

Index

A

Abbey, Antonia, 160
Abortion, 92–94
  and decision making, 146
  Greek practices, 5
  induced, 92
  Ireland practices, 5
  and the law, 130–131
  medical techniques, 93
  Roe vs. Wade, 93
  RU 486, 93–94
  spontaneous, 92
Abstinence, 80
  and preventing HIV transmission,
    200, 202
Abstinence only until marriage
  definition, 206
  research, 284
  sexuality education, 32, 37, 133
Acquired Immune Deficiency
    Syndrome, See AIDS
Active listening
  during conflict resolution, 108–9
Adame, David Daniel, 282, 283
Adams, Patricia F., 222
Adolescent Family Life Act, 130
Adolescents
  and sexual health, 7
  statistical information regarding
    sexual behavior, 180
Age
  and the decision to engage in
    sexual intercourse, 102
  and sexual intercourse, 102
  and sexuality, 7–8, 12
  as a sociological aspect of
    sexuality, 122–24
Aggressiveness, 194
AIDS, 4, See also HIV/AIDS,
    HIV/AIDS education
  and condom use, 81
  definition of, 197
Alan Guttmacher Institute, 30, 103, 283
Albanese, Robert, 258, 263
Allgeier, Elizabeth Rice, 153
Allstetter, Billy, 88

Allukiah, Myron, 93
Alter, Judith, 16, 30, 237
Alternative sexual behavior
  bestiality, 156
  bisexuality, 156
  continuum of classification, 155
  exhibitionism, 155–56
  fetishism, 156
  frottage, 156
  masochism, 156
  nymphomania, 156
  sodomy, 156
  transsexualism, 156
  transvestism, 156
  troilism, 157
  voyeurism, 157
American Association of Sex
    Educators, Counselors, and
    Therapists (AASECT), 30,
    241–42, 245
  certification of sexuality educators,
    57, 58–60
American Civil Liberties Union, 89
American Federation for Sex
    Educators, 29
American Purity Alliance, 29
American Social Health Association, 29
Amniocentesis, 90
Andre, Thomas, 21
Annon, Jack, 245
Archer, Dane, 101
Assertiveness
  definition, 194
  training, 194–95
Avoiding, conflict control method, 263

B

Bachey, 103
Balog, J.E., 284
Bandura, Albert, 98
Barrios, Michael, 101
Bartley, Gene L., 282
Beck, Kenneth H., 88, 89
Bell, Robert R., 153
Bensley, Loren B., 43, 45, 256
Berenson, Bernard G., 245

Bernstein, 125
Bestiality, 156
Biological systems
  in sexuality, 5–6
Birth control pill, 84–85
  advantages of, 84
  contraindications for use, 85
  disadvantages of, 84
  effectiveness, 84
  as emergency contraception, 85
  hormones in, 84
  mini-pill, 85
Birth process, 91–92
  alternative sites for delivery, 92
  complications of, 91–92
  rooming in, of infant, 92
  stages of labor, 91
Bisexuality, 156
Blacklisting
  by opposition groups, 37
Blake, S.M., 285
Blended families, 114, See also under
    Family life
Blumstein, Philip, 113
Body image, 52–53
Brainstorming, as instructional
    strategy, 188–89
Breech birth, 91
Brick, Peggy, 7, 285
Bruess, Clint E., 55, 80, 85, 101, 110,
    111, 119, 150, 158, 202, 244
Bullis, Ronald K., 130
Bullough, V.L., 5
Burchell, R. Clay, 99
Bush, President George W., 206
Buzz groups, as instructional
    strategy, 190–91
Byler, Ruth, 231

C

Calendar method, of natural family
    planning, 80
Call, V., 154
Carkhuff, Robert R., 245
Carnegie, Dale, 258
Caron, S.L., 5

Carrera, Michael D., 29
Carter, Jimmy, 52
Carton, Jacqueline, 282, 283
Carton, John, 282, 283
Case studies, as instructional
        strategy, 188
Catholicism, and HIV/AIDS
        education, 208
Centers for Disease Control and
        Prevention (CDC), HIV/AIDS
        education, 207
Certification, definition of, 57
Cervical cap, 83
Cheng, Y., 21
Child Study Association, 29
Chilgren, R.A., 282
Chorionic villi sampling, 90
Christian Coalition, 35
Christian Crusade, 36
Christianity, influences on sexuality, 24
Cietsch, Christine, 21
Citizens Concerned for Our Youth, 47
Citizens groups, opposition to
        sexuality education, 36–37
Clearie, Andrew F., 282, 283
Clitoris, 72
Cloud, J., 161, 162
Cluster marriage, 128
Coalition for Adolescent Sexual
        Health, members, 37
Cohabitation, 111–13
    considerations regarding, 113
    as a lifestyle, 127
    rates of, 111
    reasons for, 113
Collins, Janet, 207
Combination Strategy, and decision
        making, 145
Communes, 128
Communication, 109–11
    agreement, beginning discussion
        with, 110
    "and" and "but," use of, 110
    as a component of marital sexual
        behavior, 154
    communication effectiveness, 175
    discussion, planning time for, 110
    "I" statements, 110
    improving communication, 175
    listening, 110
    models of, 174
    nonverbal, 109–10, 174
    skills needed for sexuality
        education, 173–74
        building trust, 175
        listening skills, 173–74
        nonverbal communication, 174
    "why" questions, avoidance of,
        110–11

Community, handling concerns,
        262–63
Comprehensive sexuality education,
        206–207
Comstock, Anthony, 27
Condoms, 80–82
    and AIDS, 81
    correct use of, 81
    criticisms of, 80
    as a display at the World Fair, 153
    definition of, 80
    female condom, 81
    and preventing HIV
        transmission, 202
    television advertising, 203
    use by teenagers, 222
    yearly sales, 82
Conflict resolution
    active listening, 108–9
    brainstorming, 109
    family life, 107–9
Congenital condition
    association with pregnancy, 90
Conflict resolution, 261–62
Confronting, conflict control
        method, 263
Continuum of classifying alternative
        sexual behavior, 155
Contraception, 79–90
    abstinence, 80
    birth control pill, 84–85
    cervical cap, 83
    choosing method of, 88–90
    condoms, 80–82
    Dalkon Shield, 83
    definition of, 79
    Depo-Provera, 85
    diaphragm, 82–83
    emergency contraception, 85
    female condom, 81
    hormonal implants, 85
    intrauterine devices, 83
    natural family planning, 80
    newer methods, 87–88
        contraceptive patch, 88
        Essure, 88
        Implanon, 88
        Jadelle, 88
        Lea's Shield, 88
        male contraceptive patch, 88
        NuvaRing, 87
    reasons for not using, 89
    sales and advertising, 130
    spermicidal agents, 83
    spermicidal sponge, 84
    sterilization, 86–87
    use of contraception during
        coitus, 88
    withdrawal, 80

Contraceptive sponge, 84
    risk of toxic shock syndrome, 84
Contract marriage, 114, 128–29
    prenuptial agreement, 129
Core-Gebhart, Pennie, 279, 284
Cost-benefit, 275–76
Cost-effectiveness, 275–76
Counseling, See Sexuality counseling
Cowper's gland, 69
Coyle, K., 284
Critical incident, as instructional
        strategy, 188
Cross, Richard J., 123
Cultural factors
    of the Chinese Republic, 5
    in sexuality, 5
Culture
    as a dimension of sexuality, 5
    and sexuality education, 238
    and the sexuality educator, 55
Cunnilingus, 150

D

Dalal, A., 130, 131
Dalkon Shield, 83
Danoff, D.S., 244
Darroch, J., 180, 230
Date rape, 160–61
    and adolescents, 160
    drugs associated with, 160–61
        GHB, 161
        Ketaject, 161
        Rohypnol, 161
    prevention strategies, 161
    prevention techniques, 160
    statistical information
        regarding, 160
Dating, 111–12
    reasons for, 111
Decision making
    abortion, 146
    about marriage, 103
    about parenthood, 104–5
    about sexual intercourse, 102
    about sexuality, 144
    improving the process, 144–46
        combination strategy, 145
        escape strategy, 145
        safe strategy, 145
        wish strategy, 145
    scope of, 7
    steps involved, 145
Dehydroepiandrosterone, 74
De La Vega, E., 238
De Mauro, Diane, 17, 37, 42, 144, 255,
        266, 282, 286
Depo-Provera, 85
Development, 9

characteristics of learners, 229–31
latency period, 11
and masturbation, 9–10
Dewey, J., 181
Diaphragm, 82–83
Dintiman, George B., 74, 93, 181
Divide and conquer, use by
opposition groups, 38
Donnerstein, Edward, 155
Dorman, St. M., 207
Drake, Dr. Gordon V., 36
Drummond, T., 130
Dyspareunia, 244

E

Educational process, of evaluation, 271
Eisen, Marvin, 283
Ejaculation, 70
Elderly persons
attitude, importance of, 123
dispelling myths, 122–23
and implications for educators, 124
rules regarding, 123–24
and sexuality, 122–124
sexuality education for, 237
and sexual relations, 237
Ellis, Altis L., 282
Ellis, Havelock, *Studies in the
Physiology of Sex*, 27
Emergency contraception, 85
Epididymis, 69
Erectile dysfunction, 243
Erikson, Erik
parenthood, 104
psychosexual development, 98
sexual guilt, 99
Escape Strategy, and decision
making, 145
Estrogen, 74
Ethics
definition of, 139
rule ethics, 140
and sexuality, 139–41
in sexuality, 5–6
situation ethics, 140
Ethnicity, 55
Evaluation of sexuality education
programs
categorization of, 270
cost-benefit/cost-effectiveness,
275–76
educational process, 271–72
evaluation process, 270
extrinsic motivation, 269
formative evaluation, 270
objectives, 273–74
school based versus community
based, 269–70

and the sexuality educator, 273
summative evaluation, 270
Evaluation of sexuality education
research, 280–81
Excitement phase, of sexual
response, 77
Exhibitionism, 155–56
Extended families, 113
Extremist Groups, 39
Extrinsic motivation, 269

F

Fallopian tubes, 74
Family life
cohabitation, 111–13
communication, 109–11
conflict resolution, 107–9
dating, 111–12
dual-career families, 114
evolving family structure, 113–15
blended families, 114
"boomerang" children, 114
contract marriage, 114
group families, 114
family roles, 107
marriage, 113
nuclear family, 113
parenthood, 115–17
single-parent families, 117–18
Fear-based sexuality education
program, 284
Federal Drug Administration, and
contraceptives, 85, 86, 87
Fellatio, 150
Female condom, 81
Female reproductive system, 70,
71–74
fertilization of ovum, 73–74
parts of, 70, 71–74
Females, in the workforce, 101
Femininity, 52
Fertility cults, 23
Fetishism, 156
Fishbowls, as instructional strategy, 192
Fisher, W.A., 282
Flax, Ellen, 11, 132
Follicle-stimulating hormone (FSH)
in females, 75
in males, 74
Fong, Kevin, 238
"Foot in the door" argument, as an
opposition tactic, 39
Force-field analysis, 259
Forcible sexual behavior
incest, 157–58
necrophilia, 157
obscene telephone calls, 157
pedophilia, 157

rape, 158–61
sexual harassment, 161–62
Formative evaluation, 270
Forrest, Jacqueline D., 85, 130
Freedman, A.M., 23, 24, 25
Freedom, definition of, 172
Fretz, Bruce R., 282
Freud, Sigmund, 27
psychosexual development, 97–98
sexual guilt, 99
Front groups, as opposition to
sexuality education, 38
Frottage, 156
Fulton, Gere B., 46

G

Gag rule, 130
Gaming, as instructional strategy, 191
Garrard, Judith, 282
Gelatt, 145
Gendel, Evalyn S., 46
Gender, 55
Georges, E., 5
Gerner, Jennifer, 103
Gilgun, Jane, 47
Girls Incorporated, 283
Goldfarb, E.S., 284, 285
Gonadotropic hormones, 75
Goodson, P., 32
Gordon, Sol, 37, 47
Graafian follicle, 75
Graham, C.A., 7
Grant, I., 282
Gravatt, Arthur E., 282
Greeks, ancient, and sexuality, 23–24
Greenberg, Jerrold S., 5, 55, 74, 80, 85,
93, 99, 101, 110, 111, 117, 142,
150, 151, 158, 181, 191, 193, 202,
244, 261, 262, 270
Greenhouse, L., 132
Group families, 114
Group marriage, 128
Grunseit, A., 285
*Guidelines for Comprehensive Sexuality
Education*, 235–37
Guilt, and sexual behavior, 99

H

Haas, A., 244
Haas, K., 244
Hackett, Thomas, 238
Hadorn, D., 282
Haffner, Debra W., 16, 17, 19, 20, 22,
37, 42, 80, 85, 101, 110, 111,
117, 129, 130, 131, 133,
143–44, 150, 158, 202, 244,
255, 266, 282, 284, 285, 286

Hardy, Ann M., 222
Hargis, Reverend Billy James, 36
Harlap, Susan, 85
Harmin, Merrill, 141, 193
Harvey, P.D., 155
Hatcher, Robert A., 82, 83, 84
Health Protection Branch of Health
        Canada, 4
    concept of sexuality education, 16
Hemophilia, 200
Herman, Robin, 94
Heterosexual behavior, 153–54
    determining readiness to have
        sex, 153
    marital sexual behavior, 154
        frequency, 154
        importance of
            communication, 154
    premarital sexual behavior, 153
High Schools and Sex Education, 29
History and sexuality, 22–29
    ancient cultures, 23–24
    Christianity, 24
    15th–16th century, 24
    19th century, 26–27
    prehistoric times, 23
    17th–18th century in America, 26
    17th–18th century England, 24–26
    20th–21st century in America,
        27–29
    Witchcraft, 24
HIV
    and abstinence, 200
    and condom use, 202
    definition of, 197
    myths and facts regarding, 223–24
    prevention, 200–2
HIV/AIDS
    and death, 200, 201
    and minority populations, 200–1
    as a social and behavioral
        problem, 203
    statistical information regarding,
        198–200
    in the United States, 198–200
HIV/AIDS education
    abstinence-only-until-marriage, 206
    Centers for Disease Control and
        Prevention, 207
    comprehensive sexuality
        education, 206–7
    considerations for different levels
        & populations, 207–8
    for individuals with
        disabilities, 211
    instructional strategies, 222–26
    and the law, 132–33
    and prevention, 200, 202

principles of behavior change, 202
program assessment, 212–222
prohibition efforts, 203
religious settings, 208, 211
research, 285
and risky behaviors, 202
strategies for prevention, 204–5
teaching suggestions, 212
Hoch, Loren Lee, 282
Homosexuality
    and adolescence, 11
    as an alternate sexual behavior,
        150–53
    experimentation, 10–11
    heterosexual-homosexual rating
        scale, 171
    laws pertaining to, 129–30
    myths regarding, 150–52
    statistical information
        regarding, 180
Hormonal implants, 85–86
    advantages, 86
    considerations for use, 86
    disadvantages, 86
    Norplant, 85
    side effects, 86
Hormones
    female, 74, 75–76, 90
    male, 74–75
Hornstein, S., 282
Hughes-McLain, C., 161
Human chorionic gonadotropin, 90
Human Immunodeficiency Virus,
    See HIV
Hymen, 72

I

Identity diffusion, 98
Illness and sexuality, 125–26
    cardiac patient, 126
    medical personnel, 126
    surgery, effects of, 126
Incest, 157–58
    common forms, 157
    help for victims, 158
    identifying behaviors of
        victims, 158
    prevention strategies, 158
Infiltration, by opposition groups, 39
Inhibited sexual desire (ISD), 242–43
Instructional media, as instructional
        strategy, 195
Instructional strategies
    assertiveness training, 194–95
    assuming responsibility, 226
    brainstorming, 188–89
    buzz groups, 190–91

case studies, 188, 222–23
critical incident, 188, 223
fishbowls, 192
gaming, 191
of HIV/AIDS education, 222–26
instructional media, 195
learner-centered activities, 195
lesson plans, 185
resistance skill training, 225–26
resource speakers, 193–94
role-playing, 189–90, 225
scales and questionnaires, 223
sentence completion, 192, 225
unit plans, 185, 186
values clarification, 192–93
Interactions of sexuality educators
        with others, 54–55
Intimacy, sexual, 7
Intrauterine devices, 83
    dangers of Dalkon Shield, 83
Irwin, Charles E., 202
*Is the School House the Proper Place to
    Teach Raw Sex,* 36
IUDs, *See* Intrauterine devices

J

Jews
    ancient, and sexuality, 23
    and HIV/AIDS education, 208
John Birch Society, 36
Johnson, Virginia E., 28, 75, 77, 173,
        243, 245
Johnson, Warren R., 282

K

Kaeser, L., 284
Kann, Laura, 222
Kaplan, Helen Singer, 23, 24, 25, 245
Karpen, M.L., 282
Kates, J., 198
Katz, D., 244
Keenan, Faith, 86
Kemper, M.E., 9
Kenney, Asta, 130
Kilander, H.F., 176, 270
Kilpatrick, Dean G., 282
Kimes, Debra D., 101
Kinsey, Alfred C., 28, 170
Kirby, Douglas, 16, 19, 30, 282, 283,
        284, 285
Kirkendall, Lester, 141
Knowlton, Roberta, 37, 40
Kolodny, Robert C., 75, 173, 245
Kost, Kathryn, 85
Krebs, M., 160
Kreinin, T.A., 124

L

Labeling, by opposition groups, 37
Labia majora, 70
Labia minora, 70
Lamaze, Fernand, 92
Lamaze method, 92
Landray, D.J., 230, 284
Language, sexual
    importance of acceptable
        terminology, 176
    problems with different cultures, 238
    terms in, 177–80
Latency, 11
Latency period, 97
Laumann, E.O., 157, 180
Law, and sexuality, 129–133
    access to treatment and services,
        130–32
        abortion, 130–31
        condom distribution, 131
        contraception, 130
        minors, 130
        reproductive health care
            in schools, 131–32
        sexually transmitted
            infections, 131
    education about sexuality &
        HIV/AIDS, 132–33
    legal regulations, 129
        homosexuality, 129–30
    sexual discrimination, 132
        and the Internet, 132
            Online Protection Act, 132
Learner-centered activities, as
        instructional strategy, 195
Learner developmental
        characteristics, 229–31
    early elementary, 230
    lower secondary, 230
    preschool, 230
    upper elementary, 230
    upper secondary, 230–31
Learners
    adolescents, 180
    developmental characteristics,
        229–31
    differences in sexual behavior,
        180–81
    evaluation of, 272–73
    involvement in research, 280
    and the learning process, 181
    questions of school-aged children,
        231–32
    sexuality education for, 232–37
    and use of language, 181
Learning environment, and
        research, 280

Learning objectives, 183
    criterion of, 183–84
    validity of, 183
Leboyer, Frederick, 92
    recommendations for
        childbirth, 92
Ledray, L.E., 161
Lee, Deborah, 238
Leibee, Howard, 29
Leigh, B.C., 88
Lepkowski, J., 202
Lesson plans, 185–87
Levine, M.I., 283
Lewin, Kurt, 98, 258
Lewis, Gertrude, 21, 231
License, 172
Lichenstein, Grace, 245
Life cycle, and sexuality, 7
Lifestyles, 126–129
    cluster marriage, 128
    cohabitation, 127
    communes, 128
    contract marriage, 128–29
    group marriage, 128
    marriage, 126–27
    non-parenthood, 127
Linz, Daniel, 155
Lipke, L.A., 282
Little, L., 258
Long, V.E., 88
Lubrication, of vagina, 72
Lundberg, G., 84
Luteinizing hormone (LH)
    females, 75
    males, 74
Lyman, S.A., 161
Lyons, C., 208

M

McAlister, Alfred L., 283
McCary, James L., 75, 99, 282
Machen, R.B., 282
Male reproductive system, 69–70
    ejaculation, 70
    parts of, 69–70
Manley, Helen, 30
March of Dimes/National
        Foundation, 115
Marcotte, David B., 282
Marriage
    among homosexuals, 113
    attractions of, 103
    cluster, 128
    cohabitation, 127
    common-law, 113
    communes, 128
    contract, 114, 128–29

decision making about, 11–12,
        103–4, 113
    and family life, 113
    group, 128
    as a lifestyle, 126–27
    statistical information about, 113
Martin, Clyde E., 170
Marx, David, 279, 284
Masculinity, 52
Masochism, 156
Masters, William H., 7–8, 28, 75, 77,
        173, 243, 245
Masturbation, 9–10, 99, 150, 155
    statistical information regarding, 180
Mazur, Ronald M., 283
Means, Richard K., 29, 30
Measurement, of evaluation of sexuality
        education programs, 270
Menopause, 75
    and sexuality, 123
Menstruation, 75–77
Mentally disabled
    and sexuality, 125
    sexuality education for, 125
Mid-Century White House Conference
        on Children and Youth, 30
Miller, Heather G., 111, 202
Mims, F., 282
Monography, serial, 114
Moorman, R., 161
Morality, 55, 139
    and sexuality, 139–41
Morning after pill, 93
    effectiveness, 93
    mechanism of action, 93
    side effects, 93
Morrison, Eleanor S., 193
Moses, Lincoln E., 202
Mosher, W.D., 88, 202
Movement to Restore Decency
        (MOTOREDE), 36
Mullen, Kathleen, 55, 110
Mudd, Helen P., 283
Munson, Howard E., 56
Murphy, C., 285
Murphy, G., 130, 198

N

Nash, E., 130, 131
National Christian Right, groups,
        and opposition to sexuality
        education, 37
National Clearinghouse on Child
        Abuse and Neglect
        Information, 157
National Coalition to Support
        Sexuality Education, 44

National Commission on Adolescent Sexual Health, views on sexual health, 9
National Congress of Parents and Teachers, 29
National Council on the Aging, Love, and Life, 237
National Education Association, 29–30, 44
National Foundation/March of Dimes, 115
National Guidelines Task Force, 142
National Health and Social Life Survey, 157
National Parent-Teachers Association, 115
National Survey of Family Growth, 202
Natural Family Planning, 80
    calendar method, 80
    ovulation methods, 80
    sympto-thermal method, 80
Necrophilia, 157
Neill, A.S., 172
Neutens, James J., 263
Newman, Lon, 47
Nocturnal emissions, 11
Non-assertiveness, 194
Nonverbal communication, 174
Norplant, 85, *See also* hormonal implants
Nuclear family, 113
NuvaRing, 87
Nymphomania, 156

O

Objectives
    importance of, 273–74
    outcome, 273
    process, 273
Obscene telephone calls, 157
Ogletree, Roberta J., 88
Old Testament, views on sexuality, 23
Olson, David H., 282
Online Protection Act, 132
Opposition to sexuality education
    background of, 36
    citizens groups as, 36–37
    court cases, 46
    defense against extremist attacks, 43–47
    extremist groups, stages of attack, 39
    logical approach to opposition, 45–47
    logical responses to opposition attacks, 40–43
    national advocacy organizations as, 37

national patterns of, 36
non-extremist opponents, 40
opponents' arguments, 40–43
and public meetings, 45
tactics of opponents, 37–39
Orgasm, 79
    nocturnal emissions, 11
Orgasmic dysfunction, 244
Orgasmic phase, of sexual response, 77
Ova, 74
Ovaries, 74
Ovulation, 75–77
Ovulation method, of natural family planning, 80

P

Packard, Vance, 114
Papadopoulos, Chris, 124
Parenthood, 115–17
    decision-making about, 104–5
    education programs, 115
    non-parenthood, 127
    single parent families, 117
    training programs, 115
Parent Notification Proposal, 130
Parents without partners, 117
Patterson, J., 86
Pawlowski, Wayne, 152
Pedophilia, 157
Penile erection, in newborns, 7
Penrod, Steven, 155
Physically disabled, and sexuality, 125
Piccinino, L.J., 88, 202
Pickerel, Catherine, 208
Plateau phase, of sexual response, 77
PLISSIT, approach to sexual therapy, 245
Pluralism, sexual, 42
Pomeroy, Wardell B., 170
Poponoe, D., 127
Pornography
    and aggressive behavior, 155
    child pornography, 155
    mainstream pornography, 155
    and sexual behavior, 155
Postpartum depression, 91
Pregnancy, 90–91
    and the birth process, 91–92
    complications of, 90
    hormones, 90
    prenatal care, 90
    pre-pregnancy state, importance of, 90
    postpartum depression, 91
    teenage pregnancy, 103
    testing for, 90

Premature ejaculation, 243
Prenuptial agreement, 129
Price, Mila Underhill, 193
Progesterone, 74
Prostate gland, 69
Prostitution, 154–55
    adolescent, 155
    and HIV, 202
    therapy programs, 155
Psychological factors of sexuality, 5–6
Psychosexual development theories, 97–99
Public meetings, tips for success, 45
Puritans, views of sexuality, 25
Putnam, Paul, 44

R

Race, 55
    and myths regarding sexuality, 124–25
Rape, 158–61
    assistance for victims, 160
    date rape, 160, *See also* Date rape
    definition of, 158, 159
    incidence of, 158
    myths regarding, 158
    statistical information regarding, 158–59
Raths, Louis E., 141, 193
Redfearn, S., 87
Refusal skills, 194
Reiss, Ira, 42, 153
Religion and sexuality, 143–44
Reproductive systems
    of females, 70
    of males, 69–71
Reschovsky, J., 103
Research, of sexuality education, *See* Sexuality education research
Resistance skills
    definition of, 225
    training, 225
Resolution phase, of sexual response, 77
Resource speakers, as instructional strategy, 193–94
Rhynard, J., 160
Richards, C.L., 284
Risk-taking, behaviors related to, 202
Rivara, F.P., 283
Roe vs. Wade, 93, 131
Role-playing, as instructional strategy, 189–90
Rome, ancient, and sexuality, 23
Rose, Andrew, 208
Rothenberg, Debra L., 126
Rotter, Julian, 98

RU 486, 93, *See also* Morning after pill, abortion
Ruan, F.F., 5
Russell, Uclaf, and morning after pill, 93

S

Sabini, John, 99
Sadock, Benjamin J., 23, 24, 25
Safe strategy of decision-making, 145
Sanger, Margaret, 28
Sawyer, Robin G., 88, 89
Scales, Peter, 16, 30
Schiavi, Raul C., 124
Schiller, Patricia, 30
Schulz, Esther D., 23
Schwartz, Pepper, 113, 154
Scrotum, 69
Secondary sex characteristics
   females, 75
   males, 74
Sedway, Mark, 35, 37, 39
Self-esteem, 99
Seminiferous tubules, 69
Sentence completions, as
      instructional strategy, 192
Serial monogamy, 114
Sex flush, 78
Sexuality Information & Education
      Council of the United States
      (SIECUS), 16, 22, 30, 36,
      41–42, 115, 206, 235, 256
   definition of sexuality, 4
Sex role stereotyping, 100–2
   causes, 102
   common stereotypes for males and
      females, 100–1
   definition, 101
   disadvantages, 101
Sexual attitudes, 99–100
Sexual behavior, 53–54
Sexual counselor
   characteristics needed, 245–46
   comparison with educator, 246
   function of, 242
   overview, 241
Sexual desires, 51
Sexual dysfunctions
   dyspareunia, 244
   erectile dysfunction, 243
   orgasmic dysfunction, 244
   premature ejaculation, 243
   sexual unresponsiveness, 244
   treatment for, 245
   vaginismus, 244
Sexual harassment, 161–62
   hostile environment, 161
   problems with defining, 161

quid pro quo, 161
statistical information regarding, 162
Sexual intercourse
   decision to engage in, 102–3
   rates among high school
      students, 103
Sexuality
   definition of, 4
   dimensions of, 4–5
Sexuality counseling, 241–42
   by the educator, 247
   referral process, 247–48
   requirement for certification,
      241–42
   techniques involved in, 247
   training, 241
Sexuality education, 12
   abstinence-only-until-marriage,
      32, 133
   advocates' successes, 47
   for college-aged and adult learners,
      235–37
   comprehensive programs, 16–17
   controversies about, 32, 35
   for coronary patients, 238
   for culturally varied groups, 238
   current trends, 30–32
   definition of, 15
   goals of, 15–17
   history of, 29–30
   justification for programs, 15, 20
   national support for, 20–21
   objectives of, 15–17
   for older adults, 237
   opposition to, *See* Opposition to
      sexuality education
   reasons for, 20–22
   rights of individuals receiving, 17
   for school-aged learners, 232–35
   scope of, 18
   steps to show support for, 257–58
   traditional reasons for, 19–20
   values of, 142
Sexuality education program
   avoiding confusion during, 263–66
   and change process, 258–60
   communication skills, 173
   community concerns, handling of,
      262–63
   components of, 271
   comprehensive education, 206–7
   evaluation, *See* Evaluation of
      sexuality education programs
   fear-based, 284
   gaining support for, 255–57
   and group dynamics, 260–62
   implementation of, 256, 263–66
   implementation, steps in, 256

implications for conducting,
      285–86
   learning strategies for, *See*
      Instructional strategies
   rules surrounding communication
      in, 169–73
      availability, 171
      disclosure, 169–70
      feelings, 172
      humor, 173
      input, 172–73
      language, 169
      questions, 170–71
      respect for diversity, 173
      topics, 171
Sexuality education research
   content, 280
   difficulty of, 279–80
   educational strategy, 280
   encouraging findings, 282–86
   evaluation, 280–81
   examples of studies, 282–85
   and learners, 280
   learning environment, 280
   permission to conduct, 281–82
   and sexuality educators, 280
*Sexuality Education Within
      Comprehensive School Health
      Education*, 235
Sexuality educators
   as advocate for responsible sexual
      behavior, 89
   age factors, 54
   body image of, 52–53
   certifications of, 56–57
   communication effectiveness, 175
   culture and, 55
   evaluation of, 273
   handling alternative sexual
      behavior, 149
   and HIV/AIDS, 198
   interactions with others, 54–55
   parents as, 57, 60
   qualifications of, 56–57
   and research, 280
   sense of humor of, 54
   sexual behavior of, 53–54
   sexual experiences of, 53–54
   sexuality of, 51–54
   sexual responsibility of, 55–56
Sexual lifestyles, 126–29
Sexually transmitted infections,
      19–21
   and access to care, 131
   statistics, 20
Sexual maturity, 99
Sexual orientation, 10–11, *See also*
      Homosexuality

Sexual pluralism, 42
Sexual response
    comparison of male and female
        responses, 77–79
    phases, 77
    physiological reactions during, 78
Sexual responsibilities, 56
Sexual thoughts, acceptance of, 51–52
Sexual unresponsiveness, 244
Shapland, C., 257
Shaw, Kenneth A., 260, 261
Sherwin, Barbara B., 124
Simon, Sydney B., 141, 193
Simpson, Katherine M., 211
Singh, S., 180, 230
Single-parent families
    problems associated with, 117
    statistical information regarding, 117
    suggested guidelines for, 117–18
Situational homosexuality, 170
Sivin, I., 88
Smith, E.J., 7, 9
Smith, William, 47, 206
Smoothing, conflict control
        method, 263
Social Learning Theory, and
        psychological development,
        98–99
Societal mores, 55
Sociological aspects of sexuality
    age, 122–24
    illness, 125–25
    law and sexuality, 129–33
    lifestyles, 126–29
    mentally disabled, 125
    physically disabled, 125
    race, 124–25
Sodomy
    as an alternative sexual behavior, 156
    laws pertaining to, 130
Sohn, W., 202
Solot, D., 111
Sonenstein, F.L., 88
Sonfield, A., 130, 131
Sowers and Associates, tips for
        dealing with negative
        resistance, 45
Spermicidal agents, 83–84
Spermicidal sponge, 84
Spermicide, 83–84
Splitting, conflict control method, 263
Sprecher, S., 154
"Squeal Rule," 130

Stein, J., 155
Sterilization, 86–87
    electrocoagulation, 86
    hysterectomy, 86
    tubal ligation, 86
    vasectomy, 86–87
Stiggall, Lynne, 211
Stout, J.W., 283
Suegroff, S., 12
Summative evaluation, 270
Suplee, C., 93
Suppressing, conflict control
        method, 263
Sweden, criticisms and defense of
        sexuality education programs,
        46–47
Sympto-thermal method of natural
        family planning, 80

T

Taylor, Mary E., 88
Teachable moment, 186
Teenage pregnancy, statistical
        information regarding, 103
Tepper, M.S., 232
Testosterone, 69, 75
Theoretical effectiveness
    of contraceptives, 79–80
    definition of, 79
Thomas, Lucinda L., 282
Thompson, G., 161
Thyroxin, 74
Torres, Aida, 130
Totman, Ruth, 231
Transsexualism, 156
Transvestism, 156
Trevor, C., 35
Troilism, 157
Trudell, Bonnie, 284
Tubal ligation, 86
Turner, Charles F., 202

U

Unintended pregnancy, 79, 104
Unit plans, 185–86
User effectiveness, of contraceptives, 80
Uterus, 73

V

Vagina
    definition of, 72

lubrication of, 72
    in newborns, 7
Vaginismus, 244
Vaitkus, Aldona, 282
Values, 145
    behavioral principles related to,
        141–42
    and decision-making, 145
    and sexuality, 140–41
    in sexuality education programs, 142
    subprocesses related to, 141
    values clarification, 141
Values clarification, as instructional
        strategy, 192–93
Vasectomy, 86–87
Vincent, Murray L., 282, 283
Voyeurism, 157

W

Wagoner, 20
Wang, Min Qi, 283
Ward, S.K., 160
Watkins, S.A., 200
Webster, Claudia L., 211
Wellington, S., 101
West, Elizabeth N., 283
Whatley, Marianne, 284
Whitehead, B.D., 127
White House Conference on Child
        Welfare, 29
Whitson, James A., 46
Wiechman, Gerald H., 282
Williams, Sally R., 231
Wish strategy of decision-
        making, 145
Witchcraft, and sexuality, 24
Withdrawal, as birth control, 80
Woodworth, Robert T., 43
Workforce, statistical information
        regarding, 101–2

Y

Yarber, W.L., 279
Yeaworth, R., 282
YMCA and YWCA, 29
Young, Michael, 284

Z

Zellman, Gail L., 283
Zygote, 75

Photo Credits

p. 1, © Rubberball Productions; p. 4, © Kent Knudson/PhotoLink/Photodisc; p. 9, © Image Source/Creatas; p. 16, © Frederic Cirou/PhotoAlto/PictureQuest; p. 20, © Bill Aron/Photoedit; p. 21, Courtesy Jerrold Greenberg; p. 25, © RubberBall Productions/Alamy Images; p. 28, © AP Photo; p. 31, © Michael Newman/Photoedit; p. 36, © Michael Newman/Photoedit; p. 38, © Sanford Weinstein; p. 44, © PhotoLink/Photodisc; p. 52, © David Young-Wolff/Photoedit; p. 55, © Vincent Thian/AP Photo; p. 57, © Keith Brofsky/Photodisc; p. 67, © T. Baxter/Photodisc/Getty Images; p. 79, © Marcio JoseSanchez/AP Photo; p. 83, © SIU/Visuals Unlimited; p. 93, © Meryl Levin; p. 102, © Rim Light/Photo Light/Photodisc; p. 103, Courtesy Jerrold Greenberg; p. 109, © Creatas; p. 111, © Rubberball Productions; p. 116, (TL) © Brand X/Creatas, (TR) © PhotoDisc/Getty Images, (BL) © Steve Mason/Photodisc, (BR) © Ryan McVay/PhotoDisc/Getty Images; p. 121, © Photodisc/Getty Images; p. 123, © Photodisc/Getty Images; p. 124, © Steve Mason/Photodisc; p. 125, © D. Berry/Photolink/Photodisc; p. 132, © Nicola Sutton/LifeFile/Photodisc; p. 137, © Rubberball Productions; p. 140, © Michael Newman/Photoedit; p. 143, © The Diamondback; p. 143, © AbleStock; p. 145, © Michael Newman/Photoedit; p. 152, © ThinkStock/Creatas; p. 153, © Rubberball Productions; p. 159, © Christopher Brown/Stock Boston; p. 162, © Richard Hutchings/Photoresearchers; p. 167, © PhotoLink/Photodisc; p. 170, © PhotoLink/Photodisc; p. 170, © The Diamondback; p. 174, © Stockbyte; p. 181, © Rachel Epstein/Photoedit; p. 184, © PhotoLink/Photodisc; p. 189, © John A. Rizzo/Photodisc/Getty Images; p. 194, © Aneal Vohra/Unicorn Stock Photo; p. 197, © Kevin Lamarque/Reuters/Landov; p. 206, © Rubberball Productions; p. 225, © Tom McCarthy/Photoedit; p. 233, © The Diamondback; p. 237, © Chuck Savage/Corbis; p. 242, © Nancy P. Alexander/Photoedit; p. 246, © Michelle D. Bridwell/Photoedit; p. 247, © James Shaffer/Photoedit; p. 253, © PhotoLink/Photodisc; p. 256, © Paul Springett/Up the Resolution/Alamy Images; p. 262, © Jacobs Stock Photography/Photodisc/Getty Images; p. 270, © Spencer Grant/Photoedit; p. 272, © Jack Hollingsworth/Photodisc/Getty Images; p. 275, © Photodisc; p. 284, © Rubberball Productions; p. 287, © Mel Curtis/Photodisc/Getty Images.